THE HEALTH EFFECTS OF
Asbestos

An Evidence-based Approach

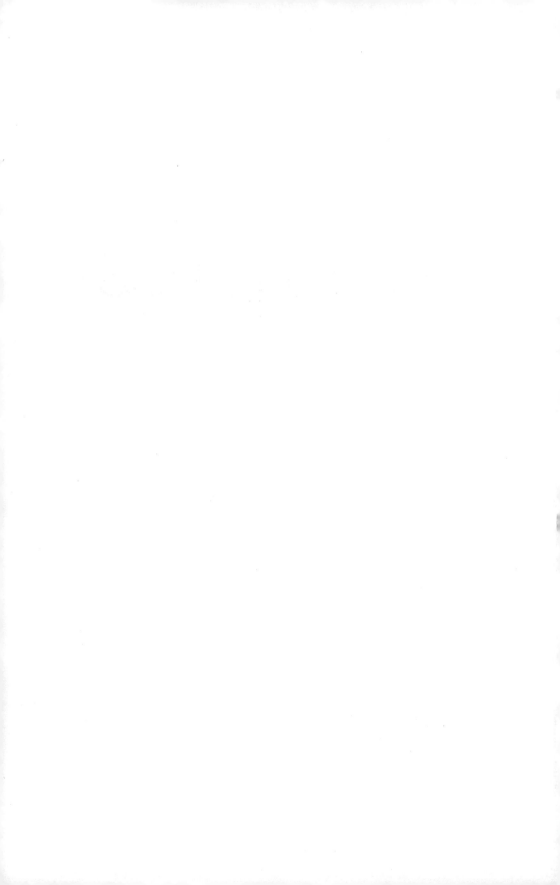

THE HEALTH EFFECTS OF
Asbestos
An Evidence-based Approach

Dorsett D. Smith MD, FCCP, FACP, FACOEM
Clinical Professor of Medicine, Division of Respiratory
Diseases and Critical Care, University of Washington
Medical School, Seattle, Washington, USA

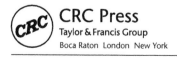

CRC Press
Taylor & Francis Group
Boca Raton London New York

CRC Press is an imprint of the
Taylor & Francis Group, an **informa** business

CRC Press
Taylor & Francis Group
6000 Broken Sound Parkway NW, Suite 300
Boca Raton, FL 33487-2742

First issued in paperback 2020

© 2016 by Taylor & Francis Group, LLC
CRC Press is an imprint of Taylor & Francis Group, an Informa business

No claim to original U.S. Government works

ISBN 13: 978-0-367-57538-0 (pbk)
ISBN 13: 978-1-4987-2838-6 (hbk)

Visit the Taylor & Francis Web site at
http://www.taylorandfrancis.com

and the CRC Press Web site at
http://www.crcpress.com

This book is dedicated to John Butler MB, CHB, past Professor of Medicine, Pulmonary Disease, and Physiology at the University of Washington Medical School, Seattle, in gratitude for his encouragement in the study of asbestos-related disorders, and to the library staff of the Providence Medical Center in Everett and Spokane, Washington, for their tireless support for more than 40 years.

Contents

Introduction

Asbestos is a miracle mineral with worldwide usage because of its heat and acid resistance. It is the most studied occupational agent known to man, with more than 12,000 bibliographic references on Medline, the National Library of Medicine database, that begins primarily in 1965, and more than 14,000 references for mesothelioma. More than 600 articles were published in the older medical literature prior to 1965. Unfortunately, a large amount of interest in asbestos, asbestosis, and mesothelioma has been related to litigation against asbestos manufacturers, suppliers, and providers of asbestos-containing products. The physician expert is placed in the awkward position of not just treating and diagnosing the patient with an asbestos-related disorder, but *assigning blame* for a cancer or other asbestos-related disorder. Scientifically, medical certainty is an expression of a >95% probability that an association exists between an asbestos exposure and causation of a particular disorder. The legal standard in the United States is "more likely than not," or 51% probability of causation with a given exposure. This very unscientific standard places the medical expert in an untenable position as a scientific expert. This book is written to provide the reader with a perspective on the many complex issues related to asbestos exposure.

A Rand Report in 2002 stated that asbestos litigation is the longest-running mass tort litigation in the U.S. history. Through 2002, approximately 730,000 individuals in the United States who had been exposed to asbestos brought claims against some 8400 business entities, and almost as many future claims are likely. Defendants and insurers spent a total of $70 billion on asbestos litigation through 2002 and the total likely exceeds well over $100 billion through 2014. Claimants "and defendants" litigation expenses consumed more than half of these costs. Approximately 31 cents was spent on defense costs and 27 cents was spent on plaintiff attorneys and other related costs per dollar. When both defense and plaintiff law firms are making billions in legal fees, it makes it virtually impossible in the U.S. political system to arrive at a more equitable system of compensating plaintiffs for asbestos-related injuries. At least 73 corporations filed for bankruptcy through 2004, the most important being the Johns Manville Corporation bankruptcy in 1982. It was estimated that bankruptcy fillings resulted in losses of around 52,000–60,000 worker jobs and a loss to workers of $25,000–50,000 over the workers' lifetimes. (*Asbestos Litigation*, Rand Corporation Report [ISBN: 0-8330-3078-7].)

I am a clinician who graduated from the University of Pennsylvania Medical School in 1963 and trained in internal medicine, infectious disease, and pulmonary disease at the Johns Hopkins Medical Institutions for the next 4 years and then returned to be Chief Resident in Medicine at the University of Pennsylvania Presbyterian Medical Center in 1967. I moved to Seattle in 1972 to direct the Chest Clinic at the University of Washington Hospital. I was originally requested in 1978 by the United States Department of Labor to review all questionable cases of asbestos-related disease in District Six as part of my role as Director of the Chest Clinic at the University of Washington Medical School and Hospital. Later, at the U.S. Labor Department's request, I became a National Institute of Occupational Safety and Health (NIOSH)-certified B-Reader in 1980 and have been sequentially recertified from 1980 to 2014. I also formed the Northwest Cardiopulmonary Panel, at the Department of Labor's request, to panel asbestos-related claims in 1980. Over the years, I have examined over 1000 patients with asbestos-related claims, mostly from Puget Sound shipyards, and have reviewed more than 200 cases of mesothelioma and reviewed several thousand chest x-rays and computed tomography scans as a NIOSH-certified B-Reader. I have offered numerous depositions and trial testimonies primarily for the defense in asbestos torts and provided many positive reports in plaintiff cases.

This book is unique because it is not written by pathologists but by a pulmonologist with a large experience in evaluating patients with asbestos-related disorders and who has been required to defend his diagnosis and opinions many times before the best and brightest asbestos tort attorneys in the United States, as well as my scientific peers. I am grateful for this experience since it has required me to go to the scientific literature to evaluate the truth claims used as evidence for a variety of opinions by various authors. The book contains my carefully referenced analysis of the medical literature on the health effects of asbestos. I have tried my best to make sure that all my opinions are supported by reference to the published medical literature. I have attempted to present the important literature on asbestos without bias from both the plaintiff and defense positions. I have tried to avoid "cherry picking" or selecting only articles that support my personnel bias on a subject.

Gradually, over the years, I have read most of the important published medical articles on asbestos-related disease. I have catalogued approximately 5000-plus articles that I have read and saved as reprints in my office over a 40-year period. These are available as a supplement bibliography to this book. I have tried to make this book readable and have avoided more detail than necessary in explaining basic cell mechanisms that produce fibrosis and neoplastic change. The book contains a critical review of the medical published literature. I have not intended to slander or insult any medical authors, but some of the asbestos literature makes truth claims that cannot be supported by evidence. I have made an effort to provide analysis of all the important scientifically based articles on the health effects of asbestos exposure in the literature referenced by the National Library of Medicine PubMed database up to December 2014.

Chapter 2, "Limitations of epidemiologic exposure studies on the health effects of asbestos," promises to be helpful to the reader who is struggling to understand conflicting reports that claim to be evidence based on the effects of asbestos exposure.

Unfortunately, some experts' hermeneutic or method of interpretation is to "proof text" or take selected portions from various published articles out of context to prove their hypothesis. The medical literature cannot be understood by quoting from all or just parts of selected articles. The basic rule of hermeneutics is "context is king"; without the understanding of both the socioeconomic bias as well as the scientific context and bias of historical medical publications, an interpretation is impossible. I have attempted to provide a broad overview of the medical literature, largely from a historical perspective, as understood by the contemporaneous scientists at the time to provide the context of those medical articles of historical interest. In addition, a review of the pertinent clinical, radiologic, pathological, toxicological, mechanistic, and epidemiologic issues that commonly confront the occupational physician or respirologist are explored in depth. (Cooper MW. Is medicine hermeneutics all the way down? *Theor Med* 1994;15(2):149–80.)

For instance, most experts agree that Wagner's 1960 article on mesothelioma was the seminal and first major article that other scientists in retrospect have relied on as proof that a specific type of South African Cape crocidolite asbestos exposure causes mesothelioma. The medical community's response to this heretofore unknown South African pathologist's claims, supported by only three complete autopsies out of 33 cases, was slow and many of Wagner's contemporaries in the 1960s were very skeptical of his claims that only a certain type of crocidolite asbestos, not amosite, chrysotile, or crocidolite mined in other areas of South Africa, caused mesotheliomas. This issue is discussed in detail in the chapter on mesothelioma with appropriate references. Scientists question data and wait for confirmation through animal studies, toxicological and mechanistic research, and publication of confirmatory data. It may take many years for scientific acceptance of a new hypothesis; for example, the good epidemiologic data on cigarette smoking was published in Germany in the late 1920s, in the United States in 1950 by Wynder, and in Great Britain in 1952 and 1954 by Doll, yet general acceptance in America of the fact that cigarette smoking causes lung cancer did not occur until the 1964 report by the Surgeon General of the United States Public Health Service. Hopefully, the reader will find here up-to-date and useful information, as well as a historical perspective on asbestos-related disease.

Various experts have combed the historical medical literature to find the earliest case reports mentioning a specific hazard from asbestos exposure. Their implication is that the general medical community and asbestos manufacturers should have been aware of this hazard much earlier than the general medical community and therefore manufacturers should have warned end users of the risk related to their products. For instance, the first case reports of lung cancer in individuals with asbestosis was in 1935 by Lynch and Smith in the United States and Gloyne in Great Britain. Numerous other case reports followed, such as the study by Sir Richard Doll in 1955 of the relationship of asbestosis-related lung cancer with a specific crocidolite-using asbestos textile plant. The cohort consisted of those heavily exposed to asbestos prior to the 1933 British dust standard. The American medical community largely ignored the work of Doll on asbestos and cancer, just as they ignored Doll's work on cigarette smoking as a cause of lung cancer. General acceptance of the relationship between asbestosis and lung cancer by the general medical community did not occur until the mid-1960s, based on the work of Selikoff and Hammond. This issue is explored in greater detail in the chapter on asbestosis and lung cancer. The subject of what experts actually understood about the health effects of asbestos versus what should they have known is explored, as well as when a general scientific consensus was established to the point at which some type of regulatory action or warnings were required. This issue is explored in greater detail in the text. All of my opinions in this treatise are authored within a reasonable degree of medical and scientific certainty. There will inevitably be some redundancy of references and text in this book.

Finally, I have chosen to put brackets around many of the important references. The bibliography is so long that the diversion of looking up references would interrupt the flow of the text. Hopefully, this slightly unorthodox bibliographic technique will make this book more readable. Some references are placed at the end of a paragraph to enhance readability. Every important statement needs foundation and is supported by references to the medical literature somewhere in this book.

For additional subject reading please see the extended reading list at www.crcpress.com/9781498728386/downloads.

1

How to critically read and find truth in the medical scientific literature

Pilate said to Him, "What is truth?"

(John 18:38)

The grand hope of the scientific method, which is a model of hypothetical deductivism, is purified objectivity and truth. This hypothetical model leaves out the human factor of bias, which realistically recognizes that pure objectivity is a goal that is never completely achieved. Many sources of error are inherent in epidemiologic studies and the goal of the clinician/scientist is to present data honestly, admitting the limitations of any study while minimizing any possible error, bias, confounding, or chance. In the laboratory, we often use a homogeneous population of white rats specially bred to be as genetically close as possible and cloistered in a toxin-free clean environment. In human studies, we study the effects of asbestos on humans with marked genetic diversity with multiple unknown or unappreciated exposures to many different toxins in a polluted environment. Humans are very complex, which makes the interpretation of scientific studies suboptimal because there may be unknown genetic or environmental factors that affect the results.

The interpretation of a study requires knowledge of the population studied, including how they were recruited for the study, such as unions, plaintiff lawsuits, or from a sentinel case of a death of a coworker. How the information was obtained (i.e., questionnaires, phone calls, medical records, next of kin, etc.) is important, as well as whether the method of acquisition has been adequately verified with a known sensitivity and specificity for the population under evaluation. The validity of accurate smoking histories in firemen, for example, cannot be used for a population of asbestos insulators. Statistics for cigarette smoking in the general population are not valid either as a comparison in asbestos insulators. Epidemiological research is an imperfect tool because of the human elements of memory, lust for financial reward by plaintiffs, and promotional and financial needs of investigators.

Our quest for truth is infinitely more complicated than can be reached with a simple questionnaire. Humans are fantastically more complicated than we realize and the tools of epidemiological studies are constantly changing. New causes of disease such as the role of human papillomavirus in laryngeal cancer are evolving and it is likely that many more viruses will be discovered that cause cancers. Keats wrote, "Beauty is truth and truth beauty." The joy of science is getting to the truth about causation.

The scientific literature is increasing at an exponential rate. Between 1978 and 1985, nearly 272,344 articles were published annually and listed in Medline. Between 1986 and 1993, this number reached 344,303 articles per year, and between 1994 and 2001, the figure had grown to 398,778 articles per year. To be up to date with current knowledge, a physician practicing general medicine has to read 17 articles a day, 365 days a year. There were 682,121 articles recorded in PubMed in 2005. If clinicians, trying to keep up with the medical literature, were to read two articles per day, in just 1 year they would be over nine centuries behind in their reading! Despite the volume of medical literature, fewer than 15% of all articles published on a particular topic are useful for clinical practice. Peer review is a mechanism that is far from perfect, and it does not guarantee that the published article is without flaw or bias. Publication biases are inherent in any process, despite an adequate peer-review process. Studies showing statistically significant results (see Chapter 2) and having larger sample sizes are more likely to be accepted and published than are nonstatistically significant, but equally important studies. William F Miser MD has published perhaps the best general article on evaluating the medical literature and he concludes, "Articles published in the most prestigious journals are far from perfect. The average quality score of clinical trials over the past 2 decades is less than 50%. Trials with negative results may take twice as long to be published as do positive trials. Finally, no matter how good the peer review system, fraudulent research, although rare, is extremely hard to identify." (Miser WF. Finding truth from the medical literature: How to critically evaluate an article. *Prim Care Clin Office Pract* 2006;33:839–62; Subramanyam RV. Art of reading a journal article: Methodically and effectively. *J Oral Maxillofac Pathol* 2013;17(1):65–70.)

Unfortunately, many physicians lack the tools of critical appraisal of published scientific data to dispute an author's conclusions. The words "statistically significant" are overused in order to get papers published and research funded. (du Prel JB, Rohrig B, Bletter M. Critical appraisal of scientific articles. *Dtsch Arztebl Int* 2009;106:100–5.) Even in the best of studies, systematic errors can often not be excluded, such as loss of subjects to follow-up, misinformation on exposure, cigarette smoking, incorrect pathological diagnosis, alcohol use, and death certificates.

P Tharyan has succinctly stated that "The essence of scientific research, and scientific discovery, is the search for truth. Research evidence can deceive. The sobering reality is that the current research agenda is tainted by academic and financial conflicts that permeate the very foundations of what is considered research." (Tharyan P. Criminals in the citadel and deceit all along the watchtower: Irresponsibility, fraud, and complicity in the search for scientific truth. *Mens Sana Monogr* 2012;10:158–80; Tharyan P. Evidence-based medicine: Can the evidence be trusted? *Indian J Med Ethics* 2011;8(4):201–7; Tharyan P. Introducing conceptual and analytical clarity on dimensions of complexity in systematic reviews of complex interventions. *J Clin Epidemiol* 2013;66(11):1202–4.)

Scientific reproducibility has been at the forefront of many news stories and there exist numerous initiatives to help address this problem. This large problem is due to the lack of specificity about research methods and materials that are required to enable adequate research reproducibility. In particular, the inability to uniquely identify research resources, such as antibodies used in a pathological study, makes it difficult or impossible to reproduce experiments even in which the science is otherwise sound. A review of research sources has demonstrated that 54% of resources are not uniquely identifiable in scientific biomedical publications, regardless of domain, journal impact factor, or reporting requirements. For example, in many cases, the pathological stain methodology with which the experiment was performed or the source of the antibody that was used could not be identified in cancer pathologic reports. Results between laboratories can be widely divergent while claiming use of the same standardized techniques such as counting asbestos bodies in tissue. The results show that identifiability is a serious problem for reproducibility. Scientific efficiency and reproducibility depend upon a research-wide improvement of this substantial problem in science today. In various epidemiological studies, certain types of information such as patient or surrogate interviews and various physiological tests and pathologic techniques are not available for evaluation by other scientists who would like to reevaluate a patient population. (Vasilevsky NA, Brush MH, Paddock H et al. On the reproducibility of science: Unique identification of research resources in the biomedical literature. *Peer J* 2013;1:e148.)

Stephen Gelhback suggests in his book, *Interpreting the Medical Literature*, the following questions for the reader of the medical literature to critically consider:

1. Are the differences observed between the groups under study likely to be due to chance?
2. If the differences are not due to chance, do they occur because of biases or are they related to another study factor?
3. If differences are statistically significant, are they practically important?
4. If differences are not statistically significant, is it possible that a true difference has been overlooked (type II error)?
5. *Validity* is the extent to which a test such as a chest x-ray is measuring what we think it is measuring, such as the incidence of pleural plaques and asbestosis related to asbestos exposure. To determine validity, a test such as a chest x-ray needs to be compared to a gold standard, such as autopsy data. Validity needs to be tested for other data, such as questionnaires about asbestos exposure, cigarette smoking, and other information about potential confounders. The measure of diagnostic accuracy of the test used, such as a chest x-ray, is defined as the *sensitivity* or the ability to detect correctly those

with asbestos-related abnormalities divided by all subjects with asbestos-related abnormalities on autopsy to determine the number of false-negative and false-positive results. The specificity of a test correctly identifies those who do not have asbestos-related abnormalities such as false positives due to subpleural fat, muscle shadows, or changes from other nonasbestos-related causes of pleural/parenchymal disease. Once this information is known, then the *positive predictive value* or the probability of disease with a positive test can be determined, as opposed to the *negative predictive value* or the probability that the patient does not have the condition being evaluated if the test is negative. The reader will notice that the positive and negative predictive values for the chest x-ray are rarely mentioned in many epidemiologic studies. In the majority of case–control studies as well as most cohort studies, there is a glaring *lack of suitable control groups* in the published asbestos-exposed literature. This can lead to a serious misinterpretations of data.

(Egger M, Smith GD, Sterne JA. Uses and abuses of meta-analysis. *Clin Med* 2001;1:478–84; Gehlback S. *Interpreting the Medical Literature*, 5th Edition. New York: McGraw-Hill, 2006, pp. 146–56; Callcut RA, Branson RD. How to review a review paper. *Resp Care* 2009;545:1379–85; Szklo M. Quality of scientific articles. *Rev Saude Publica* 2006;40:30–5; Bletter M, Huer C, Razum O. Critical reading of epidemiological papers: A guide. *J Public Health* 2001;11:97–101; Hodgson J. Quality of evidence must guide risk assessment of asbestos, by Lenters, V; Burdorf, A; Vermeulen, R; Stayner, L; Heederik, D. *Ann Occup Hyg* 2013;57(5):670–4; Berman DW, Case BW. Quality of evidence must guide risk assessment of asbestos, by Lenters, V; Burdorf, A; Vermeulen, R; Stayner, L; Heederik, D. *Ann Occup Hyg* 2013;57(5):667–9; Berman DW, Case BW. Overreliance on a single study: There is no real evidence that applying quality criteria to exposure in asbestos epidemiology affects the estimated risks. *Ann Occup Hyg* 2012;56:869–78.)

2

Limitations of epidemiologic exposure studies on the health effects of asbestos

Occupational epidemiology is the scientific study of the effects of workplace exposure on the frequency and distribution of various diseases or injuries in a given population. Basically, an epidemiologist studies the occurrence, or *incidence or number of new cases over the sum of time individuals in the population were at risk for having that event,* such as lung cancer in a population of workers such as asbestos textile workers, and then compares the rate of disease such as lung cancer to the rate of lung cancer in the general population or another more typical reference population. The term *incidence* is defined as the fraction of a study population initially free of disease that develops a condition such as lung cancer over a period of time, commonly expressed as events/person/years. *Prevalence* is the epidemiological term used to describe the proportion of people possessing a clinical condition at a single point of time.

Epidemiologic studies are usually divided into four types:

- Cohort studies, or a *prospective* observational study, of a group that is exposed to asbestos as compared with a group not exposed to asbestos, and then following their outcomes over a defined period. The results in cohort studies are commonly expressed as the (RR; risk ratio), meaning the incidence of disease in the exposed group divided by the corresponding incidence in the unexposed group.
- Case–control studies are *retrospective studies* evaluating groups, in which a certain outcome such as mesothelioma is compared to a control group without a mesothelioma and then determining risk factors for the disease. The data are commonly expressed as the odds ratio (OR) or the odds of exposure in the group with disease as compared to the control group.
- Cross-sectional studies are observational studies that evaluate the absence or *presence of an exposure and disease at a specific time.*

- Case reports, or case series, are descriptive reports on a single case or series of cases with a specific disease and a specific exposure reported to *raise a hypothesis, but they cannot test a hypothesis* because they do not include an appropriate comparison group.

If the occurrence of disease is elevated in the exposed population as compared to the nonexposed population of workers, then a possible association between the exposure and the occurrence of lung cancer potentially can be made if the association is strong and bias has been limited by correcting for cigarette smoking and any other known causes of lung cancer in both the exposed and control population. The control population must be comparable to the study group and show no systemic discrepancies in order to achieve valid results. The common method of expressing risk in an exposed population is OR, which is the measure of the strength of an association. It is the odds of exposure among cases to the odds of exposure among the controls. The RR is the risk of disease associated with a particular exposure.

There are two types of errors that may occur in the data analysis of epidemiologic studies. The first error is called a type I error, which means that a study claims that a difference is present between the exposed and unexposed control group when a difference does not exist. This type of error is similar to a jury that finds a person guilty of a crime based on the evidence presented to them but that person did not commit any crime. A common source of error is that studies are underpowered; this is the most common error in investigational studies in which investigators are trying hard to find a difference between an exposed population and an unexposed control population. Small statistical differences may exist, but "statistically significant" does not mean that a relationship between an exposed and unexposed population is proven, causal, or "clinically significant." For instance, a small loss in lung function of 5% from 100% of predicted to 95% of predicted is not clinically significant in individuals with previously normal lung function because of the tremendous pulmonary reserve in humans that allows us to live with only one lung. However, a 5% reduction in lung function in someone with severe preexisting emphysema may be very clinically significant. The term clinically significant refers to a biological change that either likely will produce symptoms sufficient to impair functional capacity or a biological change likely to produce other types of functional or lifestyle changes in the future, such as finding premalignant or malignant changes of cancer.

The term statistically significant means that there is a probable *association* and not necessarily *causation* between two different events, conditions, or physical or biological processes. For instance, there is a highly *statistically significant association or correlation* between the morning herald of dawn and the crowing of a rooster, but the rooster is not *causative* of the early morning rising of the sun.

A type II error is just the opposite of a type I error and is like a jury finding a person innocent of a crime he did actually commit. It occurs when investigators find no difference between study groups when a difference actually exists. (Bletter M, Huer C, Razum O. Critical reading of epidemiological papers; a guide. *Eur J Public Health* 2001;11:97–101.)

The *power of a study* is related to finding a difference between populations when a difference exists. The greater the number of individuals in the study, or the power of the study, the greater the ability to discriminate true differences between populations. Many studies are underpowered to detect real differences between groups. Investigators need to report a "power analysis" in their studies. Only 32% of randomized controlled trials reported between 1975 and 1990 in the *JAMA*, *Lancet* and *New England Journal of Medicine* reported sample size populations, and on review, most of these studies had too few patients to detect real differences in populations. (Moher D, Dulberg C, Wells G. Statistical power, samples size, and their reporting in randomized control trials. *JAMA* 1994;272:122–4.)

The limitations of epidemiology are that epidemiology demonstrates only an association between exposure and a given disease. Systemic errors are more common in epidemiologic studies compared to experimental studies because of largely human factors. Workers' memories of exposure may not be accurate, creating a *recall bias*. Some workers are more concerned with safety issues and use respirators in dusty environments compared with other workers performing the same task who may never use respirators, creating an *exposure bias*.

A *dose response* between the exposure and cancer should be present. In other words, greater exposure to asbestos fibers should result in a greater incidence of lung cancer. For example, the risk of lung cancer in cigarette smokers is related to the duration and intensity of smoking. If a biological gradient between smoking and lung cancer is not present, then the proof of possible causation is not probable. This is only an association of exposure and disease, but this does not prove causation. I am not an epidemiologist but a student of clinical epidemiological methods and an experienced reviewer of many epidemiological studies submitted to clinical pulmonary and occupational medical journals. I recommend Sven Hernberg's book (*Introduction to Occupational Epidemiology*. Chelsea: Lewis Publishers, 1992) to those interested in a clear, succinct introduction to occupational epidemiology. For a clear, concise history of the epidemiology of malignant mesothelioma, read a brief review by JC McDonald. (McDonald JC. Epidemiology of malignant mesothelioma—An outline. *Ann Occup Hyg* 2010;54:851–7.) For a more in-depth review, I recommend: Gibbs G, Berry G. Epidemiology and risk assessment. In JC Craighead, AR Gibbs (Eds.), *Asbestos and Its Diseases*. Oxford University Press, 2008, pp. 94–119; McDonald JC. *Epidemiology of Work Related Diseases*, 2nd Edition. London: BMJ Books, 2000; Gardner MJ, Machin D, Bryant TN, Altman DG. *Statistics with Confidence. Confidence Intervals and Statistical Guidelines*. London: BMJ Books, 2002; Fletcher, RH, Fletcher SW. *Clinical Epidemiology: The Essentials*, 4th Edition. Baltimore: Lippincott, Williams & Wilkins, 2005; Rothman KJ, Greenland S. *Modern Epidemiology*. Philadelphia: Lippincott, Williams & Wilkins, 1998; Checkoway H, Pearce N, Crawford-Brown DJ. *Research Methods in Occupational Epidemiology*. New York: Oxford University Press, 1989 and 2004; Gehlback S. *Interpreting the Medical Literature*, 5th Edition. New York: McGraw-Hill, 2006.

There is a standard sequence of events that is typically necessary to establish certainty of a cause-and-effect relationship. A study may show statistical significance between an exposed population versus a control population. However, this does not mean that a small increase in statistical risk is relevant or of practical importance. A statistical increase in risk does not prove causality, but only an association. Epidemiologic studies may show a correlation between a toxic exposure and an effect, but *correlation does not prove causation*. In many areas of science, such as chemical effects, we may find a correlation between a chemical exposure and the incidence of cancer. However, that does not mean necessarily that the mechanisms of causation are understood.

1. Case reports are only *suggestive* of a possible cause-and-effect relationship.
2. Multiple case reports are stronger evidence of a *possible* cause-and-effect relationship.
3. Animal, toxicological, and autopsy studies that demonstrate a dose–response effect and mechanisms make *relationships much more likely*.
4. Epidemiological studies that are strongly statistically positive and have a dose–response relationship make a cause-and-effect relationship *probable*.
5. Replication of epidemiologic studies and animal studies by different authors in different countries with appropriate controls make a cause-and-effect relationship *proven*. *No single study proves anything*! (Berman DW, Case BW. Overreliance on a single study: There is no real evidence that applying quality criteria to exposure in asbestos epidemiology affects the estimated risk. *Ann Occup Hyg* 2012;56(8):869–78.)

Again, perhaps the best example of an association or correlation without causation is the morning herald of dawn by the crowing of the rooster. There is a provable, consistent *association* with rooster crowing and the rising of the sun, but *not causation*. If one wrings the neck of the rooster and eats him for dinner, dawn still comes. Many of the early physicians studied a specific disorder, such as scrotal cancer in chimney sweeps, and noted an association to a given exposure. For instance, Sir Percival Pott (*1775: Chirurgical Observations*. London: Hawes, Clarke and Collins) identified that scrotal cancer in London chimney sweeps was due to chimney soot. However, it was not until the late nineteenth and early twentieth centuries that chemical carcinogens were identified in coal soot. (Hogstedt C, Jansson C, Hugosson M, Tinnerberg H, Gustavsson P. Cancer incidence in a cohort of Swedish chimney sweeps, 1958–2006. *Am J Public Health* 2013;103(9):1708–14.) It is the identification of a specific carcinogen capable of producing cancer when applied to the naked skin of animals and humans that was necessary to prove causation, even though the epidemiologic evidence was strong. The withdrawal of the offending hazard with consequent reduction of the cancer is also strong evidence of causation. Laws were passed in England forbidding young, often naked boys from climbing down chimneys. This resulted in a reduction in the incidence of scrotal cancer, suggesting a cause-and-effect relationship.

Science demands evidence, including animal studies, large epidemiological studies with appropriate controls, plausibility, and other information, outlined nicely in a paper by Sir Bradford Hill in 1965. In his Presidential Address to the Section of Occupational Medicine of the Royal Society of Medicine, Dr. Hill outlined the nine requirements of proof to establish a cause-and-effect relationship between an environmental exposure and a specific disease. These nine requirements were

1. Strength of the association
2. Consistency in different populations or circumstances
3. Specificity or a single effect
4. Temporality or exposure precedes disease with an appropriate latency
5. Biological gradient or dose–response
6. Plausibility or that the causation is biologically plausible
7. Coherence or that the disease should not seriously conflict with what is generally known about the natural history and biology of disease
8. Experimental, or can the disease be altered experimentally by some intervention, or the condition can be replicated in an animal model
9. Finally by analogy, such as if one drug can cause cancer, then perhaps similar drugs may cause cancer
      (Hill AB. The environment and disease: Association or causation? *Proc R Soc Med* 1965;58:295–300.)

More than 50 years have lapsed since this speech was given, but it still remains the standard today by which science evaluates the relationship between an environmental exposure and a given disease. Harrington quoted Sir Bradford Hill in 1993 as saying, "All scientific work is incomplete—whether it be observational or experimental. All scientific work is liable to be upset or modified by advancing knowledge. That does not confer upon us a freedom to ignore that knowledge we already have, or to postpone the action that it appears to demand at a given time." (Harrington JM. Re: Attitudes and opinions regarding asbestos and cancer (Commentary). *Am J Ind Med* 1993;23:505–6.)

Lung cancer and mesothelioma were identified in some early case reports of workers who died of asbestosis, but the evidence for a biological explanation and positive animal studies took many decades. Case reports are not proof of a clear association or causation. Epidemiologic studies with a sufficiently sized population, with appropriate control of potential bias, are necessary to suggest an association. Once an association—controlled for confounding variables—between a particular substance of appropriate intensity and duration was found in the workplace, such as carcinogenic mineral fibers or known chemical carcinogens like cigarette smoke with a clear dose response, then proof of causation is highly likely. Generally speaking, an OR, standard mortality ratio, or RR of greater than 2 is required to strongly suggest a significant association unless the power of the study and confidence limits allow for using a lower number. (Gardner MJ, Machin D, Bryant TN, Altman DG. *Statistics with Confidence. Confidence Intervals and Statistical Guidelines*. London: BMJ Books, 2002.)

It is very important to recognize the need for data to demonstrate the minimal magnitude of exposure necessary for causation. Cigarette smoking causes lung cancer only when the exposure has been of sufficient duration and intensity. There is no risk of lung cancer to someone who tried smoking for a brief period as a teenager or in college because the exposure was not of sufficient magnitude and duration to be considered hazardous. Exposure to asbestos does not necessarily imply that the exposure was of sufficient magnitude and duration to be hazardous. It is just like cigarette smoking; exposure to cigarette smoking or asbestos must be of sufficient intensity and duration to suggest causation.

Discussions by experts on various epidemiologic studies of asbestos-exposed workers have often resulted in disagreement on the true magnitude of the exposure–effect relationships for asbestos. Many of these issues are discussed by the Chrysotile Asbestos Expert Panel in Montreal, Quebec, in November of 2007. (Chrysotile Asbestos Expert Panel, Montreal, Quebec. *Chrysotile Asbestos Consensus Statement and Summary.* November 13–14, 2007. Health Canada.) The panel listed sources of exposure misclassification or bias that have caused confusion in the interpretation of epidemiologic studies, to which I have added 17 of my own. I have defined bias as a systematic error that results in misrepresentation or departs systematically from the true values of a scientific study, and therefore leads to misinterpretation and misclassification of data. This frequently leads to conclusions that are systematically different from the truth. (Sackett DL. Bias in analytical research. *J Chronic Dis* 1979;32:51.)

A. Exposure concentrations estimated in published epidemiological studies were mostly determined by area monitoring, rather than personal monitoring, and this usually underestimates personal exposure and can miss short periods of high exposure. This produces a *measurement bias.*
B. Published epidemiologic studies differ in their frequency and time period over which sampling was conducted. Most historical sampling was for short periods and average daily or weekly exposure data are not available. Little routine sampling was conducted prior to the 1950s, when exposure concentrations were much higher than exposures that have occurred more recently. The early exposures may be estimated by extrapolation, a very uncertain process. This produces a *sampling bias.*
C. Studies vary in the degree to which various operations were directly sampled and the degree to which asbestos exposures at unmeasured operations were estimated. Industrial processes change with time and exposures are constantly changing with changing work conditions and work practices, requiring continuous monitoring of work exposures to develop an estimate of total cumulative exposures. Task-based estimates of exposure are not reliable predictors of exposure. Risk perception affects work practices and then consequently exposure. (Creely KS, Cowie H, Van Tongeren M, Kromhout H, Tickner J, Cherrie JW. Trends in inhalation exposure—A review of the data in the published scientific literature. *Ann Occup Hyg* 2007;51(8):665–78; Cherrie JW. Are task-based exposure levels a valuable index of exposure for epidemiology? *Ann Occup Hyg* 1996;40(6):715–22; Stewart-Taylor AJ, Cherrie JW. Does risk perception affect behaviour and exposure? A pilot study amongst asbestos workers. *Ann Occup Hyg* 1998;42(8):565–9.)

D. Laboratories often do not agree with one another when they measure exposures in the same environment, and this is particularly important in that it affects measurements before modern quality checks became common around 1980. (Health Effects Institute—Asbestos Research. *Asbestos in Public and Commercial Buildings: A Literature Review and Synthesis of Current Knowledge.* Cambridge: Health Effects Institute—Asbestos Research, 1991.)

Exposure estimates from before around 1970 have involved conversion from particle counts to fiber accounts, a very uncertain process whose effects will vary from environment to environment. (Ayer HE, Lynch JR, Fanney JH. A comparison of impinger and membrane filter techniques for evaluating air samples in asbestos plants. *Ann NY Acad Sci* 1965;330:274–87; Lynch JR, Ayer HE. Measurement of asbestos exposure. *J Occup Med* 1968;10(1):21–4; Edwards GH, Lynch JR. The method used by the U.S. Public Health Service for enumeration of asbestos dust on membrane filters. *Ann Occup Hyg* 1968;11(1):1–6; Timbrell V, Gibson JC, Webster I. UICC standard reference samples of asbestos. *Int J Cancer* 1968;3(3):406–8.)

SOURCES OF BIAS

1. Optical microscopy is used for counting fibers and cannot distinguish between asbestos fibers and nonasbestos materials. Cleavage fragments of various minerals are nontoxic yet counted in historical fiber measurements. Therefore, it is possible that in some particularly dusty environments, a significant amount of material counted was not asbestos. This leads to variable underestimates of risk per unit of exposure in the different environments. Also, many workers were exposed to asbestos other than the main type of asbestos used in their job compared with other workers, and this may not be apparent in the measurements. For instance, the main exposures to American insulators in using high-temperature asbestos insulation are to mixed asbestos consisting of both chrysotile and amosite. However, crocidolite was commonly used in small concentrations as a finish coat of asbestos-wrapped pipes. In some of the historical studies, the reader cannot be sure whether the observed measurements were of total dust or asbestos dust established by estimating the present asbestos in the main product and multiplying that by the total dust count.

2. Phase-contrast optical microscopy has been the standard American tool for measuring airborne asbestos since 1972. However, the optical microscope cannot count fibers thinner than 0.25 μm. It is now widely recognized that the most hazardous thin long fibers are not visible on optical microscopy. The proportion of fibers visible by optical microscopy depends on fiber type. The light microscope is able to visualize only 5% of crocidolite, 26.5% of amosite, and <14% of chrysotile fibers present in lung tissue. (Pooley FD, Ranson DL. Comparison of the results of asbestos fiber dust count in the lung tissue obtained by analytical electron microscopy and light

microscopy. *J Clin Pathol* 1986;39:313–7.) The level prior to 1968 was 5 million particles of asbestos dust per cubic foot of air or 185 particles of dust per cubic centimeter, which is approximately 30 fibers/cc according to the 1972 National Institute of Occupational Safety and Health (NIOSH) counting standard. The conversion of particles per cubic foot to fibers per cubic centimeter is a very uncertain process and is very dependent on the type of industrial process being evaluated.

Beginning in 1965, the optical microscopic methodology has changed several times. With each improvement in standardization, there has been an increase in the quality of measurement and the quantity of true asbestos fibers counted. By 1980, the measurement differences between the early methods and the modern standard method have probably increased several-fold. This means that the actual concentration of hazardous asbestos fibers present in the breathing zone in many of the historical studies published prior to 1980 were much greater than estimated. (Ogden TL, Shenton-Taylor T, Cherrie JW et al. Within-laboratory quality control of asbestos counting. *Ann Occup Hyg* 1986;30(4):411–25.) This again produces a *measurement bias*.

3. The fiber size counted by optical microscopy is not identical to the size of fibers present in the exposure. The *inability to count pathogenic fibers* (fibers <0.25 μm in diameter and >8–10 μm in length) to which the worker was actually exposed has made interpretation of various epidemiologic studies difficult to correlate to the measured dose effect of lung cancer and mesothelioma incidence, particularly for those workers in South Carolina textile mills exposed to thin long fibers visible only by electron microscopy. (Dodson RF, Hammar SP, Poye LW. A technical comparison of evaluating asbestos concentration by phase-contrast microscopy (PCOM), scanning electron microscopy (SEM), and analytical transmission electron microscopy (TEM) as illustrated from data generated from a case report. *Inhal Toxicol* 2008;20(7):723–32.)

4. Individual fiber count samples are subject to substantial random error, particularly when small numbers are counted. Most data points in a good epidemiologic study use many samples to reduce these *random errors*. There is significant lack of agreement between different laboratories in counting fibers. (Gylseth B, Churg A, Davis JM et al. Analysis of asbestos fibers and asbestos bodies in tissue samples from human lung. An international inter-laboratory trial. *Scand J Work Environ Health* 1985;11(2):107–10.)

5. Exposure level may be overestimated in workers who wear protective equipment, wet down asbestos during removal, and do not mix asbestos-containing mud in closed spaces. This is particularly likely in the dusty jobs in which individual preference and comfort may affect respirator use, creating an *exposure bias*. Many individuals have poor recall of their exposures due to a poor memory or inattention to the details of their surroundings, resulting in a *recall bias*. This is a *differential information bias* due to the difference between the true exposures and the inability to accurately replicate the exposures because of poor memory or inattention to the working

environment. This bias may be important in the "non-exposed" control population who might be unaware of prior asbestos exposure. (Checkoway H, Pearce N, Crawford-Brown DJ. *Research Methods in Occupational Epidemiology.* New York: Oxford University Press, 1989 and 2004.)

6. Some health effects are underestimated because of the nonnegligible under-estimation of adverse health effects in actual occupational cohort studies due to the *dilution effect* or the comparison bias. The dilution effect results from the inclusion of nonexposed or very-low-exposed workers in the study cohort. The *comparison bias* results from healthy hire effects at the beginning of an exposure history. The lung function of blue-collar workers is typically better than the references taken from the general population (i.e., usually over 100% predicted). This is called the *healthy worker effect*. The healthy worker effect is particularly important in the evaluation of lung function decline after heavy asbestos exposure. For instance, if a worker begins with a forced vital capacity (FVC) of 110% of predicted and loses 20% of his lung function over time, then they are left with a FVC of 90% of predicted, which is well within normal predicted limits, in spite of the fact they have had a substantial detrimental decline in lung function due to asbestos exposure. The healthy worker effect may be balanced by other workers who are smokers, drug users, or have some nonasbestos-related reason for lower lung function prior to employment. The only way to accurately measure the effect of asbestos exposure on lung function is to obtain baseline lung function prior to the period of asbestos exposure. I am not aware of a published study of serial lung function tests in an asbestos-exposed population that begins with preexposure testing. (Hernberg S. "Negative" results in cohort studies—How to recognize fallacies. *Scand J Work Environ Health* 1981;7(Suppl. 4):121–6; Baillargeon J. Characteristics of the healthy worker effect. *Occup Med* 2001;16:359–66.)

Chrysotile mine exposures produce varying incidences of lung cancer and mesothelioma, largely based on the concentration of tremolite contamination of the mine ore. Epidemiologic studies concerning chrysotile exposure are often interpretable without consideration of fiber length, amphibole (tremolite) contamination, and industrial process such as miners/millers versus textile workers. Studies that include workers with exposures from different sources with varying amounts of amphibole contamination or long versus shorter fiber length exposures produce a *selection bias*. (McDonald AD, Case BW, Churg A et al. Mesothelioma in Quebec chrysotile miners and millers: Epidemiology and aetiology. *Ann Occup Hyg* 1997;41:707–19; McDonald JC, McDonald AD. Chrysotile, tremolite and carcinogenicity. *Ann Occup Hyg* 1997;41(6):699–705.) The issue of whether chrysotile asbestos causes mesothelioma has largely been related to the studies of McDonald AD, Case BW, Churg A et al., as published in a review in the *Annals of Occupational Hygiene* (1997;41:707–19). This article summarizes the study of a cohort of miners that included 11,000 men born between 1891 and 1920 who were employed in the Quebec chrysotile production industry. The results of this long-term follow-up of these miners reveals that of 9780 men who survived until 1936, 8009 were known to have died before 1993 and 38 had probably died from mesothelioma. Thirty-three of these 38 workers were miners and five were factory workers, and the factory workers apparently had exposure to amphibole asbestos in the form of crocidolite and/or amosite. This leaves a total of 33 cases of mesothelioma out of 11,000 initial workers that were studied and about 10,000 that were followed. There appeared to be more mesotheliomas from the Thedford area of Quebec than from other areas of Quebec where there was less contamination by tremolite in the rock where the asbestos is mined. The results of these careful studies of chrysotile-associated mesothelioma indicate that there are high concentrations of tremolite asbestos, a known contaminate of these ores associated with these mesotheliomas. There have been two careful mineralogical analyses of the Cary Canadian Mine, which are unique in that they did not yield evidence of significant tremolite contamination or epidemiologic evidence of mesothelioma.

Earlier studies had suggested that perhaps chrysotile might cause mesothelioma, and there was caution during the 1960s about chrysotile as an adequate replacement for crocidolite asbestos. With time and the careful studies of McDonald and coworkers in Canada, the evidence has come forth that there does not appear to be any risk of mesothelioma associated with pure chrysotile. Many of the Quebec cohort with mesothelioma were exposed to crocidolite and amosite. McDonald has suggested that these amphibole exposures were due to work in a plant that made military gas mask filters. (McDonald AD, Case BW, Churg A et al. Mesothelioma in Quebec chrysotile miners and millers: Epidemiology and aetiology. *Ann Occup Hyg* 1997;41:707–19.)

Many research studies have been performed since the 1960s comparing tremolite-free asbestos to tremolite-contaminated asbestos as a cause of mesothelioma. The problem with many of the epidemiologic studies of chrysotile asbestos workers has been the contamination of the cohort by other amphibole exposure as summarized by Dunnigan in 1988 and Pierce in 2008. Different mining areas have different risks for lung cancer and mesothelioma based on amphibole contamination (tremolite) of the asbestiform rock, as shown in Table 2.1. (Dunnigan J. Linking chrysotile asbestos with mesothelioma. *Am J Ind Med* 1988;14:205–9; Pierce JS, McKinley MA,

Table 2.1 Disease differences between Quebec mines with higher versus lower amphibole contamination of chrysotile asbestos

Cause of death	N	Central mines "Area A"	Peripheral mines "Area B"
		Odds ratio (90% confidence interval)	Odds ratio (90% confidence interval)
Mesothelioma	21	2.55 (1.52–4.27)	1.11(0.47–2.62)
Lung cancer	262	1.98 (1.53–2.57)	1.09 (0.78–1.51)

Source: Reprinted from *Occup Hyg*, 41(6), McDonald JC, McDonald AD, 699–705, Copyright 1997, with permission from Elsevier.

Paustenbach DJ, Finley BL. An evaluation of reported no-effect chrysotile asbestos exposures for lung cancer and mesothelioma. *Crit Rev Toxicol* 2008;38:191–214.)

7. *Interpretation bias* is related to the very human condition of subjectivity or lack of scientific objectivity on the part of the reader, reviewer, editor, or interpreter of a scientific paper. Some interpretation errors by readers of scientific papers are simply related to ignorance and lack of scientific training and experience. Often, some prior experience and understanding of the subject is required. Some papers require requests to the author for more information to facilitate interpretation and clarification. Those of us who are experts in the field under study may harbor various belief systems and prejudices against institutions, medical journals, personalities, scientific methodology, and a variety of minor issues that color our interpretations when reading certain scientific papers. If we are aware of our lack of objectivity, we should ask for help from others who are more objective. *Disclosures of conflicts of interest* are critical to protecting the ethical standards of the reviewer and the medical journal. Objectivity takes self-awareness and self-discipline, which requires more time when reviewing certain papers. We must acknowledge that our best judgments are fallible. (Armstrong D. Medical reviews face criticism over lapses. *Wall St J* 2006;B1, B2.)

8. Job title is commonly used to estimate exposure when the workers are not available for interview or are deceased. The actual exposures to workers may vary considerably from the exposure estimated by job title. Job title does not take into account other exposures to asbestos-containing materials from previous or subsequent employment and creates an *information bias*. This was a particular problem in the estimation of the health effects of amosite exposure in the Paterson, New Jersey plant studied by Seidman and Selikoff, where many of the workers had had previous employment in the surrounding asbestos industries. McCullagh published a paper in the *Journal of the Society of Occupational Medicine* (1980;30:153–6) on "Amosite as a cause of lung cancer and mesothelioma in humans." He pointed out that many of the Paterson, New Jersey cohorts studied by Selikoff had previous exposure to asbestos from other manufacturing plants in the area. He felt that rather than 1/50th of the group, it seemed more likely that one-third of the group or 300 members of the Paterson cohort had been occupationally exposed to asbestos before entering the cohort.

9. Historical epidemiologic studies have focused primarily on asbestos exposure and cigarette smoking. There is always an *information bias* not only from self-reported exposures and cigarette smoking histories, but this bias also underestimates the effects of other hazardous materials in the workplace on lung cancer risk, such as nickel, chromium, cadmium exposures, diesel fumes, welding fumes, and second-hand cigarette smoke and other types of carcinogens. *Confounding information* on drug abuse, hepatitis, AIDS, and human papillomavirus (HPV), radon exposure, and other carcinogens has been largely ignored in these studies. Recent studies have demonstrated an increased risk of lung cancer in agriculture workers and other

workers exposed to inorganic and organic dust. (Baser S, Duzce O. Evyapan F, Akdag B, Ozkurt S, Kiter G. Occupational exposure and thoracic malignancies, is there a relationship? *J Occup Health* 2013;55(4):301–6.) It is very naïve to view every disease as having a single cause, but unfortunately this is the working hypothesis used in many large epidemiological studies.

The reliance on individual histories of presumed asbestos exposure is fraught with inaccuracy. Dodson reported a lung fiber analysis and found that, of 18 people reporting no history of asbestos exposure, only 7 had been unexposed and 11 were unaware that they were exposed. However, 6 individuals out of 20 who reported a history of exposure had only background levels of asbestos. The conclusion reached was that there was a lack of association between lung fiber burdens of asbestos fibers and the reported histories of exposure. (Dodson RF. 1997, 2003, 2005 quoted by Carbone M et al. 2012; Carbone M, Ly BH, Dodson RF et al. Malignant mesothelioma: Facts, myths, and hypotheses. *J Cell Physiol* 2012;227(1):44–58.) There have been attempts to create questionnaires and complicated formulae to estimate asbestos exposure, but they have produced discordant results. (Rödelsperger K, Jöckel KH, Pohlabeln H, Römer W, Woitowitz HJ. Asbestos and man-made vitreous fibers as risk factors for diffuse malignant mesothelioma: Results from a German hospital-based case-control study. *Am J Ind Med* 2001;39:262–75.) Industrial hygienists have attempted to translate job titles or job descriptions into exposure categories and then quantify exposure into "fibers/mL-years" unsuccessfully. Iwatsubo said in 1998 that "Because no measurements of airborne asbestos levels were available, all estimates of exposure parameters were based on experts subjective [sic], that is semi quantification [sic], to which we subsequently assigned weight factors. This index of cumulative exposure was expressed in terms of fiber/mL-years." (Iwatsobo Y, Pairon JC, Boutin C et al. Pleural mesothelioma: Dose response relation at low levels of asbestos exposure in French population-based case control study. *Am J Epidemiol* 1998;148:133–42.) The most objective way to quantify exposure is by measuring lung fiber burden. There is a poor correlation between fiber burden and reported exposure history. (Takahashi K, Case BW, Dufresne A et al. Relation between lung asbestos fiber burden and exposure indices based on job history. *Occup Environ Med* 1994;51:461–9.) A *voluntary response bias* or *recall bias* can arise when case subjects think they have been exposed to a dangerous product or hazardous concentrations of a mineral like asbestos. Publicity in news media and advertisements create fear and an increased number of supposedly exposed individuals compared to individuals not exposed to the media. (Sackett DL. Bias in analytic research. *J Chronic Dis* 1979;32:51–63; Lerchen ML, Samet JM. An assessment of the validity of questionnaire responses provided by a surviving spouse. *Am J Epidemiol* 1986;123:481–9; Hernberg S. Some guidelines for interpreting epidemiologic studies. In *Introduction to Occupational Epidemiology*. Chelsea: Lewis Publishing, 1992, pp. 201–3.)

Certainly, one of the big issues in evaluating epidemiologic studies has been the issue of the unreliability of certain information obtained from patients or an *information bias*. This is a trickier problem in smokers, who often deny they smoke or reduce the amount they smoke, particularly when they are confronted with the possibility of a smoke-related disease such as emphysema, lung cancer, or heart disease. Now, with the advent of the computerized medical record, information about alcohol use, drug use, cigarette smoking, and sexually transmitted diseases is potentially available to insurance companies, which might disqualify some individuals from certain types of life and health insurance or raise their premiums. A recent article in the *Wall Street Journal* on Tuesday, February 19, 2013, by Sumathi Reddy, entitled "I don't smoke, Doc, and other patient lies," points out that patient lies, which vary from half-truths to boldly blatant lies, are surprisingly common. In a 2009 survey, 28% of patients surveyed acknowledged sometimes lying to their healthcare provider or omitting information. The healthcare providers surveyed suspected worse and 77% said that one-fourth or more of their patients submitted incorrect facts or lied, and 28% of healthcare providers estimated that it was more than half of their patients. In a survey conducted by General Electric with the Cleveland Clinic and the Ochsner Health System of 2000 people and more than 1200 doctors, it was concluded that patients aged 25–34 years were more likely to lie than older patients. Men were two times as likely to get caught lying compared to women. Some patients lie out of embarrassment or fear of disappointing a doctor. Others worry about electronic medical records or information being communicated to employers, insurance companies, or authorities. (Wallner-Liebmann SJ, Grammer TB, Siekmeier R et al. Smoking denial in cardiovascular disease studies. *Adv Exp Med Biol* 2013;788:35–8.)

Doctors themselves may shade the truth for a variety of reasons, and in a study published in the *Journal of Health Affairs*, it was found that one-tenth or more of 1800 physicians surveyed had told patients something untrue in the previous year. More than half said they described a prognosis in a more positive manner than warranted and approximately 20% admitted to not fully disclosing a mistake to a patient due to fears of litigation. Often, the history of asbestos exposure is problematic because laypersons often cannot identify asbestos products accurately and cannot accurately quantify hazardous dust exposures. Therefore, retrospective epidemiologic studies that rely on patents' histories are fraught with error and are not accurate estimates of exposure to asbestos or specific asbestos-containing products. American physicians may be pressured into *cost shifting* by reporting a disorder as work related in order to shift the cost of care away from certain low-paying insurance programs or self-insurance to better-paying, more comprehensive workers' compensation health insurance programs.

10. *Latency bias* due to the long latency of mesothelioma has resulted in an underestimation of the true incidence of mesothelioma, particularly in very heavily exposed populations in which many of the workers who would likely develop a mesothelioma die prematurely from asbestosis and lung cancer, or they die prematurely from degenerative conditions such as stroke and heart disease. Many workers who were older at the time of exposure never had sufficient remaining years of life expectancy to develop a mesothelioma.

Today, the average age of diagnosis of a mesothelioma is about 70 years. The time from initial exposure to asbestos to the diagnosis of the disease has been slowly increasing over the years from about 30 years to now about 50 years. This is thought to be related to lower levels of exposure in individuals living in the twenty-first century compared to the historical cohorts with heavier exposures and shorter latency times in the twentieth century. (Roggli V, Vollmer R. Twenty five-years of fiber analysis: What have we learned? *Hum Pathol* 2008;39:307–15; Bianchi C, Giarelli L, Grandi G, Brollo A, Ramani L, Zuch C. Latency periods in asbestos-related mesothelioma of the pleura. *Eur J Cancer* 1997;6:162–6; Newman V, Günthe S, Mülle KM, Fischer M. Malignant mesothelioma—German mesothelioma register 1987–1999. *Int Arch Occup Environ Health* 2001;74:383–95.)

11. Persons coming to autopsy are not representative of persons who die in the general population, producing a *selection bias*. Also, death certificate classifications of causes of death are often inaccurate. (Wagner JC, Berry G, Pooley FD. Mesothelioma and asbestos type in asbestos textile workers: A study of lung contents. *Brit Med J* 1982;285:603–6; Baker D. Limitations in drawing etiologic inferences based on measurement of asbestos fibers from lung tissue. *Ann NY Acad Sci* 1991;645:61–73; Selikoff IJ, Seidman H. Use of death certificates in epidemiological studies, including occupational hazards: Variations in discordance of different asbestos-associated disease on best evidence ascertainment. *Am J Ind Med* 1992;22:481–92; Selikoff IJ. Death certificates in epidemiological studies, including occupational hazards: Inaccuracies in occupational categories. *Am J Ind Med* 1992;22:493–504; Percy C, Stanek E 3rd, Gloeckler L. Accuracy of cancer death certificates and its effect on cancer mortality statistics. *Am J Public Health* 1981;71:242–50.)

12. An *immortal time bias* refers to a span of time in the observation or follow-up of a cohort during which the outcome under study could not have occurred. It usually occurs with the passing of time before a subject has been exposed. While a subject is not truly immortal during this time span, the subject necessarily had to remain event free until the start of the exposure to be classified as exposed. Bias occurs from incorrect consideration of prior exposures. The design or analysis of a cohort trial leads to what is called an immortal time bias. A good example is the study of Seidman and Selikoff of New Jersey amosite workers who were exposed in a specific factory making amosite-containing insulation. (Seidman H, Selikoff IJ, Gelb SK. Mortality experience of amosite asbestos factory workers: Dose–response relationships 5–40 years after onset of short-term work exposure. *Am J Ind Med* 1986;10:479–514.) The authors assumed that asbestos exposures were only from this Paterson, New Jersey plant, only to amosite asbestos, and exposure began at employment. Others have concluded that a significant percentage of these workers had previous employment in other asbestos manufacturing plants in northern New Jersey prior to employment at the Paterson, New Jersey plant. McCullagh published a paper in the *Journal of the Society of Occupational Medicine* (1980;30:153–6) on "Amosite as a cause of lung cancer

and mesothelioma in humans." He pointed out that many of the Paterson, New Jersey cohorts studied by Selikoff had previous exposure to asbestos from other manufacturing plants in the area. He felt that rather than 1/50th of the group as reported by the authors, it seemed more likely that one-third of the group or 300 members of the Paterson cohort had been occupationally exposed to asbestos before entering the cohort. (Suissa S. Immortal time bias in pharmaco-epidemiology. *Am J Epidemiol* 2008;167:493–9.)

13. Epidemiology evidence is important, but does not trump other important evidence such as dose response, animal data, mechanistic data, and often, the inability to control for confounding by other important occupational exposures or viral infections such as HPV in carcinoma of the larynx, and simian virus 40 in mesothelioma. Robert Sataloff reminds us that "Medicine is replete with assumptions and myths based on faulty reasoning. It is important for all of us to be aware of this problem and diligent about assessing evidence to draw the best possible conclusions. One of the most frequent errors results from *post hoc ergo propter hoc* reasoning. This classic error in logic assumes that because Event B happens after Event A, Event B is caused by Event A. Proof of causation requires considerably more rigorous evidence." In more simplistic terms, an *association does not prove causation*. There is an association between the cock heralding the coming of dawn but the crowing of the cock does not cause the morning rising of the sun. (Ahmed SM, Sataloff RT. Asbestos exposure and laryngeal cancer: Is there an association? *Ear Nose Throat J* 2009;88:1140–2.)

14. P Boffetta, Chief epidemiologist of the International Agency for Research on Cancer in Lyon, France, has wisely rebuked his fellow epidemiologists as follows: "False-positive results are inherent in the scientific process of testing hypotheses concerning the determinants of cancer and other human illnesses. Much of what is known about the etiology of human cancers has arisen from epidemiological studies, epidemiology has been increasingly criticized for producing findings that are often sensationalized." Boffetta calls for humility regarding findings in epidemiology that would go a long way to diminishing the detrimental effects of false-positive results. Type I errors reject the null hypothesis that there is no difference in different groups and purports a difference when one does not exist. Unfortunately, academic medicine is financed through biomedical research that demands positive results or encourages type I errors and the "publish or perish dilemma" subtly states that bad or sloppy published research is better for academic advancement than no publication of research. (Boffetta P, McLaughlin JK, La Vecchia C, Tarone RE, Lipworth L, Blot WJ. False-positive results in cancer epidemiology: A plea for epistemological modesty. *J Natl Cancer Inst* 2008;100(14):988–95.)

15. Always remember that there may be an "elephant in the room." By this comment, I am referring to unaccounted for, or unappreciated causes of disease such as HPV infection as a major cause of laryngeal and other head and neck cancers. Genetic factors will likely be the "elephant in the room" in the future. Once new causes of disease have been established, previous

epidemiologic studies without correction for this new information confounding produces a selection and information bias that makes these earlier
studies invalid for use in meta-analysis.

16. Meta-analysis is the statistical analysis of a collection of studies used to
determine whether combining different studies results in further clarity of
relationships between a potential cause and effect. In the current medical
knowledge hierarchy, systematic review articles take precedence over nar-
rative or unsystematic ones. The systematic nature of collection and quality
assessment is meant to ensure that all relevant works are included and
adequately evaluated. This is the somewhat naïve view of many physicians.
This idea emerged in medical publishing during the 1980s, and has become
a core element of a movement that somewhat broadly is referred to as
evidence-based medicine. In preparation for a meta-analysis study, variables
that could affect outcome need to be controlled, such as confounders like
cigarette smoking, alcohol use, para-occupational exposures, socio-economic
factors, age, race, and sex. Exposures need to be similar, such as not using
data from insulators mixed with data from electricians and carpenters. The
quality of the studies used in the meta-analysis of asbestos health effects
should be determined by whether or not the evidence is based and graded in
a similar fashion to the Cochrane evidence-based grading system.

Fiber type, fiber size, and dose need to be similar or homogeneous for
comparison purposes. For instance, the incidence of lung cancer is very different in chrysotile miners and millers versus South Carolina textile workers
because of exposure to more carcinogenic thin, long asbestos fibers in textile
plants. Various meta-analysis studies have been performed to evaluate the
risk of lung cancer and mesothelioma from chrysotile exposure. A legiti-
mate study of lung cancer incidence in chrysotile asbestos workers cannot
include subjects from textile production and chrysotile mining and milling
in the same study because of the large proportionate effect of long chrysotile fiber length on the risk for lung cancer. In a similar fashion, the risk for
lung cancer and mesothelioma in chrysotile asbestos miners and millers
is related to amphibole contamination. This nullifies the ability to evaluate
risk for mesothelioma and lung cancer from chrysotile exposure by consoli-
dating cohorts from all chrysotile miners and millers with different levels of
amphibole contamination in the study population. This type of *confounding*,
by including chrysotile workers with varying amphibole exposure, makes a
helpful analysis impossible. Meta-analysis studies are thought by many to be
an impartial method for pooling data to increase sample sizes and increase
statistical power. The ability to collect large sample sizes may make even
miniscule differences statistically significant, but this does not make these
findings relevant or necessarily true.

Meta-analysis is the darling of some statisticians and epidemiologists,
but the potential bias in case selection makes interpretation impossible
in some studies. Wilkens and coworkers from Hamburg, Germany, performed a meta-analysis on lung function in asbestos-exposed workers. They
identified 542 papers on Medline and found 46 others by manual searching

congress reports that mentioned lung function and asbestos exposure. They then selected 289 articles for detailed evaluation. They found 30 articles for inclusion in their meta-analysis, 15 of which had a high-resolution computerized tomography (HRCT)-based diagnosis. Why the authors mixed HRCT diagnosis analysis of asbestos-related abnormalities with much less sensitive and specific chest x-ray diagnosis of asbestos-related pleural disease is unclear. The sample sizes ranged from 19 to 3383 and included studies focused on 13 different occupations including asbestos cement workers, ironworkers, railway workers, ceiling tilers, wall boarders, sheet metal workers, constructions workers, carpenters, mill wrights, boilermakers, shipyard workers, and asbestos manufacturing and insulation workers for a total of 9921 cases for analysis. The heterogeneity of the study group is obvious. The study population differed considerably in duration of employment—from 1 year to 30 years—with major differences regarding intensity of exposure, employment type, and fiber type. There is heterogeneity in the quality of lung function tests, instrumentation, reference values, and types of diagnostic radiology. This makes accurate assessment of the issue of the effects of asbestos exposure on lung function impossible because of the heterogeneity in this meta-analysis study. The disparity of evidence and the little homogeneity in meta-analysis methodologies introduces an unresolvable bias in this systematic review article, even though the methodology may be adequate. This produces an appearance of better external validity than the primary studies would allow. (Wilkens D, Garrido MV, Manuwald U, Baur X. Lung function in asbestos-exposed workers, a systematic review and meta-analysis. *J Occup Med Toxicol* 2011;6:1–16; Santaguida P, Oremus M, Walker K et al. Systematic reviews identify important methodological flaws in stroke rehabilitation therapy primary studies: Review of reviews. *J Clin Epidemiol* 2012;65:358–67; Manterola C, Astudillo P, Arias E, Claros N. Systematic reviews of the literature: What should be known about them. *Cir Esp* 2013;91(3):149–55.)

In reality, there is a great *selection bias* created in deciding which studies are included or not included in the pooled data analysis. An author can choose to include only studies that favor their bias and then use various favorable selected studies to strengthen their view on causation by excluding less favorable studies from inclusion in the pooled data analysis. The strength of a pooled data analysis is entirely related to the quality, validity, homogeneity, and inclusiveness of the epidemiologic reports used in the analysis. The inappropriate inclusion of poor studies in meta-analysis results in an inexorable conclusion of the aphorism "garbage in, garbage out"!

The advantage of pooled data is that they increase the statistical power of the study by including large numbers of subjects. Large studies usually have narrow confidence limits and claim greater precision. Unfortunately, studies with sufficient power and narrow confidence limits are not necessarily useful or truthful because of selection bias and heterogeneity. *Statistical certainty is not synonymous with biologic certainty, nor does it indicate the importance of the result.*

17. Small studies suffer from a *small sample bias*. Small sample bias is mainly determined by the sample size ratio, which is defined as the ratio of the sample size to the number of disease categories in the reference population. A recently published proximate mortality ratio (PMR) analysis of radiation and mesothelioma resulted in a PMR overestimation of 22.5%. (Zhou JY. Bias in the proportionate mortality ratio analysis of small study populations: A case on analyses of radiation and mesothelioma. *Int J Radiat Biol* 2014;90(11):1075–9.)

18. Publication bias reflects the bias of scientific editorial boards in either refusing to publish or encouraging the publication of scientific papers that support the bias of the editorial board of that particular scientific journal about asbestos. This leads to a systematic distortion in the body of scientific knowledge, since many negative studies are not published. Some authors have financial interests in their publications. Some medical journal editors are reluctant to ban some authors for fear they will publish important papers elsewhere. (Armstrong D. Medical reviews face criticism over lapses. *Wall St J* 2006;B1, B2.)

    Asbestos litigation has become a multi-billion dollar industry and governmental agencies have been pressured by outside interests. Medical journals are inundated with articles about asbestos. If certain peer-reviewed journals refuse to publish their articles, then some of these authors start their own medical journal and choose like-minded experts to be on their editorial board. Some poor-quality papers are published in certain "peer-reviewed" journals that would not withstand editorial appraisal in journals with a high-quality review process.

    A good example of *publication bias* is shown in the of news about global warming and the favorable treatment of certain authors submitting positive papers in favor of global warming to certain scientific journals. Scientists need financial support from public and private institutions to support their research. Research projects are more likely to be funded if the purpose of the scientific study is likely to support the scientific bias of the funding institution. Negative results are more difficult to publish and are less likely to receive further research grant support in the future. Unfortunately, many environmental issues have been heavily politicized; not only asbestos, but also global warming, as discussed by many of the authors listed below. (Akerlof K, Rowan KE, Fitzgerald D, Cedeno AY. Communication of climate projections in US media amid politicization of model science. *Nat Climate Change* 2012;2:648–54; Brysse K, Oreskes N, O'Reilly J, Oppenheimer M. Climate change prediction: Erring on the side of least drama? *Global Environ Change* 2013;23(1):327–37; Easterbrook D (Ed.), *Evidence-Based Climate Science: Data Opposing CO$_2$ Emissions as the Primary Source of Global Warming.* Oxford: Elsevier, 2011; Gould LI. Man-made 'global warming' (AGW): A critical thinking approach to exposing some of its scientific and methodological flaws. *Bull Am Phys Soc* 2012; Keller EM. Re-constructing climate change: Discourses of the emerging movement for climate change [Master's Thesis]. Queen's Research & Learning Repository, Queens

University, Kingston, Ontario, Canada, October 2012; Ritter SK, Mann M. Global warming and climate change: Believers, deniers, and doubters view the scientific forecast from different angles [cover story]. *Chem Eng News* 2009;87(51):11–21; Van der Sluijs JP. Uncertainty and dissent in climate risk assessment: A post-normal perspective. *Nat Cult* 2012;7(2):174–95; Van der Sluijs JP, van Est R, Riphagen M. Beyond consensus: Reflections from a democratic perspective on the interaction between climate politics and science. *Curr Opin Environ Sustain* 2010;2(5–6):409–15.)

19. *Governmental agency bias* is related to the assumption that governmental agencies must be ultra-conservative in their estimates of risk calculation in order to perform their due diligence to protect the public from illness or injury. This policy may produce unnecessary fear in the uninformed population because of exaggerated fears of risk for cancer based on government risk evaluation. Governmental agencies use a linear model based on logistic regression back to zero exposure to calculate risk, as opposed to a biological model of no effect below a threshold dose that assumes a minimal threshold dose to determine risk. The issues of risk determination and government policy are discussed in more detail in Chapters 15 and 16. Government agencies also tend to support trendy research and research that supports government political agendas, such as the research on global warming.

20. The important issue in all cancer epidemiologic studies is *confounding*. It is difficult to control for confounders such as *Helicobacter pylori* infection, atrophic gastritis, and diet in gastric cancer, or esophageal reflux in esophageal and laryngeal cancer. Some subtypes of cancer, such as lung cancer, may have different confounders, such as the role of HPV in the causation of squamous cell cancer of the lung, oropharynx, and rectum. Radon exposure is the second leading cause of lung cancer in the United States, but is seldom mentioned in epidemiologic studies. Race, ethnicity, sex, age at the time of first exposure, genetic susceptibility, tobacco exposure, and socio-economic factors are important. Many important confounders have not been identified. Exposure information such as heavy prolonged or intermittent heavy exposure are often confused. Information on fiber type, fiber length, and fiber diameter is usually not reported. Many authors report "asbestos exposure" as if any and all asbestos exposure has equal carcinogenicity! For instance, exposure to occasional brake or clutch dust is often included as a significant asbestos exposure in various epidemiologic studies, in spite of the fact that this is not supported in the scientific medical literature. Other authors assume that any asbestos exposure is a significant exposure. The difficulty in distinguishing between gastrointestinal neoplasms and epithelial peritoneal mesotheliomas is not mentioned in many published papers. The reader needs to be aware of papers in which potential or incomplete lists of confounders are missing or ignored. This creates a bias, which is a *type of lack of information about confounder bias* due to an absence or lack of inclusion of potential confounders. Confounding is particularly important when there are only small differences between those exposed versus nonexposed populations to asbestos, such as in carcinoma of the larynx. There are at

least 15 different causes of carcinoma of the larynx (Chapter 11), which makes data interpretation of epidemiologic studies very difficult when there is no correction for confounding.

21. When I review a paper to be published or already published, I carefully review the bibliographic references used to support the author's paper. Often, only references that support the conclusions of the paper are referenced, with little or no discussion of other papers that do not support the author's conclusion. This *bibliographic bias* is a red flag to me that suggests an agenda rather than fair, unbiased presentation of scientific data. A good scientific paper always discusses papers that have reached different conclusions and then explains why his or her paper has reached a different conclusion from other scientists. Some authors purposely omit reference to older literature that has reached the same conclusion to make their paper appear to present new information. (Smith DD. Earlier study on asbestos workers, ILO scores, and oxygenation more comprehensive. *Occup Environ Med* 2003;60(8):611.)

22. *Imprecision*; random errors occur because of the lack of precision of the instrument (lack of random error) used in an epidemiologic study, such as the chest x-ray, HRCT scans, autopsy material such as asbestos body and fiber counts, etc. A good example is the use of the chest x-ray to evaluate the prevalence of pleural plaques or asbestosis in a population of workers. The precision or accuracy of the instrument will vary with the prevalence of the disorder under study in the population studied, causing a *sampling error* or *sampling variation error.* Autopsy studies have been performed to evaluate the ability of chest x-rays to visualize pleural plaques. Most pleural plaques found at autopsy are not seen radiologically by standard posterior anterior (PA) chest x-rays. Hourihane et al. found that 85% of pleural plaques found at autopsy were invisible by chest x-ray. (Hourihane DOB, Lessof L, Richardson PC. Hyaline and calcified pleural plaques as an index of exposure to asbestos: A study of 100 cases with consideration of epidemiology. *BMJ* 1966;1:1069–74.) Chest x-ray diagnosis of pleural plaques lacks the precision to be useful based on the poor correlation between autopsy findings and chest x-rays. (Meurman L. Asbestos bodies and pleural plaques in a Finnish series of autopsy cases. *Acta Pathol Microbiol Scand* 1966;(Suppl. 181):1+.) Study after study has been performed trying to correlate chest x-ray findings thought to be due to pleural plaques with lung function and risk of thoracic malignancy. Because of the imprecision of chest x-ray diagnosis of pleural plaques, many authors have switched to HRCT in an effort to improve precision. However, HRCT cannot be considered the gold standard for the detection of pleural or parenchymal disease based on the very limited autopsy data comparing autopsy findings and HRCT in the detection of pleural plaques.

Sensitivity, specificity, accuracy, and positive and negative predictive values of standard chest radiographs were calculated with respect to HRCT by Neri and coworkers, who used HRCT, artificially assuming it as the gold standard, compared to the standard chest x-ray, and this resulted in, respectively, for pleural and parenchymal findings: sensitivity 89% and 40%; specificity 53% and 97%; accuracy 66% and 80%; negative predictive value 52% and 79%; and positive predictive value 89% and 86%. (Neri S, Antonelli A, Falaschi F, Boraschi P, Baschieri L. Findings from high resolution computed tomography of the lung and pleura of symptom free workers exposed to amosite who had normal chest radiographs and pulmonary function test. *Occup Environ Med* 1994;51(4):239–43.) Akira and colleagues demonstrated that postmortem HRCT findings were similar to premortem HRCT findings for parenchymal lung disease only and correlated well with the pathologic findings of asbestosis. (Akira M, Yamamoto S, Yokoyama K et al. Asbestosis: High-resolution CT–pathologic correlation. *Radiology* 1990;176(2):389–94.) These findings were similar to the findings of Aberle et al. (Aberle DR, Gamsu G, Ray CS. High-resolution CT of benign asbestos-related diseases: Clinical and radiographic correlation. *AJR Am J Roentgenol* 1988;151(5):883–91.) Further autopsy studies are necessary to determine the accuracy and precision of HRCT in epidemiologic studies. Any study that uses HRCT scans to screen workers without the use of a standardized reference system of interpretation is of little value because of *interpretation bias.* (Hering KG, Hofmann-Preiß K, Kraus T. Update: Standardized CT/HRCT classification of occupational and environmental thoracic diseases in Germany. *Radiologe* 2014;54(4):363–84.) The international system of classification (International Classification of Occupational and Environmental Respiratory Diseases [ICOERD]) is more sensitive and specific for interstitial lung abnormalities and should be used as an interpretation standard in all epidemiologic studies. (Vehmas T, Oksa P. Chest HRCT signs predict deaths in long-term follow-up among asbestos exposed workers. *Eur J Radiol* 2014;83(10):1983–7.)

Data from chest x-ray surveys have substantial inaccuracies and random errors that preclude it as a reliable tool in the investigation of asbestos-related disorders. There is a *diagnostic bias* in asbestos surveys. As an experienced NIOSH-certified B-Reader, I am more likely to over-read a chest x-ray or HRCT scan if I find pleural plaques. Conversely, I tend to under-read chest x-ray and HRCT films with minor abnormalities if the films are otherwise normal. Attempts have been made to blind B-Readers to avoid bias, but this is impossible in an asbestos-exposed population with significant x-ray abnormalities, since certain radiologic abnormalities suggest asbestos exposure. (Laurent F, Paris C, Ferretti GR et al. Inter-reader agreement in HRCT detection of pleural plaques and asbestosis in participants with previous occupational exposure to asbestos. *Occup Environ Med* 2014;71:865–70.)

Friedman and coinvestigators, who were expert chest radiologists, concluded that the "positive predictive values (the likelihood that a positive report is correct) for pleural disease were outside films 56%, inside films 79%, HRCT 100%" at their university hospital-based practice. The positive predictive values for parenchymal disease were outside films 51%, inside films 83%, and HRCT 100%, if HRCT is the gold standard. The addition of HRCT to chest radiography is most useful in eliminating false-positive diagnoses of asbestos-related pleural disease caused by subpleural fat, and false-positive diagnoses of parenchymal asbestosis in patients with extensive plaques or emphysema obscuring lung detail. These expert chest radiologists concluded, "The interpretation of chest radiographs in patients exposed to asbestos is often extremely difficult and subjective, and we recommend that positive findings (except calcified plaques) be confirmed with HRCT." (Friedman AC, Fiel SB, Fisher MS, Radecki PD, Lev-Toaff AS, Caroline DF. Asbestos-related pleural disease and asbestosis: A comparison of CT and chest radiography. *AJR Am J Roentgenol* 1988;150(2):269–75; Mizell KN, Morris CG, Carter JE. Antemortem diagnosis of asbestosis by screening chest radiograph correlated with postmortem histologic features of asbestosis: A study of 273 cases. *J Occup Med Toxicol* 2009;4:14–9.)

Even HRCT interpretation has a significant element of subjectivity, particularly when reviewing borderline studies. There is significant bias in interpreting chest x-rays by the 1980 International Labor Office (ILO) standard. (Bourbeau J, Ernst P. Between- and within-reader variability in the assessment of pleural abnormality using the ILO 1980 international classification of pneumoconioses. *Am J Ind Med* 1988;14(5):537–43.) This results in an *observer bias*. The imprecision of the chest x-ray and computed tomography scan is discussed in greater detail in Chapters 4 and 7.

23. Lack of dose response is not a source of bias by itself, but is very important in analyzing claims of health effects from exposure to asbestos. Bias occurs when authors claim a cause-and-effect relationship but omit comments about the lack of dose response. When a dose response is absent, then proof of causation is very tenuous at best.

24. Lack of a suitable control population has made the majority of radiologic surveys of asbestos-exposed workers uninterruptable since pleural and parenchymal lung changes are frequently found in the nonasbestos-exposed populations, particularly with increasing age. This is discussed further in Chapters 5, 6, and 8.

In summary, the reliability of any test is prerequisite to the validity of the results and conclusions of any study. For example, if a chest x-ray is not a reliable tool for detecting pleural plaques or asbestosis, then studies based on a chest x-ray evaluation of asbestos-exposed workers lack validity (see Chapters 4, 5, 6, and 8). The conclusion of the matter is that the scientific literature contains many articles that are flawed due to many different sources of bias, lack of a comparable control population, inadequate power, and reliance on tests that lack sufficient validity. The fact that a scientific article is published in a reputable journal is no guarantee that the data and their conclusions are valid. The reader of this book will be introduced to the deficiencies, biases, and the poor scholarship that comprises much of the asbestos literature in the hope of developing tools to be used in evaluating all scientific literature.

3

Clinical toxicology of asbestos

MINERALOGY

Asbestos is not a mineralogical term, but a generic and regulatory term for commercially useful fibrous silicate mineral fibers of a crystalline nature (chrysotile, amosite, crocidolite, tremolite, anthophyllite, and actinolite). The National Institute of Occupational Safety and Health (NIOSH) has recognized that imprecise terminology and mineralogical complexity have affected progress in research. "Asbestos" and "asbestiform" are two commonly used terms that lack mineralogical precision. "Asbestos" is a term used for certain minerals that have crystallized in a particular macroscopic habit with certain commercially useful properties. These properties are less obvious on microscopic scales, so a different definition of asbestos may be necessary at the scale of the light microscope or electron microscope, involving characteristics such as chemical composition and crystallography. The lack of precision in these terms and the difficulty in translating macroscopic properties to microscopically identifiable characteristics contribute to miscommunication and uncertainty in identifying toxicity associated with various forms of minerals like asbestos. (Case BW, Abraham JL, Meeker G et al. Applying definitions of "asbestos" to environmental and "low-dose" exposure levels and health effects, particularly malignant mesothelioma. *J Toxicol Environ Health B Crit Rev* 2011;14(1–4):3–39.)

The word asbestos means "inextinguishable" since it was used in ancient times to make oil lamp wicks. The word chrysotile comes from the Greek words *chrysos* or golden and *tilos* or fiber. Chrysotile is actually an off-white color and amosite asbestos has brown fibers and crocidolite asbestos has bluish fibers. Commercial asbestos contains iron, sodium, magnesium, and calcium silicates. NIOSH 2011 states, "Asbestos is a term used for certain minerals that have crystallized in a particular macroscopic habit with certain commercially useful properties." These commercially useful fibrous minerals have been differentiated by their crystalline structure. Various forms of fibrous silicate minerals of an asbestos type are found all over the world. They are commonly called "naturally occurring asbestos" or asbestiform minerals. These minerals, such as erionite, winchite, richterite, fluoro-edenite, balangeroite, and antigorite, may be equally fibrogenic and equally or more carcinogenic than various forms of commercial asbestos.

Many areas of the world have asbestiform rock outcroppings, which have resulted in asbestos fiber contamination of the biosphere by wind and water erosion of these rock formations. The movement of continental and oceanic tectonic plates produces, in some parts of the world, serpentines in the lower layer of the oceanic plate to push up as it moves into the continental plate and forms the so-called ophiolites. Ophiolites consist of soil and rocks containing serpentine-type asbestos, mostly chrysotile asbestos, with variable amounts of tremolite/actinolite and anthophyllite. Silica is the most common mineral on earth and asbestos is a type of magnesium silicate. More recent studies in the polar ice cap have indicated that airborne concentrations of asbestos fibers have been present in the atmosphere for thousands of years. Certain countries have more environmental exposure to asbestos and asbestiform minerals then others, such as Turkey, China, Russia, New Caledonia, Corsica, Cyprus, Greece, Italy, South Korea, South Africa, Pakistan, Bolivia, Brazil, Finland, Bulgaria, Rhodesia (Mumbai), Australia, and various areas of the United States and Canada. (Kohyama N. Airborne asbestos levels in non-occupational environments in Japan. Non-occupational exposure to mineral fibers. *IRAC Pub* 1989;90:262–76.) All human beings have been exposed to some level of environmental asbestos from atmospheric contamination, and fiber analysis of the older human lungs demonstrates asbestos fibers in nearly everyone. (Sporn, T. Mineralogy of asbestos. In: A Tannapfel (Ed.), *Malignant Mesothelioma; Results in Cancer Research* 2011;189:1–11.) Asbestos fibers are present in all adult lungs and background levels of asbestos are equal or below 1,000,000 fibers per gram of dry lung in the population in Australia, the United Kingdom and North America. (Berry F, Roger J, Pooley FD. Mesothelioma, asbestos exposure and lung burden. *IARC* 1989;90:486–96.)

Asbestos particles found in natural mineral deposits do not have fixed dimensions but form as parallel aggregations of long crystalline fibrils or fibers. In natural mineral formations, these fibers can be up to several centimeters long. They are quite brittle, and when stressed, break easily into shorter lengths. In preparing it for commercial use, asbestos-containing rock is crushed mechanically and cleaned in a process called milling. This results in an infinite variety of sizes for commercial asbestos fibers; most are less than 50 μm long, and many are shorter than 1 μm. Chrysotile is the only commercial fiber type in the serpentine group. It is also the only asbestos fiber that is curly and is often found in intertwined bundles. The crystalline structure of chrysotile consists of parallel sheets of silica and magnesium hydroxide (i.e., brucite), which give the appearance of overlapping scrolls in cross-section. The basic structural unit of chrysotile is the fibril, which is a curved sheet of this material that forms into a scroll or tube. Chrysotile fibrils have a fixed diameter of 0.02–0.04 μm, which makes them the thinnest fiber found in nature (in comparison, the diameters of a cotton fiber and a human hair are 10 and 40 μm, respectively). In nature, these chrysotile fibrils are usually found bunched together to form a chrysotile fiber with a typical diameter of 0.75–1.5 μm. Serpentine fibers derive their name from the serpentine rocks in which they are found. Asbestos forms when very hot liquid supersaturated with minerals invades fissures in serpentine rock and then slowly cools and crystallizes into veins. In natural formations, chrysotile is often found with quartz micas, fosterite, brucite, and feldspar, so commercial formulations can be contaminated with these materials. (Ross M. The geologic occurrences and health hazards of amphibole and serpentine asbestos. *Rev Mineral* 1981;9A:279–323; Guthrie GD, Mossman BT. Health effects of mineral dusts. *Rev Mineral* 1993;28; Bayram M, Bakan ND. Environmental exposure to asbestos: From geology to mesothelioma. *Curr Opin Pulm Med* 2014.)

There are two groups of these minerals, the first of which is chrysotile, which is a member of the serpentine group of minerals: chrysotile, antigorite, and lizardite (see Table 3.1; Figures 3.1 through 3.4). Chrysotile asbestos has long thin fibers suitable for the production of asbestos clothing, blankets, and gloves. It is found worldwide. The other type of asbestos is called amphibole asbestos and contains regulated minerals called crocidolite, amosite, tremolite, anthophyllite, and actinolite, plus nonregulated amphibole minerals. The iron-rich amphibole type of asbestos forms needle-like fibers, as opposed to the silky, hollow scrolls of hydrated magnesium silicate sheets that characterize chrysotile asbestos. Chrysotile asbestos is very easily degraded by body defense mechanisms and therefore is not very "bio-persistent" as compared to amphibole asbestos. If there is concurrent exposure to fine particles such as wallboard joint compound, the resulting increase in pulmonary inflammatory reactions increases the removal of the chrysotile by tenfold. (Bernstein DM, Donaldson K, Decker U et al. A biopersistence study following exposure to chrysotile asbestos alone or in combination with fine particles. *Inhal Toxicol* 2008;20:1009–28.)

The amphibole type of asbestos has high tensile strength, a high dielectric constant, and low thermal conductivity. Amosite is more resistant to corrosion from low-pH (acid) solutions and is more resistant to the corrosive effects of seawater, as well as being more tolerant of higher temperatures than chrysotile. These properties of amosite have been of particular interest to the U.S. Navy, making it the preferred pipe insulation on ships. Amphiboles are used often in the manufacturer of asbestos-containing concrete pipes. All the amphiboles have a straight, needle-like shape and are found in nature stacked in parallel rows. In crystalline structure, the amphiboles are parallel chains of silica tetrahedras, which have incorporated in them varying amounts of different metal ions, giving each type its unique chemical form. Amphiboles do not have a true fibril structure but are formed as parallel plates of crystalline material, which can shear apart to form fibers with a variety of diameters. The thinnest amphibole fibers are 0.1–0.2 μm, but more typical diameters are 1.5–4.0 μm.

Amphibole asbestos is formed by forces of heat and pressure rearranging and recrystallizing materials in existing mineral formations. Crocidolite and amosite are found in sedimentary rocks called banded ironstones. Tremolite, actinolite, and anthophyllite deposits are found as pockets in igneous, metamorphic, or sedimentary rocks. In natural mineral formations, the amphibole fiber types are often mixed with iron oxides and quartz, so commercial formulations can be contaminated with these materials; in contrast to chrysotile asbestos's silky

Table 3.1 Physical and optical properties of different asbestos fibers

Property	Chrysotile	Amosite	Anthophyllite	Crocidolite	Tremolite	Actmoilite
Tensile strength, kp/cm^2	31,000	25,000	5000	35,000	5000	5000
Flexibility	Good	Fair	Fair to brittle	Good	Fair to brittle	Fair
Temp. at max ignition loss, °C	1000	870–1000	1000	650	1000	—
Filtration properties	Slow	Fast	Medium	Fast	Medium	Medium
Electric charge	Pos.	Neg.	Neg.	Neg.	Neg.	Neg.
Fusion point, °C	1520	1400	1470	1190	1315	1390
Spinnability	Very good	Fair	Poor	Good	Poor	Poor
Resistance to acids	Poor	Good	Very Good	Good	Good	Fair
Magnetite content, %	0.5.2	0	0	3.0–5.9	0	—
Resistance to heat	Good brittle at high temp	Good brittle at high temp.	Very Good	Poor, fuses	Fair to Good	—
Color	White to light green/gray	Light gray, brown/ gray or green	Silver gray to fawn	Lavender to blue	Gray/white to greenish, yellowish, bluish	Greenish

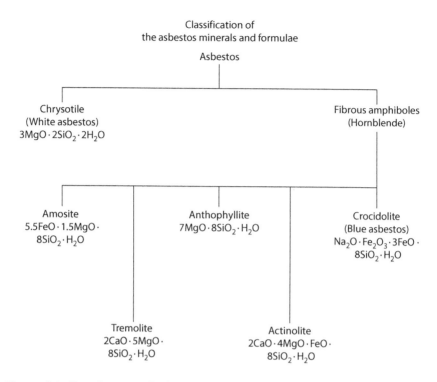

Figure 3.1 Classification of asbestos minerals.

flexible fibers, amphiboles are solid needle-like rods. There are five common types of commercial amphibole varieties: amosite (grunerite asbestos, renamed by the commercial company for Asbestos Mines South Africa to AMOSITE), crocidolite (riebeckite asbestos), tremolite asbestos, anthophyllite asbestos, and actinolite asbestos. Amphiboles are also more resistant to destruction at higher temperatures and, as previously mentioned, are more acid resistant when compared with chrysotile asbestos; therefore, they have been used in the past in high-temperature steam applications such as furnace, turbine, and pipe insulation where high-temperature (>500°) and acid resistance are important. During World War I, ship steam turbines operated at 300 pounds of pressure. World War II ships operated at 600 pounds of steam pressure, which required higher operating temperatures or superheated steam. Navy regulations required improved pipe and boiler insulation to meet the higher operating temperatures. All pipe insulation installed on high-temperature applications was required to be "85% Mag" insulation or to contain 15% amosite amphibole asbestos and various forms of silica. Recently, French researchers have discovered a significant aggravating role of concurrent silica and mineral wool exposure in potentiating the mesotheliogenic effect of asbestos exposure. (Lacourt A, Gramond C, Audignon S et al. Pleural mesothelioma and occupational co-exposure to asbestos, mineral wool and silica. *Am J Respir Crit Care Med* 2013;187(9):977–82.)

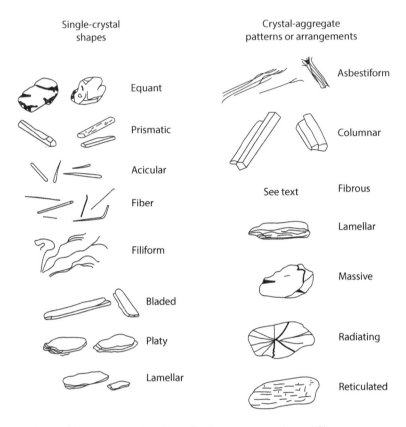

Figure 3.2 Different mineral habits of asbestos crystals and fibers.

Amphibole asbestos is very acid resistant so that it is not easily degraded by natural body defenses and fluids once it is inhaled. The resistance to degradation results in a very long residence time in the human body (bio-persistence due to bio-durability) and it is thought to play a large role in the pathogenesis of amphibole-related asbestos diseases. The pulmonary toxicity of inhaled fibers depends on several characteristics. These include fiber type, chemical and crystalline composition, fiber dimensions, aerodynamic characteristics, and bio-durability. (Warheit DB, Driscoll KE, Oberdorster G et al. Contemporary issues in fiber toxicology. *Fundam Appl Toxicol* 1995;25:171–83.)

Erionite fibers are a type of noncommercial fiber that are the most carcinogenic fibers of all asbestiform mineral fibers. The incidence of mesothelioma in the erionite areas of Turkey is more than 135 times the rate of mesothelioma in males in Sweden (see Table 3.2).

It is the ability of the body to dissolve and destroy asbestos fibers that seems to be the critical factor in mesotheliogenesis (see Figure 3.5). Carbone and coworkers in his laboratory studied the effects of chrysotile bio-persistence on the cellular transformation of mesothelial cells. Among asbestos fibers, crocidolite is considered the most and chrysotile the least oncogenic. Chrysotile accounts for more

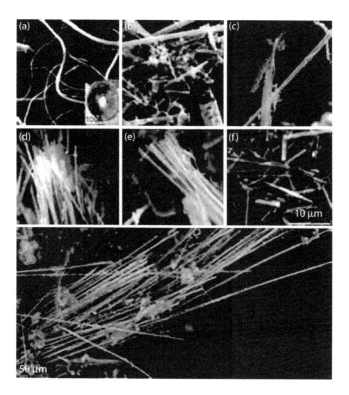

Figure 3.3 Scanning electron microscopy of different asbestos fibers.

than 90% of the asbestos used worldwide, but its capacity to induce malignant mesothelioma is still debated. Carbone found that chrysotile and crocidolite exposures have similar effects on human mesothelial cells. Morphological and molecular alterations suggestive of epithelial–mesenchymal transition, such as E-cadherin down-regulation and β-catenin phosphorylation followed by nuclear translocation, were induced by both chrysotile and crocidolite. Gene expression profiling revealed high-mobility group box-1 protein (HMGB1) as a key regulator of the transcriptional alterations induced by both types of asbestos. Crocidolite and chrysotile induced differential expression of 438 out of 28,869 genes interrogated by oligonucleotide microarrays. Out of these 438 genes, 57 were associated with inflammatory and immune responses and cancer, and 14 were HMGB1-targeted genes. Crocidolite-induced gene alterations were sustained, whereas chrysotile-induced gene alterations returned to background levels within 5 weeks. Similarly, HMGB1 release *in vivo* progressively increased for 10 or more weeks after crocidolite exposure, but returned to background levels within 8 weeks after chrysotile exposure. Continuous administration of chrysotile was required for sustained high serum levels of HMGB1. These data support the hypothesis that differences in bio-persistence influence the biological activities of these two asbestos fibers (see Figures 3.6 through 3.8). (Qi F, Okimoto G,

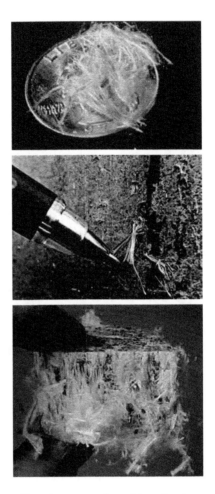

Figure 3.4 Raw chrysotile asbestos as found in asbestos ore.

Jube S et al. Continuous exposure to chrysotile asbestos can cause transformation of human mesothelial cells via HMGB1 and TNF-α signaling. *Am J Pathol* 2013;183(5):1654–66.)

Once adequate information on the adverse health effects of asbestos was provided in various commercial settings, asbestos consumption fell rapidly after

Table 3.2 Mesothelioma in Turkey: Karain born cohort average annual mesothelioma incidence rates (AMIR; per 100,000)

	AMIR	Ratio to Sweden	Ratio to world
Male	298.1	135.5	229.3
Female	400.9	1336.3	2004.5

Source: From Metintas M et al. *Eur Resp J* 1999;13:523–6. With permission.

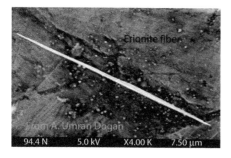

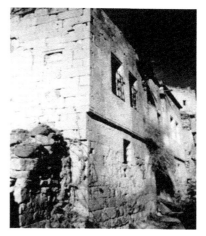

• Houses constructed with bricks
  containing erionite fibers

Figure 3.5 Sharp, needle-like erionite fiber found in Turkey is particularly pathogenic for mesothelioma.

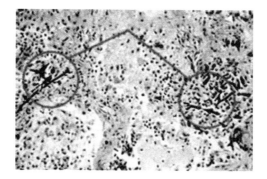

Figure 3.6 Asbestos bodies in lung tissue.

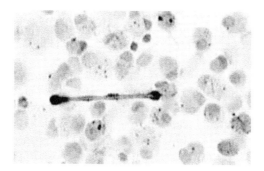

Figure 3.7 The relationship of asbestos-related disorders with amphibole and Quebec chrysotile contaminated with tremolite.

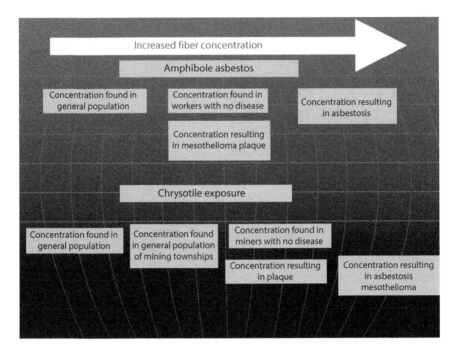

Figure 3.8 Median lung fiber concentration responsible for disease based on fiber type- and exposure-matched workers between chrysotile and amphibole exposure. Based on the work of Andrew Churg MD.

the mid-1970s. The risk of mesothelioma continued to rise due to the long latency from initial exposure to amphibole asbestos to the development of disease (see Figure 3.9).

Inhalation

Inhalation of asbestos fibers is the only significant route of exposure leading to adverse health effects. Asbestos appears to exert its effects either by direct contact with terminal lung airways and alveoli or by stimulating an acute and chronic inflammatory reaction in lung tissue (as in asbestosis). Asbestos fibers in the lungs do not become directly absorbed into the blood. There is no true systemic effect, although the fibers that can mechanically penetrate into lung tissue also find their way into the lymphatics, where they may be transported to the heart and then small amounts of asbestos may be found in other organs. Total lifetime ambient background exposure (combined indoor and outdoor) to asbestos varies substantially according to geographic location (near shipyards or asbestos manufacturing or mining facilities versus pig farming in Iowa). Work type (farmer versus office worker) and other factors are important. Generally, the average lifetime exposure for most people is a little below 1 fibers/cc year, but may be more than an order of magnitudes higher in some asbestos mining

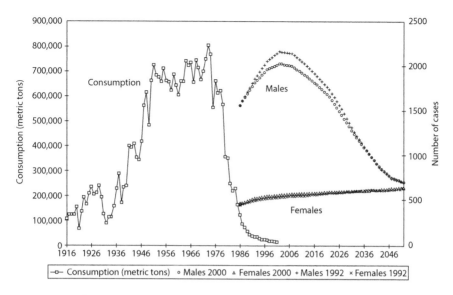

Figure 3.9 The relationship between asbestos consumption and the incidence of mesothelioma between males and females. (From Price B, Ware A. *Am J Epidemiol* 2004;159:107–12. With permission.)

communities, such as Thedford, Quebec (Table 3.3). (National Academy of Sciences/National Research Council. *Asbestiform Fibers: Nonoccupational Health Risks*. Washington, DC: National Academies Press, 1984; Camus M, Siemiatycki J, Meek B. Nonoccupational exposure to chrysotile asbestos and the risk of lung cancer. *N Engl J Med* 1998;338(22):1565–71.)

Table 3.3 Exposure levels: Ambient and regulatory

United States Public Health Service (USPHS)	1938	30 fibers/cc
American Conference of Governmental Industrial Hygienists (ACGIH)-proposed standard	1968	12 fibers/cc
ACGIH-proposed standard	1970	5 fibers/cc
ACGIH-proposed standard	1972	2 fibers/cc
ACGIH-proposed standard	1983	0.5 fibers/cc
ACGIH-proposed standard	1986	0.2 fibers/cc
ACGIH-proposed standard	1990	0.1 fibers/cc
Urban ambient air		0.0001 fibers/cc
Building with asbestos containing material (ACM)		0.0002 fibers/cc
Quebec mining towns		0.01 fibers/cc
Historic epidemiology (EPI) studies		1–5 fibers/cc

Source: From Homa DM et al. *J Epidemiol* 1994;139:1210. With permission.

INGESTION

The primary source of ingestion of asbestos fibers is from inhaled asbestos, which is captured in respiratory mucus and then swallowed. Trace amounts of asbestos are also ingested in drinking water and food. Most authorities believe that ingestion of asbestos fibers does not lead to adverse health effects. Asbestos fibers in the gut have been found to penetrate the gastrointestinal mucosa, especially about the cecum. However, there is no systemic absorption of these asbestos fibers, and they do not appear to stimulate an inflammatory reaction, cancer, or any other adverse effect. (Chouroulinkov I. Experimental studies on ingested fibers. Non-occupational exposure to mineral fibers. *IARC* 1989;90:113–33.)

SKIN CONTACT AND OTHER ROUTES OF EXPOSURE

Asbestos fibers have no adverse effects on contact with the eyes, intact skin, or wounds, and asbestos is not absorbed through the skin. *Asbestos fibers may burrow subcutaneously and cause a mild foreign body reaction called an asbestos corn.* Proper safety practices for working with asbestos do include protective clothing to keep asbestos fibers off the skin and clothes, but this is to avoid carrying fibers out of the workplace where they may later be reintrained in the air and inhaled. Other than inhalation, there are no other routes of exposure for asbestos that appear to cause adverse health effects.

ASBESTOS FIBER TOXIC MECHANISMS

Because of the increasing evidence of the toxicity of asbestos fibers, scientists began in 1931 to evaluate the basic mechanisms of pathogenicity. (Gardner L, Cummings D. Studies on experimental pneumokoniosis. VI. Inhalation of asbestos dust: Its effect upon primary tuberculosis infection. *J Ind Hyg* 1931;13:65–81, 97–114; Vorwald A, Durkan T, Pratt P. Experimental studies of asbestosis. *Arch Ind Hyg Occup Med* 1951;3:1–40.) Asbestos is not a mutagen and is a poor carcinogen with the exception of mesothelioma carcinogenesis. Asbestos is primarily a promoter of lung cancer and an initiator in high doses, but it is both a promoter and initiator of neoplastic change for mesothelioma at lower doses. Since asbestos is not fatally toxic to pulmonary macrophages, the macrophages release inflammatory cytokines that recruit other macrophages and neutrophils, and cause airway epithelial cell proliferation. The inflammatory reaction is dose dependent and fiber specific, and related not only to fiber dimensions, distribution, durability aerodynamic characteristics, chemical and crystalline composition, and shape, but also fiber type. Mineral fibers that are acid resistant and have long residency times in the lung are not only more fibrogenic, but also carcinogenic, largely due to the long fiber persistence time in the lung, producing a perpetual inflammatory condition, which in turn allows time for a variety of genetic and epigenetic events to occur. The chronic inflammatory condition produced by a variety of amphibole-like mineral fibers not only produces fibrogenesis and the release of free radicles and cell cytokines, but also induces mitogenesis followed by mutagenesis. It is the chronic inflammatory condition induced not only by mineral fibers but also any cause of chronic inflammation that ultimately results in cancers of the lung and mesotheliomas. Sezgi et al. have noted that elevated acute-phase reactants and oxidative stress markers in his mesothelioma study group can be used as predictive markers for the development of asbestos-related malignant mesothelioma. (Sezgi C, Taylan M, Sen HS et al. Oxidative status and acute phase reactants in patients with environmental asbestos exposure and mesothelioma. *Sci World J* 2014;2014:902748.)

Oxidative stress appears to be localized to areas of high fiber concentration. Suzuki and Koyama found that fibrosis was a precondition of mesothelioma induction by implanted minerals. (Suzuki Y, Koyama N. Malignant mesothelioma induced by asbestos and zeolite. *Environ Res* 1984;35:277–92.) Kevin Browne has noted that there is a threshold dose in experimental animals and humans for the production of lung cancer. The implication is that a sufficient amount of fibrogenesis in the lung is necessary to induce mutagenesis. This appears to be true for lung cancer. The data also suggest a threshold dose for mesothelioma, but this dose is much lower than the dose required to produce lung fibrosis or asbestosis. (Browne K. A threshold dose for asbestos related cancer. *Brit J Ind Med* 1986;43:556–8; Browne K. Is asbestos or asbestosis the cause of the increased risk of lung cancer in asbestos workers? *Brit J Ind Med* 1986;43:145–9; Hughes JM, Weil H. Asbestosis as a precursor of asbestos related lung cancer: Results of a prospective mortality study. *Brit J Ind Med* 1991;48:229–33.) There is no evidence that this asbestos induced carcinogenic and fibrotic process results in cancers outside of the lung and pleura. This is discussed elsewise in this book. (Browne K. Asbestos related malignancy and the Cairns hypothesis. *Brit J Ind Med* 1991;48:73–6; Warheit DB, Driscoll KE, Oberdoerster G et al. Contemporary issues in fiber toxicology. *Fundam Appl Toxicol* 1995;25:171–83; Timbrell V. Review of the significance of fiber size in fiber-related lung disease: A centrifuge cell for preparing accurate microscopic-evaluation specimens from slurries used in inoculation studies. *Ann Occup Hyg* 1989;33:483–505.)

DEPOSITION AND CLEARANCE OF ASBESTOS FIBERS

As with any inhaled particles, the pattern of initial deposition of asbestos fibers in the lungs is determined by particle size and shape, the principles of aerodynamics (i.e., the settling time of fibers and air flow dynamics), and the physical structure and protective mechanisms of the respiratory system (see Figure 3.10). A fiber is defined as a particle with a length-to-diameter ratio of over 3:1. The settling time of fibers is inversely related to the square of its diameter. For an atypical asbestos fiber 5 μm long and 1 μm in diameter, the settling time in still air is about 4 hours. Air turbulence from a person walking into a room can reintrain settled asbestos fibers into the air, so that free asbestos particles in an area should be assumed to be airborne by persons entering that space. When asbestos is inhaled, wide heavy fibers over 10–20 μm long tend to be filtered out in the upper airways or collide with the walls of the conducting airway in the lungs,

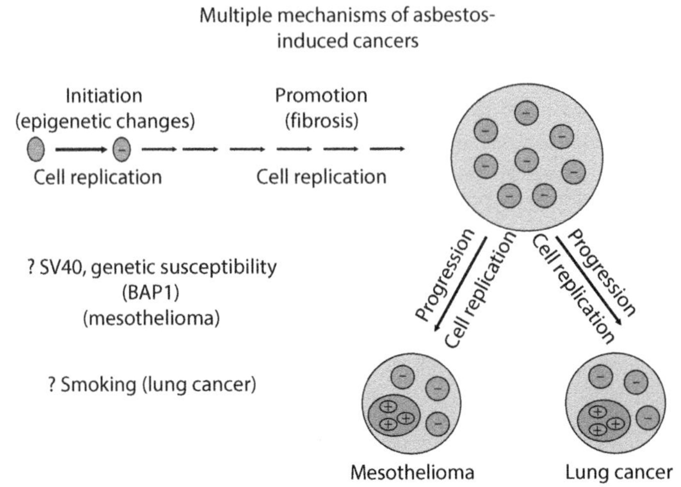

Multiple mechanisms of asbestos-
induced cancers

Initiation
(epigenetic changes)

Promotion
(fibrosis)

Cell replication

Cell replication

? SV40, genetic susceptibility
(BAP1)
(mesothelioma)

? Smoking (lung cancer)

Progression
Cell replication

Progression
Cell replication

Mesothelioma

Lung cancer

Figure 3.10 Multiple mechanisms of asbestos-induced cancers. There is a strong association between development of mesothelioma and amphibole types of asbestos fibers, but other factors such as radiation, simian virus-40 (SV40) infection, and genetic susceptibility as shown by mutations in BRCA-associated protein-1 and other tumor-suppressor genes may also be causal or facilitate mesotheliomas. As opposed to somatic driving mutations, epigenetic changes involving histone modification and microRNAs appear to be driving forces in mesothelioma development that are augmented by cell replication, which may perpetuate these changes in daughter cells. The genetic signatures of lung cancers that are primarily observed in asbestos workers who smoke as well as in individual mesotheliomas are different. (Courtesy of Brooke Mossman. With permission.)

where they are captured in the respiratory mucus. Short fibers (<5 μm) reach the alveoli but are short enough to be ingested by the natural lung defense, the alveolar scavenger cell called the alveolar macrophage, and then removed by the mucociliary elevator and swallowed. Thin (0.2 μm) and long fibers (8–50 μm) will reach the alveoli and these thin long fibers are called "Stanton fibers," named after Dr. MF Stanton at the National Institutes of Health, who did experiments in rats that demonstrated that only long fibers (>8–10 μm) that were also very narrow (<0.2 μm) where carcinogenic for mesothelioma. These long thin fibers are the most likely to cause lung cancers and mesothelioma. These fibers are attacked by alveolar macrophages that try unsuccessfully to engulf these long fibers. These "frustrated macrophages" release a variety of cytotoxic products that are thought to be the primary cause of malignant change in the surrounding cells. Occasionally, fibers up to 100 μm long are seen in the lungs, especially if they are draped over a branch point of conducting airways in a saddle-like effect. Asbestos fibers less than 10–20 μm long are more likely to stay in the center of the air stream and eventually reach the alveoli. Large fibers captured in respiratory mucus are then coughed up or swallowed. (Stanton MF, Wrench C.

Mechanisms of mesothelioma induction with asbestos and fibrous glass. *J Natl Cancer Inst* 1972;48(3):797–821; Donaldson K, Seaton A. A short history of the toxicology of inhaled particles. *Part Fibre Toxicol* 2012;9:13; National Toxicology Program. Asbestos. *Rep Carcinog* 2011;12:53–6; Vietti G, Ibouraadaten S, Palmai-Pallag M et al. Towards predicting the lung fibrogenic activity of nano-materials: Experimental validation of an *in vitro* fibroblast proliferation assay. *Part Fibre Toxicol* 2013;10:52; Xu J, Alexander DB, Futakuchi M et al. Size- and shape-dependent pleural translocation, deposition, fibrogenesis and mesothelial proliferation by multiwalled carbon nanotubes. *Cancer Sci* 2014;105(7):763–9.)

The experimental demonstration that dangerous or potentially cancer-causing fibers need to be long and thin has been critical in understanding asbestos fiber pathogenesis. Many commercial products contain short, <5-μm asbestos fibers, which are not pathogenic. Dr. JM Davis in 1986 did studies with short versus long amosite fibers and found that short fibers were better retained by the lung than long fibers but did not cause lung cancers, mesotheliomas, or lung fibrosis. Long fibers caused lung fibrosis, and many lung cancers and mesotheliomas. (Davis JM, Addison J, Bolton RE et al. The pathogenicity of long versus short fibre samples of amosite asbestos administered to rats by inhalation and intraperitoneal injection. *Br J Exp Pathol* 1986;67(3):415–30; Davis JM. Mineral fibre carcinogenesis: Experimental data relating to the importance of fibre type, size, deposition, dissolution and migration. *IARC Sci Publ* 1989;(90):33–45. Review.)

AG Wylie from the Department of Geology at the University of Maryland confirmed that wide fibers >1 μm in width are not pathogenic. Evidence from human epidemiology, experimental animal implantation and inoculation studies, and lung burden studies show that fibers with widths >1 μm are not implicated in the occurrence of lung cancer or mesothelioma. Furthermore, she points out that it is generally believed that certain fibers thinner than a few tenths of a micrometer must be abundant in a fiber population in order for them to be a causative agent for mesothelioma. "These conclusions are fully consistent with the mineralogical characteristics of asbestos fibers, which, as fibrils, have widths of less than 1 micron and, as bundles, easily disaggregate into fibrils. Furthermore, the biological behavior of various habits of tremolite shows a clear dose–response relationship and provides evidence for a threshold between fiber width and tumor experience in animals." Unfortunately, the wide fibers are often counted by the NIOSH phase-contrast optical microscopy (PCOM) 7400 method. (Wylie AG, Bailey KF, Kelse JW et al. The importance of width in asbestos fiber carcinogenicity and its implications for public policy. *Am Ind Hyg Assoc J* 1993;54(5):239–52.)

Autopsy specimens suggest that amphiboles tend to persist in the alveoli for many years, while chrysotile fibers clear rapidly in days and months. The concentration of chrysotile fibers in the lung remains low unless there has been heavy exposure. Chrysotile fibers are more easily removed from the alveolar spaces by respiratory macrophages because they are not resistant to an acid environment produced by cellular cytokines. Asbestos fibers can be found in bronchial washing obtained by bronchoscopy, but it is difficult to estimate the amount of asbestos deposited in the lung using this technique. Asbestos fibers deposited in the alveoli can undergo a variety of fates. They can remain in place in the alveoli, penetrate the alveolar walls, enter the interstitial fluid, or be cleared by the lymphatic drainage and deposited in the perihilar nodes. Other fibers, especially amphiboles, may penetrate the lung parenchyma and enter the pleural place or peritoneal space via the diaphragm. Some asbestos fibers in the alveoli are engulfed by respiratory macrophages with varying results. Chrysotile appears to be susceptible to degradation by macrophages, which may explain why this is the least toxic of the fiber types and is found in smaller amounts in autopsy specimens. Amphibole fibers over 10 μm are not easily degraded by macrophages and tend to persist in the alveoli. Some of these larger fibers become partially engulfed by macrophages but are not degraded. Instead, the macrophage dies, leaving a brown *iron-containing* proteinaceous coating about the fiber; this is known as an *asbestos body* and can be seen in light microscopy of lung tissue or sputum, preferably *after an iron stain has been performed*. Although asbestos bodies in the sputum or lung washings do indicate prior exposure, they do not signify disease nor suggest the extent of exposure. The number, size, and type of asbestos fibers deposited in the lung have been studied extensively in specimens from autopsy and open lung biopsy. This involves treating the specimen with a chemical that dissolves the tissue but leaves the asbestos fibers intact. Fibers are then counted using standard techniques, with results reported as the number and type of fibers per gram of dried lung. Asbestos fiber counts can be done on lung tissue specimens obtained by biopsy or at autopsy. This involves treating a weighed amount of dried lung with Clorox bleach to dissolve the tissue; the asbestos fibers remain intact. The number and types of asbestos fibers present can be used as a rough estimate of cumulative asbestos exposure. This technique has been used extensively to study dose–response relationships for asbestos-related diseases. (Smith MJ, Naylor B. A method for extracting ferruginous bodies from sputum and pulmonary tissue. *Am J Clin Pathol* 1972;58(3):250–4.)

There appears to be a background level of asbestos in the lungs in the general population in the United States of less than *1,000,000 fibers per gram of dried lung* or less than *100 asbestos bodies per gram of wet lung.* (Churg 1983; Churg and Wiggs 1984; Churg 1993.) Individuals with a history of some type of occupational asbestos exposure have at least three times this number of fibers in the lungs, while those with asbestosis have over 100 times the background level. This method for estimating exposure suggests a dose–response relationship between asbestos exposure and disease. Very high concentrations of asbestos fibers and asbestos bodies are consistent with an exposure sufficient to cause lung cancer *and asbestosis.* Mesothelioma is associated with significant increases in fiber burden compared to a nonexposed population. (Roggli VL, Oury TD, Sporn TA. *Asbestos-Associated Diseases,* 2nd Edition. New York: Springer, 2004; Churg A, Green FHY. *Pathology of Occupational Disease,* 2nd Edition. Baltimore: Williams & Wilkins, 1998; Churg A. Current issues in the pathologic and mineralogic diagnosis of asbestos-induced disease. *Chest* 1983;84:275–80; Churg A, Wiggs B, Depaoli L et al. Lung asbestos content in chrysotile workers with mesothelioma. *Am Rev Respir Dis* 1984;130:1042–5; Churg A. Asbestos, asbestosis, and lung cancer. *Mod Pathol* 1993;6:509–11; Lotti M, Bergamo L, Murer B. Occupational toxicology of asbestos-related malignancies. *Clin Toxicol (Phila)* 2010;48(6):485–96.)

The guiding principle of all toxicology is that toxicity is relative to dose alone: *sola dosis facet venenum*; "the dose alone makes the poison." For instance, arsenic is a deadly poison but not harmful in low doses and is present in low doses in drinking water from wells in many areas of the United States. Approximately 40% of the land mass in North America contains rock contaminated with asbestos. All adults over the age of 50 years have substantial amounts of asbestos fibers in their lungs without evidence of disease. Asbestos health effects, like arsenic-related disease, only occur with elevated levels of exposure.

The guiding principle of toxicology

Exposure resulting in increased lung fiber burden to asbestos is related to several factors, including fiber type, fiber dimension, fiber concentration, breathing pattern, bronchial anatomy, fiber clearance (which is reduced by cigarette smoking), rate of dissolution of fibers, distance from exposure, duration of exposure, respirator usage, and ventilation of area (related to whether this is a confined or open space) (see Figures 3.11 through 3.13).

- Amphibole fibers are more harmful than chrysotile fibers
- Chrysotile fibers are cleared from lungs at a more rapid rate
- The needle-like shape of amphibole asbestiforms may make them more prone to migration
- *Four types of asbestos-related lung diseases:*
  Asbestosis
  Asbestos-related pleural disease } Fibrotic

  Lung cancer
  Mesothelioma } Neoplastic

Figure 3.11 Asbestos-related lung diseases.

Toxicology tells us:

1. Exposure is important—
   i.e. nature, character, duration

2. Dose is important—magnitude and duration

3. Thresholds do exist and they are important

4. Size, shape, length, diameter, iron content, biopersistence, fiber type, and surface area are important

Figure 3.12 What does toxicology tell us? (Courtesy of Brooke Mossman. With permission.)

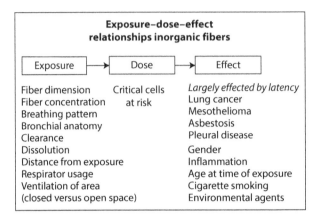

Figure 3.13 Exposure–dose–effect relationships. Effect may be moderated by other factors as well as dose.

Use of asbestos-containing products

The physical properties of asbestos make it a unique and commercially useful material. These include resistance to degradation by heat and chemicals, strength, durability, and fibrous structure (which allows it to be made into cloth or felt and to act as a good binder in ceramic materials). Asbestos has been used extensively in the industrialized world since the exploitation of large commercial deposits in Quebec in the 1860s and South Africa in the 1890s. Asbestos has over 3000 commercial uses. The majority of asbestos used commercially has been in the construction of buildings, ships, power plants, chemical plants, oil refineries, steel mills, and other industrial facilities. The largest single use of asbestos has been as a binder in cement pipes and cement panels. Asbestos has also been used extensively in all types of insulation and fireproofing, including pipe and boiler insulation and steel beam building insulation, where loose asbestos fibers mixed with water were often applied as a "mud" or "limpet" spray on fireproofing of ceilings and exposed structural beams. Asbestos has been incorporated into a variety of building products, including house siding, wallboard, floor and ceiling tiles, and acoustical insulation. Asbestos cloth has been used in fire-resistant clothing and fire and welding blankets, as well as theater curtains. When pressed into a felt, asbestos is used in pipe gaskets, and it is also used as a binder in plastics and paper. As a filtering material, asbestos has been used in gas masks and a variety of chemical processes, such as in the membranes of hydrolytic cells in chlorine production plants. Finally, asbestos has been used extensively in friction products, such as auto-brake shoes and clutches. Domestic uses of asbestos have included ironing board covers, cooking mats, hairdryers, ceiling tiles, asbestos paper, wallboards, wallboard joint compounds, floor tiles, roofing products, attic insulation and more than 1000 other domestic products.

Industrial uses for asbestos include high-temperature applications as used in boiler and steam pipe insulation, insulating blankets, some industrial paints, fireproof clothing, siding and roofing and, most importantly, in drainage and water piping. Large amounts of asbestos have been used in the past in shipyards, power plants, chemical plants, steel mills, and refineries.

Chrysotile asbestos has been the most commonly used form of asbestos in the United States. Small amounts of chrysotile have been mined in Arizona, California, Vermont, and other states. Approximately 90% of chrysotile used in North America has been produced from mines in Quebec. Russia is the world's largest producer of chrysotile asbestos today. Small amounts of amosite asbestos and crocidolite asbestos have been imported to the United States from South Africa. Large amounts of South African crocidolite asbestos were imported historically into Great Britain and Europe. Asbestos consumption per capita reached a peak in 1951 in the United States and gradually declined until 1973, when it started to drop rapidly. Almost all U.S. manufacturers of asbestos-containing products removed asbestos from most of their products by 1975. Asbestos is still used in less developed nations in the manufacture of asbestos cement pipes used for water or sewage transport, since asbestos cement pipes are very durable and less expensive than alternative plastic or steel pipes. Asbestos cement pipes may contain crocidolite, amosite, or chrysotile asbestos.

Chrysotile has been used in the past in wallboard joint compounds. Sanding dry joint compounds or mixing dry joint compounds is a dusty activity and exposures were not well characterized until the mid-1970s. Dust concentrations of asbestos fibers were estimated to be in excess of the respective current but not historical threshold limit values prior to the removal of asbestos from these compounds in the mid-to-late 1970s. Many of these joint compounds contained nonpathogenic short fiber asbestos from Coalinga, California, or pure chrysotile from the Carey Canadian mine in Quebec, which has no significant amphibole asbestos contamination. Cumulative exposure estimates for chrysotile fibers from drywall finishing are expected to result in few, if any, mesothelioma or excess lung cancer deaths according to recently published risk assessments. (Boelter FW, Xia Y, Dell L. Comparative risks of cancer from drywall finishing based on stochastic modeling of cumulative exposures to respirable dusts and chrysotile asbestos fibers. *Risk Anal* 2014.)

Chrysotile asbestos has been used in the past in the manufacture of automobile and truck brakes and clutches. There has been a great deal of controversy about the health consequences of exposure to asbestos-containing friction products. The plaintiff's experts have summarized their position and evidence used to support their position in a paper by Laura Welch in 2007 suggesting that asbestos-containing friction products cause mesothelioma, as did Richard Lemen in 2004. (Welch LS. Asbestos exposure causes mesothelioma, but not this asbestos exposure: An amicus brief to the Michigan Supreme Court. *Int J Occup Environ Health* 2007;13:318–27; Lemen RA. Asbestos in brakes: Exposure and risk of disease. *Am J Ind Med* 2004;45(3):229–37.) I will not discuss asbestos exposure from brakes, clutches, or asbestos-containing floor tiles and mastic further, since I do not believe the evidence indicates significant risk for asbestos-related cancer from these exposures. I have provided enough current references to allow the reader to reach his or her own conclusion. Some authors have reported asbestos-related pleural plaques in heavy vehicle mechanics without any increased risk of mesothelioma or lung cancer. (Cely-García MF, Torres-Duque CA, Durán M et al. Personal exposure to asbestos and respiratory health of heavy vehicle brake mechanics. *J Exp Sci Environ Epidemiol* 2015;25(1):26–36; Finley BL, Pierce JS, Paustenbach DJ et al. Malignant pleural mesothelioma in US automotive mechanics: Reported vs. expected number of cases from 1975 to 2007. *Regul Toxicol Pharmacol* 2012;64(1):10; Paustenbach DJ, Finley BL, Lu ET et al. Environmental and occupational health hazards associated with the presence of asbestos in brake linings and pads (1900 to present): A "state-of-the-art" review. *J Toxicol Environ Health B Crit Rev* 2004;7(1):25–80; Kakooei H, Hormozy M, Marioryad H. Evaluation of asbestos exposure during brake repair and replacement. *Ind Health* 2011;49(3):374–80; Paustenbach DJ, Finley BL, Sheehan PJ et al. Re: Evaluation of the size and type of free particulates collected from unused asbestos-containing brake components as related to potential for respirability. *Am J Ind Med* 2006;49(1):60–1; author reply 62; Paustenbach DJ, Sage A, Bono M et al. Occupational exposure to airborne asbestos from coatings, mastics, and adhesives. *J Exp Anal Environ Epidemiol* 2004;14(3):234–44; Lange JH. Airborne exposure during asbestos abatement of floor tile, wall plaster, and pipe insulation. *Bull Environ Contam Toxicol* 2005;74(1):70–2; Lange JH. Type and amount of asbestos in floor tile and mastic. *Bull Environ Contam Toxicol* 2006;77(6):807; Kopelovich LM, Thuett KA, Chapman PS et al. History and evolution of warning labels for automotive friction products. *Regul Toxicol Pharmacol* 2014;68(3):402–411; Bernstein DM, Rogers R, Sepulveda R et al. Evaluation of the deposition, translocation and pathological response of brake dust with and without added chrysotile in comparison to crocidolite asbestos following short-term inhalation: Interim results. *Toxicol Appl Pharmacol* 2014;276(1):28–46; Ameille J, Rosenberg N, Matrat M et al. Asbestos-related diseases in automobile mechanics. *Ann Occup Hyg* 2012;56(1):55–60; Hessel PA, Teta MJ, Goodman M et al. Mesothelioma among brake mechanics: An expanded analysis of a case-control study. *Risk Anal* 2004;24:547–52; Goodman M, Teta MJ, Hessel PA et al. Mesothelioma and lung cancer among motor vehicle mechanics: A meta-analysis. *Ann Occup Hyg* 2004;48:309–26; Wong O. Malignant mesothelioma and asbestos exposure among auto mechanics: Appraisal of scientific evidence. *Regul Toxicol Pharmacol* 2001;34:170–7.)

Chrysotile asbestos has also been used in the past in various electrical products. The question has been whether there is sufficient chrysotile exposure to cause lung cancer or mesothelioma. Various epidemiology studies indicate chrysotile asbestos has a threshold below which does not cause mesothelioma or lung cancer. A critical review was conducted to determine whether electricians are at increased risk for these cancers and, if so, whether their exposure to chrysotile in electrical products could be responsible. Goodman et al. found that most, but not all, epidemiology studies indicate electricians are at increased risk for both cancers. Studies that evaluated electricians' exposure to asbestos during normal work tasks have generally reported low concentrations in air; an experimental study showed that grinding or drilling products containing encapsulated chrysotile resulted in exposures to chrysotile fibers far below the Occupational

Safety and Health Administration (OSHA) permissible exposure limit (PEL) and the cancer no observed adverse effect level (NOAEL). Studies of other craftsmen who often work in the vicinity of electricians, such as insulators, reported asbestos (including amphibole) exposures that were high. "Overall, the evidence does not indicate that exposure to chrysotile in electrical products causes mesothelioma or lung cancer in electricians. Rather, the most likely cause of lung cancer in electricians is smoking, and the most likely cause of mesothelioma is exposure to amphibole asbestos as a result of renovation/demolition work or working in the proximity of other skilled craftsmen." (Goodman JE, Peterson MK, Bailey LA et al. Electricians' chrysotile asbestos exposure from electrical products and risks of mesothelioma and lung cancer. *Regul Toxicol Pharmacol* 2014;68(1):8–15.)

OCCUPATIONAL EXPOSURES AND REGULATIONS

In the United States, millions of individuals have had significant workplace exposures to asbestos since the beginning of the twentieth century, with the most extensive exposures occurring in the three decades during and after World War II. Limited information is available on historical levels of asbestos exposure for U.S. workers prior to 1965–1970. The Dreesen study in 1938 and Fleischer drinker report in 1946 suggested that existing protection standards were adequate to provide protection from asbestosis at the time of their studies. This was largely due to inadequate measurements of exposure prior to the use of the new technology of personal sampling using membrane filters rather than area samplers and midget impingers. In many industries, airborne asbestos levels were over 100 fibers/mL (this is 1000 times higher than the current OSHA PEL of 0.1 fibers/mL). Historically, workers in the United States who had the highest asbestos exposures were in the mining and milling of asbestos, and primary manufacturing (i.e., use of asbestos as a raw material to make products such as textiles, concrete pipes, floor tiles, and insulation). The risk to end users of asbestos-containing insulation was not recognized until the mid-1960s by Selikoff. The next highest exposures were for workers in secondary manufacturing (i.e., incorporating asbestos-containing materials into manufactured items) and construction and shipbuilding workers who were not insulators. In the United States, the shipbuilding and construction industries have had the largest cohorts of workers with heavy asbestos exposures (it is estimated that in shipyards alone, more than 1 million workers have had significant exposure). In both of these industries, insulators have had twice the rate of asbestos-related diseases compared with workers in other trades. At the other end of the spectrum, workers whose only exposure to asbestos was in changing auto-brake shoes and clutches containing asbestos have shown no increased incidence of any asbestos-related disease. The reason for this is unclear, although one theory suggests that high heat from friction on the brake shoe transforms the asbestos into fosterite, a nontoxic material that does not cause disease. By the mid-1960s, it was apparent that certain types of asbestos products were a serious health hazard and could cause asbestosis, lung cancer, and mesothelioma. Workplace regulation of asbestos exposure has become increasingly more stringent in the United States since passage of the

OSHA Act of 1970 and the promulgation of regulations in 1972. Since the early 1970s, there has been a rapid decline in the commercial use of asbestos, and by 1975, almost all asbestos-containing manufactured products in the United States had been removed. This along with the increased use of industrial respirators and the required identification and labeling of all asbestos-containing materials, as well as the use of asbestos-abatement procedures, resulted in markedly reduced worker exposures by the mid-1970s. Heavy unprotected asbestos exposures are now very rare in the United States and most developed countries in the world.

Since most epidemiologic studies of asbestos-related disease are based on occupational groups who had heavy exposures prior to 1970, the risk estimates derived from these studies may not reflect the health risks for similar jobs today. However, because diseases caused by asbestos often have latency periods of 40 or more years, many workers who were heavily exposed in the past have already died or outlived the perceived risk. Many workers have been ignorant of the health hazard. The risk of mesothelioma has been falling for several years due to the diminution of the heavily exposed populations. Asbestos present in existing structures, plants, ships, and equipment will also remain a potential hazard for workers who demolish, repair, or refurbish these items without adequate respiratory protection. In addition, asbestosis and other asbestos-related diseases may continue to be significant problems in many rapidly industrializing third-world countries where occupational exposures are not well controlled and asbestos-containing concrete pipe is the only financially feasible product for various purposes.

Epidemiologic studies of asbestos-exposed workers have generally focused on cumulative lifetime exposure as the most important risk factor for asbestos-related diseases. These exposures estimated for individuals are based on either: (a) years worked in specific job categories multiplied by estimated exposures for these jobs or (b) asbestos fiber counts from lung tissue specimens. Exposure estimates based on work history can be inaccurate since historical data on exposure levels and fiber mixes are seldom known and probably vary greatly over the working life of an individual. Retrospective studies often lack good work histories. The differential toxic effects of specific fiber types have been investigated in many studies. These have looked at groups whose lifetime exposures appeared to be predominantly from a single fiber type, such as chrysotile miners in Quebec, gas mask assemblers in Canada and England (who worked primarily with crocidolite), and those living near anthophyllite outcroppings in Finland. Typically, these studies have found crocidolite to be most toxic in causing asbestos-related diseases; amosite has intermediate toxicity, and chrysotile is least toxic. It takes more than twice the amount of chrysotile asbestos exposure to cause a mesothelioma than asbestosis in chrysotile miners and millers (Table 3.4). However, recent studies suggest that the supposedly "pure" forms of chrysotile asbestos seem to be contaminated with small amounts of amphibole fiber types. This makes it difficult to draw conclusions about the unique effects of a specific fiber type. For example, chrysotile from several mines in Quebec, which was previously thought to be pure, was found to contain small amounts of tremolite, which

Table 3.4 Median fiber concentration found in age and exposure period-matched workers with chrysotile or amphibole (amosite) exposure

	Mesothelioma (10^6 fibers/g of dry lung)	Asbestosis (10^6 fibers/g of dry lung)
Chrysotile workers	290	110
Amosite workers	0.7	26

Source: From Churg A, Wiggs B. *Am J Ind Med* 1986;9(2):143–52. With permission.
Note: Chrysotile workers require 400 times the lung burden of asbestos as do amphibole-exposed workers to develop a mesothelioma.

is the major cause of toxicity for this material. Further discussion on government regulations is contained in Chapter 15.

ASBESTOS EXPOSURES TO BUILDING OCCUPANTS

In the past decade, there has been public concern about health risk from exposures to low levels of airborne asbestos among occupants in schools and other public buildings. Asbestos has been used extensively in these buildings since World War II for boiler and pipe insulation, spray-on insulation, and fireproofing for ceilings and structural beams, and as a component in wallboard and floor or ceiling tiles. It is estimated that 20% of all building in the United States have some asbestos-containing material. The Environmental Protection Agency (EPA) regulates the disposal of asbestos as a hazardous waste and its release into the atmosphere as an air pollutant. Although it can issue advisory statements, the EPA does not have legal authority to regulate asbestos exposures to students in schools or other occupants of public buildings. No government agency regulates asbestos exposures to individuals inside their own homes. Since 1984, the EPA has required all school districts to survey their buildings for asbestos, and many purchasers of commercial and residential real estate are requiring similar inspections. This has resulted in a sizable effort to remove or encapsulate asbestos materials in these buildings. Although the EPA has not set a PEL or required any remedial action, many school districts that found asbestos have removed it or encapsulated it in place. Surveys of airborne asbestos fibers in public buildings and schools known to contain asbestos found mean levels of 0.0004–0.0010 fibers/mL, even when damaged asbestos-containing material was present. These levels of exposure are 200–500 times lower than the OSHA PEL and more than 10,000 times lower than the heavy exposures prior to 1970 experienced by those workers who have been the subjects of most epidemiologic studies of asbestos-related disease. In addition, recent studies have shown that levels of airborne asbestos fibers in school buildings are sometimes actually higher after asbestos-containing materials have been removed. (*Asbestos in Public and Commercial Buildings: A Literature Review and Synthesis of Current Knowledge*. Cambridge: Health Effects Institute – Asbestos Research, 1991; *Asbestiform Fibers: Nonoccupational Health Risks*. Washington, DC: National Academies Press, 1984; Corn JK. *Environmental Public Policy for*

Asbestos in Schools: Unintended Consequences. Boca Raton: CRC Press, 2000; Ontario Ministry of the Attorney General. *Report of Royal Commission on Matters of Health and Safety Arising from the use of Asbestos in Ontario,* Volumes 1–4. Toronto, 1984.)

ASBESTOS EXPOSURES IN OUTDOOR AMBIENT AIR

Asbestos fibers can be found in the outdoor ambient air in all industrialized and urban areas (Table 3.5). These fibers come from a variety of sources, including worn or damaged asbestos-containing building materials, demolished buildings, worn auto-brake shoes, and improper disposal of asbestos waste. In many areas, asbestos also enters the atmosphere from the weathering of natural rock formations or surface wastes of mines. Levels of asbestos found in the ambient atmosphere in industrialized areas in the United States are low and not considered significant health risks. Carl Mangold, a certified industrial hygienist (CIH), measured the ambient air concentration in the San Francisco area in 1983 at 0.02 fibers/cc. This is similar to the 10-day average in downtown Seattle of 0.024 fibers/cc measured in 1982 by Mangold. Joseph Wendlick, another CIH, measured ambient air concentrations in Newport News, Norfolk, and Portsmouth, Virginia, at 0.01–0.02 fibers/cc.

These levels are also similar to those levels of 0.01–0.02 fibers/cc noted by NIOSH in the *NIOSH Revised Recommended Asbestos Standard,* (DHEW) NIOSH Publication 77-169, December 1976.

ASBESTOS IN DRINKING WATER AND FOOD

Asbestos is found in very low concentrations as a normal contaminant in drinking water in many areas of the United States. Much of this comes from water passing over natural formations of asbestos-containing rock, and some may come from asbestos cement pipes. Asbestos fibers are also found in trace amounts as a contaminant in some processed foods. These exposures to asbestos

Table 3.5 Asbestos fiber burden in the general population of Vancouver, British Columbia: Asbestos bodies and fibers per gram of dry lung

Fiber type	Mean (10^6 fibers/g of dry lung)	Median (10^6 fibers/g of dry lung)	95th percentile
Chrysotile	0.3	0.2	1.1
Tremolite	0.4	0.2	1.2
Amosite and crocidolite	0.001	0.0	0.01

Source: From Churg A, Warnock ML. *Am Rev Respir Dis* 1980;122(5):669–78; Churg A. *Chest* 1983;84(3):275–80; Churg A, Wiggs B. *Am J Ind Med* 1986;9(2):143–52. With permission.

Note: Divide these numbers by 10 to get the number of asbestos bodies/fibers per gram of wet lung.

fibers in drinking water and food are not considered significant health hazards. The city of Everett, Washington, gets its drinking water from the snow-melt in the Cascade Mountains. The snow-melt is captured in a reservoir and then piped to the city. The water contains the highest amount of asbestos of any city in the United States, the population of the city and surrounding area has been monitored for many years for any increased risk of cancer, particularly gastrointestinal cancer and ovarian and abdominal (peritoneal) mesothelioma. The drinking water has been found to be safe. (Lange JH, Hoskins JA. Asbestos in drinking water does not cause mesothelioma. *Int J Gynecol Cancer* 2004;14(5):1048–9.)

4

History of asbestos commercial use and discovery of adverse health effects: Asbestosis

Various forms of asbestos have been used since the antiquities. Small amounts of asbestos were used to make cremation cloths and both the Chinese and Egyptians wove asbestos into mats. The word asbestos is a Greek word, which means "inextinguishable" or "unquenchable," referring to its fire resistance. Benjamin Franklin returned from Europe with a purse made out of what was called salamander skin or woven asbestos. The term salamander skin was named after an ancient mythical fireproof creature. Asbestos was discovered in the Ural Mountains of Russia in the early part of the eighteenth century and later in Italy in the early part of the nineteenth century. It had been used in pottery in Finland as early as 2500 BC. It was discovered near St. Joseph Québec around 1860 and mining started in Canada in 1878. Blue crocidolite asbestos was discovered in South Africa in 1815 and amosite was discovered in 1917. PG Harries states that asbestos has been used in naval ships since 1880 in England (Harries PG. Asbestos dust concentrations in ship repairing: A practical approach to improving asbestos hygiene in naval dockyards. *Ann Occup Hyg* 1971;14:241–54), but that the "full extent of the hazard with asbestos was not appreciated, and adequate preventive measures were not introduced into the English Naval Dockyards until 1967." Asbestos was initially used for packing steam glands and steam stanchions and then later for boiler and pipe insulation. Asbestos cement roofing was used in Europe beginning in 1896 and asbestos cement pipes were first manufactured in Italy in 1913. Amphibole asbestos is found only in specific areas and geologic formations in various countries. The major source of crocidolite and amosite asbestos has been South Africa. Crocidolite has also been mined principally outside of South Africa in Western Australia and China. Chrysotile asbestos occurs wherever there is serpentine rock and is found all over the world. Most of the chrysotile asbestos used in the United States has been mined in Quebec, Canada, and is contaminated with small percentages of amphibole tremolite asbestos. Various areas in eastern Quebec have different percentages of contamination by amphibole tremolite asbestos. In some areas of Quebec, such as the Carey Canadian mine, there is no significant amphibole contamination. There is also no amphibole in the New Idria serpentine chrysotile found in Coalinga, California. This Coalinga fiber is short and consists of a soft, powdery, pellet-like material that is not known to be carcinogenic because of its fiber size and length, and the fact that there is no contamination with amphibole asbestos fibers.

Anthophyllite asbestos is a commercial form of amphibole asbestos mined in Finland with little distribution outside of Scandinavia. It is, however, a contaminant when combined with other silicate materials, such as chrysotile asbestos and New York State talc deposits. It is a much wider fiber than other types of commercial asbestos and was not thought to usually produce mesotheliomas, but only pleural plaques, until 1989. (Tuomi T, Segerberg-Konttinen M, Tammilehto L, Tossavainen A, Vanhala E. Mineral fiber concentration in lung tissue of mesothelioma patients in Finland. *Am J Ind Med* 1989;21:247–54; Phillips J, Murray J. Malignant mesothelioma in a patient with anthophyllite asbestos fibers in the lung. *Ann Occup Hyg* 2010;54:412–16.) Since 1989, a few cases of mesothelioma have been reported in anthophyllite-exposed workers, but the overall incidence of mesothelioma in exposed individuals remains extremely low. The incidence of pleural plaques in Finland related to environmental anthophylite exposure has been high. In the Kuusjaevi district of Finland, 69% of the screened population had pleural calcifications but no reported mesotheliomas. (Kiviluoto R. Pleural calcification as a roentgenologic sign of non-occupational endemic anthophyllite-asbestos. *Acta Radiol (Stockh.)* 1960;Suppl. 194:1–67; Kiviluoto R. *Br J Radiol* 1966;39:133.) The very low incidence of mesothelioma in this group of anthophyllite-exposed individuals is most likely due to the thickness of anthophyllite fibers.

It has been reported by Selikoff and others that the health effects of asbestos were originally reported as early as 2500 BC. These reports were a mistranslation of the original Greek manuscripts, and there really is no reported information on any adverse health effects from asbestos until the beginning of the twentieth century. In 1899, the Chief Inspector of the Factories of Great Britain, Miss Deane, reported the results of an analysis of the year 1898, at which time she mentioned that there were very dusty exposures in asbestos textile plants, and that these plants might be potentially injurious. This was later mentioned in 1902, and in 1907, when Montague Murray reported to the Departmental Committee on Compensation for Industrial Diseases in Great Britain, the history of a 33-year-old man who died of interstitial lung disease, presumably asbestosis. He first saw this young man in 1899, and did a postmortem examination in April of 1900 at Charing Cross Hospital. This is the first death presumably recognized from asbestosis of a man who had worked for 14 years in what was called a carding room in an asbestos textile mill. (Murray H. Montague-testimony. *Report of Departmental Committee on Compensation for Industrial Diseases*, Minutes of Evidence. London: HMSO, 1907.) This asbestos-exposed worker evidently was the only survivor of ten people that began work in an asbestos factory room at approximately the same time as he did, and presumably they all died at somewhere around 30 years of age. Murray's patient, evidently, was supposedly reported in a medical journal published by the Charing Cross Hospital called the *Charing Cross Gazette* in 1901, but I have never been able to find a copy of that paper. (Murray R. Eighty years of occupational disease. *Med Law* 1987;6:593–9; Selikoff IJ. Historical developments and perspectives in inorganic fiber toxicity. *Environ Health Perspect* 1990;88:269–76.) This and earlier studies, as well as reports in 1906 from France by Auribault (Auribalt M. Note sur l'hygiene d'amiante. *Bull Insp Trav Paris* 1906;14:120–132) and Scarpa from Italy in 1908 (Scarpa LG. Industria dell'amianto e tubercolosi. *XVIII Congor D Soc Ital Di Med Int*, Roma, 1908, p. 34) were generally considered as curiosities, and did not raise much concern. Again, warnings were made in 1910 by Collis and others that these dusty trades were potentially dangerous. (Collis. *Dusty Processes Factories and Workshops: Annual Report for 1910.* 1911, p. 188.)

There were mixed reports on the health hazards of asbestos during the 1910s, and in an inquiry performed in 1912 of practitioners in Thetford in Quebec, some practitioners felt that asbestos dust had a weakening effect on the lungs, while other practitioners felt that there was no ill affect. (Selikoff IJ. Historical developments and perspectives in inorganic fiber toxicity. *Environ Health Perspect* 1990;88:269–76.)

Frederick Hoffman, Vice President of the Prudential Life Insurance Company in 1918, published a report entitled "Mortality from respiratory diseases and dusty trades." He urged further research to be done on the health effects of asbestos and stated "there were no medical observations on record in regards to the possible injurious results experienced in mining and manufacturing of asbestos materials." He went on to mention that American and Canadian insurance companies were declining to provide insurance policies for asbestos workers on account of "assumed health-injurious conditions of the industry."

Dr. Pancoast of the University of Pennsylvania in 1917 examined x-rays of individuals exposed to asbestos dust, and it was the general impression that these exposures were associated with abnormal chest x-rays, but this was thought to be related to silica contamination of the asbestos, and this was thought to be perhaps a form of silicosis. (Pancoast HK, Miller G, Landis RM. A roentogologic study of the effects of dust upon the lungs. *Am J Roentgen* 1918;5:129–36.) The health effects of asbestos were reviewed by the Factory Inspectorate in 1917 and according to Merewether, published in his article "A memorandum on asbestos" in *Tubercle* (1933;15s;72), "no further evidence incriminating asbestos had come to light either home or abroad and therefore no further action could be taken."

It was not until 1924 that Cooke first reported a woman by the name of Nellie Kershaw, who worked in the asbestos textile industry and who had died of diffuse fibrosis of the lungs, as well as tuberculosis. He suggested that this fibrotic condition was related to the inhalation of asbestos dust, but the contribution of tuberculosis could not be excluded. This was published in 1924, and a further analysis of the same case was published in 1927, at which time he termed this condition "pulmonary asbestosis." (Cooke WE. Fibrosis of the lungs due to inhalation of asbestos dust. *Br Med J* 1924;2:147; Cooke WE. Pulmonary asbestosis.

Br Med J 1927;2:1024–25; Selikoff IJ, Greenberg M. A landmark case of asbestosis. *JAMA* 1991;265:898–901.) Again, Pancoast and Pendergrass, in reviewing the x-rays of these workers in 1927, thought that what was called asbestosis in 1926 was some type of silicosis. (Pancoast HK, Pendergrass EP. *Pneumoconiosis (Silicosis): A Roentgenological Study.* New York: Paul B Hoeber, Inc., 1926.)

Initially, the role of tuberculosis as a contributing cause or the cause of a fibrosis associated with asbestos exposure was a source of much confusion. Dr. Ian MD Grieve reported on a series of patients from Leeds in the late 1920s, who worked in a local factory that produced insulation mattresses for steam engines. These were made from blue asbestos or crocidolite asbestos. In his thesis, he mentioned that the asbestosis was predominately in the bases of the lungs and was associated with diffuse pleural adhesions. In 9 of his 15 cases, he was unable to find any evidence of tuberculosis, and therefore his conclusion was that pulmonary tuberculosis was not the ultimate cause of death in these patients. Seiler, from South Africa, has usually been given the credit for describing the first case of asbestosis unassociated with tuberculosis in 1928. (Seiler HE. A case of pneumoconiosis. *Br Med J* 1928;2:982.) Drs. Stewart and Haddow, also from Leeds, in 1929 were the first to describe peculiar bodies from patients with pulmonary asbestosis as demonstrated by lung puncture and in the sputum, and they coined the term "asbestosis bodies." (Stewart M, Haddow A. Demonstration of the peculiar bodies of pulmonary asbestosis ("asbestos bodies") in material obtained by lung puncture and in sputum. *J Path Bacteriol* 1929;32:175.)

These papers prompted the British government to embark on a study of asbestos textile factories in 1929. This study was published in 1930 by Drs. Merewether and Price, entitled *Report on Effects of Asbestos Dust on the Lungs and Dust Suppression in the Asbestos Industry* (London: HSMO). This was a classic study of 363 workers in a British asbestos textile factory, and was extremely well done, generally proving once and for all to the medical community that asbestos dust exposure in textile plants can cause a dose-related pulmonary fibrotic condition called pulmonary asbestosis. The data were sufficient to show that there was a cause-and-effect dose-related relationship, and therefore dust suppression methods were necessary and likely to control the disease. Merewether and Price predicted "the almost total disappearance of the disease, as the measures for the suppression of dust are perfected."

Merewether's study on the dose response of exposure to asbestos and the risk of asbestosis has subsequently been repeated many times over the years and most recently by a group in China who again performed a quantitative analysis of the dose response between chrysotile exposure and asbestosis. Attempts at meta-analysis of the dose response of asbestos exposure data have been fraught with potential error when comparing dose–response data from different exposures, such as chrysotile asbestos mines in Quebec, China, India, Greece, Brazil, and South Africa, where amphibole contamination is very different and fiber lengths may also be different. Similarly, we now appreciate that the large differences in lung cancer risks between miners and millers in Quebec and chrysotile asbestos textile workers in South Carolina are largely related to fiber length and not tremolite contamination. Epidemiologic studies need to provide evidence of dust measurement techniques, fiber size, length, and diameter, as well as amphibole contamination before one dose–response study can be compared with another. Apples must be compared with apples and not apples with oranges! (Wang X, Courtice MN, Lin S, Qiu H, Yu IT. Asbestosis and exposure levels in a Chinese asbestos worker cohort. *Occup Environ Med* 2014;71(Suppl. 1):A58; Loomis D, Dement J, Richardson D, Wolf S. Asbestos fiber dimensions and lung cancer mortality amounts workers exposed to chrysotile. *Occup Environ Med* 2010;67(9):580–4; Hein MJ, Stayner LT, Lehman E, Dement JM. Follow-up study of chrysotile textile workers: Cohort mortality in exposure-response. *Occup Environ Med* 2007;64:616–25.)

The question is: Why did it take 30 years for the hazard of asbestos to become recognized by the British medical community? This is best answered by Dr. Merewether in his report to Parliament in 1930, in which on page 17 he stated,

1. Significant commercial exploitation of asbestos was relatively new.
2. The asbestos industry was small and employed comparatively few workers, particularly in dusty processes.
3. The disease developed slowly and unobtrusively.
4. The disease was easily confused with tuberculosis.
5. Affected workers left the industry and therefore fell out sight of factory inspectors.
6. Medical research on the effects of dust inhalation had concentrated on dusts containing free silica.

Recommendations were made to the British parliament, and these recommendations on dust control went into effect on January 1, 1933. It was hoped at that time that the dust control measures instituted would be sufficient to prevent future cases of asbestosis. Merewether established the concept of a dose–response relationship to asbestosis. He estimated doses by job title and relative dustiness of that particular occupation. Later scientists would estimate doses by measurement of both total dust and later calculation of asbestos fibers as a percentage of total dust.

The first case of pulmonary asbestosis in the United States was reported by Mills in *Minnesota Medicine* in July 1930. (Mills RG. Pulmonary asbestosis: Report of a case. *Minnesota Med* 1930:495–7.) While there were reports of abnormal x-rays by Sparks and others from North Carolina, the interest in this disease in the United States was not further stimulated until 1935 when Lanza, McConnell, and Fennel reported on the effects of the inhalation of asbestos dust on the lungs of asbestos workers in 1935. (*U.S. Public Health Report.* 1935;50:1–12.) Dr. Lanza was Assistant Medical Director of the Metropolitan Life Insurance Company and had been asked in 1929 by asbestos industry officials to ascertain whether asbestos dust was an occupational hazard. He stated in an article in the *Journal of the American Medical Association* in 1936 that "in our studies of asbestos mines and fabricating plants, the clinical picture of asbestosis was milder than that of silicosis," and later he stated, "All of the patients working with asbestos that were detected, were with one exception, working steadily at their trades." Also, "One feature that has impressed us is that the British investigators found asbestosis more menacing then we did." Furthermore, "In both countries, energetic steps have been taken to control dust so that it is probable that future cases of disabling asbestosis will be rare." (Lanza AJ, Asbestosis. *JAMA* 1936;106:368–9.) Lanza has been accused of being a biased industry spokesman, but in reality, his statements were consistent with the knowledge and sentiment of the British and American medical communities at that time.

Ellman, in 1933, described the natural history of his observed cases, and noted the slow asymptomatic progression over 5–15 years, with some patients not developing symptoms until many years after exposure. He felt that those patients with asbestosis had a more aggressive disease than silicosis, but he was unable to determine the dose response between exposure and latency for symptomatic disease. Actually, earlier studies by Merewether had demonstrated a dose response between exposure and latency for asbestosis. (Ellman P. Pulmonary asbestosis: The clinical, radiological, and pathological features and associated risk for tuberculosis infection. *J Ind Hyg* 1933;25:165–83.)

Nearly 30 years later, Knox stated that it had been thought that after implementation of the British dust control measures in 1933, future cases of asbestosis would not develop. It was also felt that if asbestosis could be prevented, then asbestos-related neoplasms would not develop. (Knox JF, Doll RS. Hill ID. Cohort analysis of changes in incidence of bronchial carcinoma in a textile asbestos factory. *Ann NY Acad Sci* 1965;132:526–35.) The most important occupational concern in the medical community was silicosis. Compared to silicosis, deaths from asbestosis were not significant. The Annual Report of the Chief Inspector of Factories of Great Britain in 1956 reported that, between 1949 and 1956, there were 17,328 work-related deaths, most of which were from silicosis. Only 123 deaths were from asbestosis, or 1/140th of the total.

This publication and the publications by Lynch, Smith, and others in the mid-1930s further confirmed that this problem was not limited to just textile workers in Great Britain, but included people in the asbestos textile manufacturing industry in the United States as well. (Lynch K, Smith WA. Pulmonary asbestosis III, carcinoma of lung in asbestosilicosis. *Am J Cancer* 1935;24:56–64.) Fulton, from the state of Pennsylvania, performed a nice epidemiologic study in that State that further stimulated interest by the Public Health Department in the epidemiology of asbestosis. (Fulton W, Dooley A, Matthews J, Houtz R. Asbestosis, part II & III. Bulletin—Commonwealth of Pennsylvania, Department of Labor and Industry, 1935.)

Page and Bloomfield looked at dust control methods in an asbestos-fabricating plant and published their data in November 1937. (Page R, Bloomfield JJ. A study of dust control methods in an asbestos fabricating plant. *U.S. Treasury Department Public Health Reports*, 1937:1713–27.)

Dreesen and others from the U.S. Public Health Service studied asbestos textile plants in North Carolina, with careful attention to the relationship between measurements of dust concentration and the prevalence of asbestosis. This landmark study, published in 1938, purported to show that there was a safe level of dust exposure, below which it was unlikely that people exposed to asbestos would develop disease. This level was 5 million particles of asbestos dust per cubic feet (mppcf) of air or 185 particles per cubic centimeter. (Approximately 30 fibers/cc according to the 1972 National Institute for Occupational Safety and Health [NIOSH] counting standard and >30 fibers/cc by current NIOSH counting standards.) (Dreessen [Public Health Bulletin 241] A Study of Asbestosis in the Asbestos Textile Industry, 1938.)

This study by Dreesen and the Public Health Service has often been criticized in retrospect, because many of the older workers with asbestosis had been laid off prior to the onset of the study. The remaining workforce did not have enough workers with sufficient exposure or sufficient latency to provide an accurate assessment of the health effects of exposure to asbestos. The final recommendations of the final sentence of the report were cautious:

It would seem that if the dust concentration in asbestos factories could be kept below 5 million particles...new cases of asbestosis probably would not appear.

EC Vigliani in 1940 confirmed the U.S. Public Health standard of 5 mppcf of asbestos dust as a safe level after studying four factories near Turin, Italy. (Vigliani E. *Stuio sulla asbestosi nelle manifatture di amianto.* Torino: Ediz Ente Nazionale Prevenzione Inforortuni, 1940; Vigliani EC. A glance at the early Italian studies on the health effects of asbestos. *Med Law* 1991;82:489–91.)

This value of <5 mppcf of asbestos dust was later adopted by the American Conference of Industrial Hygienists in 1946 as their standard. (*American Conference of Governmental Industrial Hygienists, Eighth Annual Proceedings.* Chicago, IL, April 1946, pp. 54–6.) It was also used by the U.S. Navy and the U.S. Government as their standard for safe asbestos exposure. Also, during World War II, the U.S. Navy commissioned a study of naval shipyards where large amounts of asbestos were used for insulation aboard ships. They studied a group of end-product users, who, as insulators were insulating pipes, bulkheads, and other areas of ships during the massive ship construction effort of World War II. Their conclusion was that the current level of 5 mppcf of asbestos dust appeared to be safe. This study, entitled "A health survey of pipe covering operations in constructing naval vessels" (*J Indus Hygiene* 1946;28:9–16) was performed under the supervision of a Harvard Professor, Philip Drinker, who was the most qualified expert on industrial hygiene and dust control of that time. The authors state on page 15 of their article: "It would appear that asbestos pipe covering of naval vessels is a relatively safe occupation." They noted "the extremely low incidence from asbestosis found, 0.29%, or three cases out of 1074 pipe coverers stands in marked contrast to the high dust concentrations found in several of the pipe covering operations." They went on to point out that certain occupations, such as band sawing and cement mixing, were associated with very high concentrations of asbestos dust, but the overall exposure averaged out at around 5 mppcf, since these individuals were exposed to high concentrations intermittently. The lack of asbestosis was thought to be related to "the lack of specialization" or the frequent change of jobs that kept the average dose to around 5 mppcf of asbestos dust. This paper was extremely important since it implied that end-users of asbestos, most importantly asbestos pipe insulators, were not at a significant risk of asbestosis. Murphy and others replicated the exact same method of dust measurement in 1966 in one of the same shipyards studied earlier by Dr. Drinker. The authors found that the measurements of Dr. Drinker were accurate, but found evidence of asbestosis at around 60 mppcf after about 13 years of employment. (Murphy RLH, Ferris BG, Burgess WA, Worcester J, Gaensler EA. Effects of low concentrations of asbestos. *N Engl J Med* 1971;285:1271–78.)

The introduction of dust control in attempting to measure the injurious dust in the air of the workplace was a significant advance in the U.S., where dust control was generally better than Britain until 1968. Some experts have questioned whether the 5 mppcf was total dust or asbestos dust (5 mppcf is equivalent to 185 particles per cubic centimeter). The standard at that time was to multiply the percentage concentration of the product by the amount of total dust (particles or fibers) measured to obtain the concentration of asbestos dust. This methodology was confirmed by Herbert E Stokinger, Chief of the Toxicology Branch, Division of Laboratories and Criteria Development of the National Institute for Occupational Safety and Health and a member of the Threshold Limit Value Committee of the American Conference of Governmental Industrial Hygienists (ACGIH) from 1951 to 1977, in an affidavit given on December 27, 1983, in Hamilton County, Ohio. The State of Washington adopted the ACGIH threshold limit values for Washington State in 1955. (*Safety Standards for Protection against Occupationally Acquired Diseases*. Olympia: Department of Labor and Industries, 1958.)

It was not until the mid-1950s that the British inspector of factories began to report an increased incidence of asbestosis in pipe fitters and end-users of asbestos products. The British occupational medicine and asbestos expert Donald Hunter stated in his 1955 edition of his textbook *The Diseases of Occupation* that "legislation has been effective in the disease of asbestos." The British used engineering controls to reduce visible dust. No dust control methods based on reducing dust levels below a directly measurable specific level were implemented until 1968 in Great Britain. Merewether had felt that if dust levels in England could be kept lower than that in spinners, then the exposures were safe. These levels were higher than those proposed by Dreesen and the Public Health Service in the United States. In general, the American medical community remained complacent and it was not until the landmark studies by Selikoff, Hammond, and others that the American medical community's sense of well-being was shattered. Certainly, part of the problem was that most of the reports in the literature were from Europe, where they used different processes and primarily used different forms of asbestos (crocidolite) compared with American factories. Most of the asbestos that was used in the United States was white asbestos or chrysotile. There were much larger amounts of blue and crocidolite asbestos used in Great Britain and in Europe, as well as amosite or brown asbestos, compared to American industrial practices. At the same time, Marr evaluated asbestos exposure during the naval vessel overhaul in 1964 and found that the asbestos levels were as reported by Fleisher and Drinker, but that there was definite asbestosis found in some of these workers. (Marr W. Asbestos exposure during naval vessel overhaul. *Am Assoc Ind Hyg J* 1964;25:264–8.)

Selikoff, Churg, and Hammond published a series of papers between 1964 and 1965 culminating in an international symposium held in New York City at the New York Academy of Sciences in October 1964. The data from the symposium in New York were finally published on December 31, 1965. Upon publication, the world medical community was alerted to the adverse health effects of asbestos, not only in terms of asbestosis, but also lung cancer and mesothelioma. (Selikoff I, Churg J, Hammond E. The occurrence of asbestosis among insulation workers in the United States. *Ann NY Acad Sci* 1965;139–55; Selikoff I, Churg J, Hammond E. Relation between exposure to asbestos and mesothelioma. *N Engl J Med* 1965;272:560–5; Selikoff I, Churg J, Hammond EC. Asbestos exposure and neoplasia. *JAMA* 1964;188:22–6.)

Since the mid-1960s, more information has been obtained on the adverse health effects from asbestosis, and in 1968, the British Occupational Hygiene Society published hygienic standards for chrysotile asbestos dust, at which time they suggested that a level of two fibers per cc would produce no more than one case in 100 of asbestosis. They felt that this level was probably safe. (British Occupational Hygiene Society/Committee on Hygiene Standards. Hygiene standards for chrysotile asbestos dust. *Ann Occup Hyg* 1968:47–69.) This paper and earlier studies stimulated the ACGIH to promulgate a recommendation that the acceptable dose of asbestosis be lowered from 5 mppcf (30 f/cc) to 2 mppcf (12 f/cc), also in 1968. In 1971, this recommendation was dropped to 5 fibers/cc, which was the initial level accepted by the Occupational Safety and Health Administration (OSHA) and became the NIOSH standard in 1972 and then lowered to 2 fibers/cc in 1976. The OSHA standard was under continuous revision until it was eventually dropped to 0.1 fibers/cc in 1994, and it has remained at that level ever since.

Asbestos was largely eliminated from most products between 1975 and 1980. The heavy industrial exposures occurred in the period of 1930–1970, largely due to shipyard exposures, since existing safety regulations focused upon asbestos miners, millers, and asbestos product manufactures, not end-users of asbestos products. The latency time from exposure to asbestos to development of asbestosis is usually less than 20–30 years. However, the actual number of patients claiming asbestosis has been increasing. This suggests that many of these patients have either been misdiagnosed with some other form of interstitial lung disease, or many of these claims are fraudulent. (Janower ML, Berlin L. "B" Readers' radiographic interpretations in asbestos litigation: Is something rotten in the courtroom? *Acad Radiol* 2004;11(8):841–2.)

Darnton et al. performed an analysis of occupational mortality in England and Wales—where there has been traditionally heavier exposure to amphibole asbestos than in the United States—during 1991–2000 based on a total of

33,751 deaths from mesothelioma and 5396 deaths from asbestosis. For both diseases, mortality showed a clear cohort effect; within birth cohorts, death rates increased progressively with age through to 85 years and older. However, the highest mortality from mesothelioma was in men born during 1939–1943, whereas mortality from asbestosis peaked in men born during 1924–1938. Notice that the total number of deaths from asbestosis was about 540 cases per year. The population of England in 2011 was 53.1 million and the population of the United States was 316.13 million in 2013, making the population of England about one-sixth of that of the United States. If exposures were equal in both countries (actually, the exposures to amphiboles, particularly crocidolite, were much greater in England), then the equivalent mortality for asbestosis would be approximately 3240 cases of asbestosis per year in the United States, and not 20,000! The actual number of asbestos cases is likely to be much lower, as discussed in Chapter 5. (Darnton A, Hodgson J, Benson P, Coggon D. Mortality from asbestosis and mesothelioma in Britain by birth cohort. *Occup Med (Lond)* 2012;62(7):549–52.) The evidence suggests that the large increase in the number of diagnosed cases of asbestosis is driven by litigation (see Figures 4.1 through 4.5.)

Gitlin and coworkers at the Department of Radiology at Johns Hopkins Hospital reviewed 551 chest radiographs read as positive for lung changes by initial "B" Readers retained by plaintiffs' attorneys, and 492 matching interpretative reports were made available to the authors representing persons alleging respiratory changes from occupational exposure to asbestos. Six Hopkins consultants in chest radiology, who were also B Readers, agreed to reinterpret

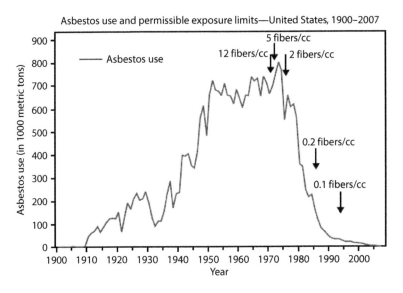

Figure 4.1 The emergence of awareness of health effects from asbestos exposure resulted in regulations to reduce exposure beginning in 1968. (Adapted from CDC. *MMWR Weekly* 2009;58(15);393–6.)

How common is asbestosis?

- In 1970: 300 hospital discharges
- 1973: 2000 cases
- 1983: 4000
- 1993: 8000
- 2000: 20,000
- One physician examined 14,000 workers and was paid $1,000,000. He found all 14,000 had asbestosis

---

Figure 4.2 The number of reported cases of asbestosis has been strongly influenced by asbestos litigation. (Adapted from CDC, *Work-related Lung Disease Surveillance Report*, 2002; ABA Standard for Non-Malignant Asbestos-Related Disease Claims, *Report of the American Bar Association*, February 2003.)

the radiographs independently, without knowledge of their provenance. The results were compared with initial readings for film quality, complete negativity, parenchymal abnormalities, small opacity profusion, and pleural abnormalities using chi-square tests and kappa statistics. The results revealed that plaintiff readers interpreted study radiographs as positive for parenchymal abnormalities (International Labor Office [ILO] small opacity profusion category of 1/0 or higher) in 95.9% of 492 cases. The six Johns Hopkins radiology consultants classified the films as 1/0 or higher in 4.5% of 2952 readings. The authors concluded that the magnitude of the differences between the interpretations by initial readers and the six consultants is too great to be attributed to inter-observer variability. The authors exposed what might be called a type

---

What does a positive x-ray mean?

- 500 qualified B readers. According to the Manville Trust, 49.6% of the tens of thousands of nonmalignancy claims are just based on 10 readers! A single physician accounted for 30,000 nonmalignancy claims over a 6-year period.
- Some readers have a "positive" finding in up to 94% of cases.
- A NIOSH audit on positive x-rays on 795 tire workers showed only 2 had any signs of parenchymal change and only 19 showed pleural changes.

Figure 4.3 The data from the American Bar Association reflect the gross overestimation of true asbestosis cases in the United States. (Adapted from ABA Standard for Non-Malignant Asbestos-Related Disease Claims, *Report of the American Bar Association*, February 2003.)

Problems with American Judicial System

- Courts are out of control. One Mississippi jury awarded $150 million to six plaintiffs with asbestos exposure who had sought redress for fear of future illness.

- 22 companies have sought bankruptcy protection since 2000.

- At risk are General Electric, Viacom, Gaf Corp, Federal Mogul Corp, Hartford Financial Services Group, and Halliburton.

- Both sides in the senate say they want reform but receive large contributions from American trial lawyers.

Figure 4.4 Problems with the American judicial system. (Adapted from *The Wall Street Journal*, CCXLII, 75, October 15, 2003.)

***Wall Street Journal* October 17, 2003**

- Tort lawyers have sued 8400 businesses.
- $70 billion in judgments.
- 90% of plaintiffs are not sick.
- 78 companies forced into bankruptcy.
- U.S. senate has proposed a $114 billion trust fund.
- Any year the asbestos fund cannot meet its obligations, the whole mess returns to court.
- The American Insurance Association "Would substitute one unaffordable, deeply flawed compensation program for another".

Figure 4.5 American courts are out of control.

of academic fraud by these unnamed plaintiff expert B Readers. (Gitlin JN, Cook LL, Linton OW, Garrett-Mayer E. Comparison of "B" Readers' interpretations of chest radiographs for asbestos related changes. *Acad Radiol* 2004;11(8):843–56; Janower ML, Berlin L. "B" Readers' radiographic interpretations in asbestos litigation: Is something rotten in the courtroom? *Acad Radiol* 2004;11(8):841–2.)

5

What is asbestosis and what is not: Radiology and pathology correlates

Asbestosis is a term describing bilateral diffuse parenchymal basilar lung fibrosis or interstitial pneumonitis, beginning in the lower basilar lobes of the lung, classically with honeycombing, in individuals with a history of heavy asbestos exposure with appropriate latency, in whom other causes of interstitial pneumonitis have been excluded. (American Thoracic Society *Ad Hoc* Statement Committee. Diagnosis and initial management of nonmalignant diseases related to asbestos. *Am J Respir Crit Care Med* 2004;170:691–715.) It is important to note that asbestosis is a bilateral diffuse bibasilar lung fibrotic condition since some physicians have called focal unilateral areas of basilar fibrosis "localized or focal asbestosis." *There is no such thing as focal or localized asbestosis.* There are many causes of focal areas of basilar pulmonary fibrosis, but by definition, asbestosis is always bilateral, initially lower lobe, and reasonably symmetrical pathologically and radiologically. Honeycombing is frequently seen. Furthermore, *there is no such thing as pleural asbestosis.* By definition, asbestosis is a lung parenchymal condition. Classically, the fibrosis is subpleural with retraction of the parenchyma at the periphery of the lung associated with thousands of asbestos bodies and large numbers of uncoated fibers by lung digestion. Ground glass opacities suggest acute inflammation and an alternative diagnosis to asbestosis, as does hilar adenopathy. Cobblestoning of the lung surface is found in a variety of interstitial lung diseases including asbestosis. Upper-lobe predominance of interstitial fibrosis suggests an alternative diagnosis. The intensity of fibrosis in asbestosis tends to be rather homogeneous without fibroblastic foci.

There is variation between pathologists in grading severity and extent of asbestos interstitial disease. Disputes often arise when the sample size is small. It is sometimes difficult to generalize that the sample is representative of a diffuse disease versus an isolated focal area of interstitial fibrosis. Efforts were made in 1982 to standardize the diagnostic criteria for asbestosis, but some variation between pathologists is inevitable. (Green FHY, Attfield M. Pathology standards for asbestosis. *Scan J Work Environ Health* 1983;9:162–8; Craighead JE, Abraham JL, Churg A et al. The pathology of asbestos-associated diseases of the lungs and pleural cavities: Diagnostic criteria and proposed grading schema. *Arch Pathol Lab Med* 1982;106:543–96; Churg A, Golden J. Current problems in the pathology of asbestos related disease. *Pathol Ann* 1982;33–66; Richman SJ. Medicolegal aspects of asbestosis for pathologists. *Arch Pathol Lab Med* 1983;107:557–61; Asbestos and the pathologist. *The Lancet* 1984;1:262; Weil H. Asbestos-associated diseases: Science, public policy, and litigation. *Chest* 1983;84:601–8; Craighead JE, Mossman BT. The pathogenesis of asbestos-associated disease. *N Engl J Med* 1982;306:1446–57; Becklake MR. Exposure to asbestos and human disease. *N Engl J Med* 1982;306:1480–2; Becklake MR. Asbestos-related diseases of the lungs and pleura. *Am Rev Resp Dis* 1982;126:187–95; Davis JMG. The pathology of asbestos related disease. *Thorax* 1984;39:801–8; Isidro MI, Abu SK, Alday E et al. Guidelines on asbestos-related pleuropulmonary disease. *Arch Bronconeumol* 2005;41(3):153–68.)

An update of the diagnostic criteria for asbestosis was made in 2010 by the report of the Asbestosis Committee of the College of American Pathologists and Pulmonary Pathology Society. (Roggli VL, Gibbs AR, Attanoos R et al. Pathology of asbestosis—An update of the diagnostic criteria: Report of the Asbestosis Committee of the College of American Pathologists and Pulmonary Pathology Society. *Arch Pathol Lab Med* 2010;134(3):462–80.)

In 1930, after inspecting British asbestos textile mills, Merewether noted that asbestosis was a dose-related disease. It was thought that if exposures could be reduced to a nonvisible level of asbestos dust, asbestosis would not occur. There must be sufficient exposure to respirable asbestos of appropriate duration and intensity to cause asbestosis as a criterion for diagnosis. In addition, the clinical/pathologic criteria require histologic evidence of at least peri-bronchial fibrosis with asbestos bodies in tissue sections. Clinical evidence documented by imaging has been less reliable. Initially, the imaging requirement suggested by the American Thoracic Society was the chest x-ray B-Reader finding of 1/1 irregular s/t, s/s opacities in 1986, which was then lowered to 1/0 in 2004; but with the advance of high-resolution computerized tomography (HRCT) imaging, and because of false-positive and negative results from standard chest x-rays, HRCT is now the standard imaging method for diagnosing all forms of interstitial pneumonitis. (Roach HD, Davies GJ, Attanoos R, Crane M, Adams H, Phillips S. Asbestos: When the dust settles—An imaging review of asbestos-related disease. *Radiographics* 2002;22:S167–84; American Thoracic Society. Medical section of the American Lung Association: The diagnosis of nonmalignant diseases related to asbestos. *Am Rev Respir Dis* 1986;134(2):363–8; American Thoracic Society Ad Hoc Statement Committee. Diagnosis and initial management of nonmalignant diseases related to asbestos. *Am J Respir Crit Care Med* 2004;170:691–715; Smith DD. Diagnosis and initial management of nonmalignant diseases related to asbestos. *Am J Respir Crit Care Med* 2005;171:665–6; Smith DD. When should you suspect asbestos-related disease? *J Respir Dis* 2005;26(11):499–510.)

The problem with the 1/0 standard suggested by the American Thoracic Society has been the lack of a standard film for comparison to the International

Labor Office (ILO) B-Reading standard. There is a significant amount of subjectivity in interpreting ILO films, which becomes more problematic without an ILO 1/0 standard film. (Ross RM. The clinical diagnosis of asbestosis in this century requires more than a chest radiograph. *Chest* 2003;124(3):1120–8; De Raeve H, Verschakelen JA, Gevenois PA, Mahieu P, Moens G, Nemery B. Observer variation in computed tomography of pleural lesions in subjects exposed to indoor asbestos. *Eur Respir J* 2001;17(5):916–21; Harkin TJ, McGuinness G, Goldring R et al. Differentiation of the ILO boundary chest roentgenograph (0/1 to 1/0) in asbestosis by high-resolution computed tomography scan, alveolitis, and respiratory impairment. *J Occup Environ Med* 1996;38(1):46–52.)

The gold standard for determining the reliability of the chest x-ray and high-resolution HRCT in the diagnosis of asbestosis is an autopsy or lung biopsy. The American Thoracic Society in 2011 produced evidence-based guidelines for the diagnosis of idiopathic pulmonary fibrosis (IPF) and stated again that the gold standard was lung biopsy, but the presence of honeycomb changes defined as dilatations of small airways giving the appearance of clumps of small cysts 3–10 mm in diameter on high-resolution computed tomography (CT) was highly predictive of mature pulmonary fibrosis. (Raghu G, Collard H, Egan JJ et al. An official ATS/ERS/JRS/ALAT statement: Idiopathic pulmonary fibrosis: Evidence-based guidelines for diagnosis and management. *Am J Respir Crit Care Med* 2011;183:788–824.) The finding of reticulation lines in peripheral and basilar distribution, without atypical features such as ground glass changes, bronchovascular distribution, nodules, air trapping, hilar or mediastinal adenopathy, or consolidation, is highly suspicious of IPF. (Raghu G, Lynch D, Godwin JD et al. Diagnosis of idiopathic pulmonary fibrosis with high-resolution CT in patients with little or no radiological evidence of honeycombing: Secondary analysis of a randomized controlled trial. *Lancet Respir Med* 2014;2:277–84; Hart SP. Understanding CT patterns in idiopathic pulmonary fibrosis. *Lancet Respir Med* 2014;2:249–50.)

The critical issue in the interpretation of HRCT scans and chest x-rays has been the effect of age. A reticular pattern is seen in 60% of individuals older than 75 years, but this is not seen in those younger than 55 years. Thickening of the interlobular septae is seen more frequently with increasing age and is often a reversible finding by imaging in the prone position. A combination of smoking, obesity, and age correlate with an increased likely of interstitial abnormalities. This means that HRCT findings are neither perfectly sensitive nor specific for asbestosis. CT findings often occupy a gray area between unequivocal health and definite disease and are increasingly problematic in the elderly. (Vehmas T, Copley SJ, Wells AU, Hansell DM. Age-related changes on thin-section CT images. *Radiology* 2009;253(1):279; Hansell DM. Thin-section CT of the lungs: The hinterland of normal. *Radiology* 2010;256(3):695–711; Vehmas T, Kivisaari L, Huuskonen MS, Jaakkola MS. Scoring CT/HRCT findings among asbestos-exposed workers: Effects of patient's age, body mass index and common laboratory test results. *Eur Radiol* 2005;15(2):213–9; Vikgren J, Boijsen M, Andelid K et al. High-resolution computed tomography in healthy smokers and never-smokers: A 6-year follow-up study of men born in 1933. *Acta Radiol* 2004;45(1):44–52;

Laurent F, Paris C, Ferretti GR et al. Inter-reader agreement in HRCT detection of pleural plaques and asbestosis in participants with previous occupational exposure to asbestos. *Occup Environ Med* 2014;71(12):865–70.)

Unfortunately, a good study comparing the clinical diagnosis of asbestosis by work history, radiology, and lung function testing with postmortem examination was not conducted until 2009, when the scientists at the University of South Alabama in Mobile, Alabama, a location of heavy historical use of asbestos in shipbuilding, evaluated 242 cases of patients with a clinical/radiological diagnosis of asbestosis who expired and were later subjected to a postmortem examination. Only 89 out of 242 (36.8%) of these cases had histologically confirmed asbestosis. This study confirms that chest radiology studies over-predict the presence of asbestosis by a wide margin. Similarly, 9.7% of this population had evidence of asbestosis not detected radiologically. This is consistent with the study of a Boston group who found 10% of pathologically diagnosed patients with some form of diffuse infiltrative lung disease to have a negative chest x-ray. (Epler GR, McLoud TC, Gaensler EA, Milkus JP, Carrington CB. Normal chest radiograms in chronic diffuse infiltrative lung disease. *N Engl J Med* 1978;298:934–9; Mizell KN, Morris CG, Carter JE. Antemortem diagnosis of asbestosis by screening chest radiograph correlated with postmortem histologic features of asbestosis: A study of 273 cases. *J Occup Med Toxicol* 2009;4:14–9.)

An autopsy study by Kipen and associates, of asbestos insulators with parenchymal asbestosis and lung cancer, found 18% to have no chest x-ray evidence of asbestosis in an era prior to the availability of HRCT. No consideration of the impact of cigarette smoking was evaluated in the association with lung cancer in this cohort of workers. Certainly, a substantial part, or the entirety of the lung cancer cases without radiologic asbestosis in the Kipen series, was related to cigarette smoking. (Kipen HM, Lilis R, Suzuki Y, Valciukas JA, Selikoff IJ. Pulmonary fibrosis in asbestos insulation workers with lung cancer: A radiological and histological evaluation. *Br J Ind Med* 1987;44:96–100.)

The diagnosis of asbestosis is now confounded by the occurrence of much more common medical conditions in an elderly population. Most manufacturers removed respirable asbestos from their products by 1972–1975. It is unlikely that asbestosis, which presents commonly within 20 years of first exposure, will present more than 40–50 years later. Most of the more heavily asbestos-exposed workers have now expired. Today, clinical asbestosis is rarely seen. From 1992 to 2003, there were 28,176,224 deaths in the United States and 175,088 decedents with pulmonary fibrosis. The average age- and sex-adjusted mortality rate was 50.8 per 1,000,000 people. (Olson AL, Swigris JJ, Lezotte DC, Norris JM, Wilson CG, Brown KK. Mortality from pulmonary fibrosis increased in the United States from 1992 to 2003. *Am J Respir Crit Care Med* 2007;176(3):277–84.) This makes more common forms and causes of pulmonary fibrosis, such as esophageal reflux, hypersensitivity pneumonitis, collagen vascular disease, respiratory bronchiolitis from cigarette smoking, or IPF, much more likely as causes of diffuse parenchymal fibrosis than asbestosis. (Barnes TW, Vassallo R, Tazelaar HD, Hartman TE, Ryu JH. Diffuse bronchiolar disease due to chronic occult aspiration. *Mayo Clin Proc* 2006;81(2):172–6; Raghu G, Freudenberger TD, Yang S et al.

High prevalence of abnormal acid gastro-oesophageal reflux in idiopathic pulmonary fibrosis. *Eur Respir J* 2006;27(1):136–42; Lee JS, Colland HR, Anstrom KJ et al. Anti-acid treatment and disease progression on idiopathic pulmonary fibrosis: An analysis of data from three randomized controlled trials. *Lancet Respir Med* 2013;1:369–76; Singh N. Reflux and autoimmunity: Common links among patients with pulmonary fibrosis? *Chest* 2007;131(3):940; Noth I, Zangan SM, Soares RV et al. Prevalence of hiatal hernia by blinded multidetector CT in patients with idiopathic pulmonary fibrosis. *Eur Respir J* 2012;39(2):344–51.)

There are more than 100 other causes of interstitial lung disease that can make it difficult to distinguish asbestosis from a variety of different fibrosing lung conditions based simply on clinical radiology. Macroscopically, asbestos-related interstitial fibrotic changes are fairly nonspecific, and cannot be differentiated from many other causes of pulmonary fibrosis unless asbestos bodies are identified in sufficient numbers to establish significant asbestos exposure associated with diffuse interstitial fibrosis. Analysis of asbestos body count in expectorated sputum, and particularly in bronchoalveolar lavage (BAL), is very helpful in quantifying exposure. (Alexopoulos EC, Bouros D, Dimadi M, Serbescu A, Bakoyannis G, Kokkinis FP. Comparative analysis of induced sputum and bronchoalveolar lavage fluid (BALF) profile in asbestos exposed workers. *J Occup Med Toxicol* 2011;6:23; Dumortier P, De Vuyst P. Asbestos exposure during uncontrolled removal of sprayed-on asbestos. *Rev Mal Respir* 2012;29(4):521–8.)

The differential diagnosis includes medical conditions such as sarcoidosis, histiocytosis X, radiation pneumonitis, mixed connective tissue disease, rheumatoid arthritis, chronic aspiration of gastric contents, genetic disorders, bronchiolitis obliterans organizing pneumonia (BOOP), inorganic pneumoconiosis, systemic lupus erythematosus, and many different drug reactions, such as interstitial lung fibrosis from antibiotics, antiarrhythmic drugs, and chemotherapeutic drugs, as well as cocaine. Bacterial, viral, fungal, and protozoan infections, lymphangetic cancer and "smoking-related interstitial lung disease" need to be excluded from causation. Berylliosis, talcosis, hard metal disease, nylon flock, textile printing aerosols, zinc oxide nanoparticles and polyvinyl chloride and didecyldimethylammonium chloride silicosis are a few of the many work-related interstitial lung disorders. (Schwarz MI, King TE, Raghu G. Approach to the evaluation and diagnosis of interstitial lung disease. In MI Schwarz, TE King (Eds.), *Interstitial Lung Disease*. London: BC Decker, 2003, pp. 1–30.)

Several case reports have demonstrated the bio-persistence of man-made mineral fibers in the lungs of workers who were exposed to rock wool or fiberglass for long periods of time and were diagnosed with interstitial pulmonary fibrosis. A 20-year follow-up study also identified refractory ceramic fibers in workers' lung tissue, with significant association between cumulative fiber exposure and radiographic pleural changes. Newly emerging man-made fiber industries appear to induce new types of occupational diseases. Insulators are exposed to rock wool, fiberglass, and a variety of other nonasbestos-containing insulation. This complicates the diagnosis of asbestosis in insulators who may have interstitial fibrosis from nonasbestos-containing insulation. (Fireman E. Man-made mineral fibers and interstitial lung diseases. *Curr Opin Pulm Med* 2014;20(2):194–8;

Lange JH, Heymann WC, Cegolon L. Other causative factors for lung diseases in populations exposed to asbestos. *Clin Respir J.* 2014;8(2):253–4.)

Other causes of diffuse interstitial fibrosis such as hypersensitivity pneumonitis can be difficult to differentiate from asbestosis. In a recent article in *Lancet Respiratory Medicine*, Morel and colleagues studied 46 consecutive patients that met the American Thoracic Society (ATS)/European Thoracic Society (ERS) 2011 criteria for a diagnosis of IPF. They all had the typical appearances of IPF on high-resolution CT, but subsequent diagnosis of chronic hypersensitivity pneumonitis was made in 20 of the 46 patients. The distinction is very important and it is generally recognized that in disorders in which inflammation precedes the fibrosis, immunosuppressive therapy can be helpful, as in hypersensitivity pneumonitis, but it is harmful in patients with IPF. (Morell F, Villar A, Montero MA et al. Chronic hypersensitivity pneumonitis in patients diagnosed with idiopathic pulmonary fibrosis: A prospective case control study. *Lancet Respir Med* 2013;1:685–94.) Hypersensitivity pneumonitis is commonly underdiagnosed by physicians because they do not ask patients about normally innocent exposures to environmental and occupational antigens such as exposures from hobbies like being a bird fancier; work exposures from farming, exposure to wood dust from woodworking, machine fluid exposures, isocyanate, zinc, or dye exposure; hot tub use, spa and indoor pool work, contaminated home or work heating and air conditioning systems; and exposure to a variety of other organic, mycobacterial, fungal, and chemical antigens. The finding of a specific antigen can be very difficult, and in my own experience, a specific antigen commonly cannot be identified in many cases. (Lacasse Y, Girard M, Cormier Y. Recent advances in hypersensitivity pneumonitis. *Chest* 2012;142:208–17; Cordeiro CR, Alfaro TM. Freitas S. Clinical case: Differential diagnosis of idiopathic pulmonary fibrosis. *BMC Res Notes* 2013;6(Suppl. 1):S1; Akashi T, Takemura T, Ando N et al. Histopathologic analysis of sixteen autopsy cases of chronic hypersensitivity pneumonitis and comparison with idiopathic pulmonary fibrosis/usual interstitial pneumonia. *Am J Clin Pathol* 2009;131(3):405–15.)

Collagen vascular diseases such as lupus, systemic sclerosis, and rheumatoid arthritis are common causes of interstitial fibrosis. Moua and others from the Mayo Clinic reviewed the serology of 386 biopsy-proven cases that were diagnosed as typical IPF and found positive serologic tests in 29%. (Moua T, Maldorondo F, Decker PA, Daniels CE, Ryu JH. Frequency and implication of autoimmune serologies in idiopathic pulmonary fibrosis. *Mayo Clin Proc* 2014;89:319–26.)

Rheumatoid arthritis-associated interstitial lung disease (RA-ILD) is common and has a prevalence in the range of 4%–42% in rheumatoid arthritis patients depending on detection methods and selection criteria. There is a correlation between rheumatoid arthritis disease activity and ground-glass appearance in the HRCT of RA-ILD patients. These results suggest a positive association between rheumatoid arthritis disease activity and lung inflammation in RA-ILD. (Pérez-Dórame R, Mejía M, Mateos-Toledo H, Rojas-Serrano J. Rheumatoid arthritis-associated interstitial lung disease: Lung inflammation evaluated with high resolution computed tomography scan is correlated to rheumatoid arthritis disease activity. *Rheumatol Clin* 2015;11(1):12–6; Zou YQ, Li YS, Ding XN, Ying ZH.

The clinical significance of HRCT in evaluation of patients with rheumatoid arthritis-associated interstitial lung disease: A report from China. *Rheumatol Int* 2012;32(3):669–73; Cavagna L, Monti S, Grosso V, Boffini N. The multifaceted aspects of interstitial lung disease in rheumatoid arthritis. *Biomed Res Int* 2013;2013:759760.) The disease tends to be indolent and less aggressive than IPF. (Song JW, Lee HK, Lee CK et al. Clinical course and outcome of rheumatoid arthritis-related usual interstitial pneumonia. *Sarcoidosis Vasc Diffuse Lung Dis* 2013;30(2):103–12.) Pathologically and radiologically, rheumatoid lung disease is very similar to IPF. (Assayag D, Elicker BM, Urbania TH et al. Rheumatoid arthritis-associated interstitial lung disease: Radiologic identification of usual interstitial pneumonia pattern. *Radiology* 2014;270(2):583–8.) The risk of lung cancer is increased in those patients with interstitial lung disease and rheumatoid arthritis with a meta-analysis incidence of 1.63 (confidence interval [CI] 1.43–1.87). Other studies have found lower risks of 1.32 and 1.44. No studies have been performed correlating the rate of progression of interstitial lung disease and the degree of interstitial fibrosis and lung cancer risk. However, there is suggestive evidence that the intensity of the inflammatory response to lung injury is the common denominator for risk of lung cancer from a variety of causes, including asbestosis. (Archontogeorgis K, Steiropoulos P, Tzouvelekis A, Nena E, Bouros D. Lung cancer and interstitial lung diseases: A systematic review. *Pulm Med* 2012;2012:315918.)

The most common cause of interstitial lung disease is IPF. The annual incidence of IPF appears to be rising, and is estimated at 5–16 per 100,000 per year in individuals; prevalence is 13–29 per 100,000. The mortality rate from IPF in the United States in 2003 was 61.2 deaths per 1,000,000 in men and 54.5 per 1,000,000 in women. IPF is more common in men, and the prevalence rises dramatically with age. IPF is sufficiently uncommon under the age of 50 years as to mandate an exhaustive search for an underlying connective tissue disease or occult environmental exposure in young patients, particularly women. In contrast, pulmonary fibrosis in patients over the age of 70 years is significantly more likely to be classified as IPF. Risk factors for IPF include age, male gender, and a history of cigarette smoking. Some radiologists assume incorrectly that diffuse pulmonary fibrosis in the presence of pleural plaques must be asbestosis. (Raghu G, Collard H, Egan JJ et al. An official ATS/ERS/JRS/ALAT statement: Idiopathic pulmonary fibrosis: Evidence-based guidelines for diagnosis and management. *Am J Resp Crit Care Med* 2011;183:788–824.)

Copley, Wells, and others have pointed out the difficulty is separating IPF from asbestosis by CT scans. These world-class radiologists and pulmonologists compared CT scans from patients thought to have IPF with others thought to have asbestosis. The problem with any study of this type is that it is difficult to be certain that each patient population is properly identified without a lung biopsy. Fortunately, the authors were able to compare a subpopulation with lung biopsies from each group and found that asbestosis patients had courser fibrosis than IPF patients with an odds ratio of 1.52. The authors claim that subtle differences are present and these differences are potentially useful in separating patient study populations. Based on my 34 years of experience as a National Institute for Occupational Safety and Health (NIOSH) B-Reader, I doubt that these subtle differences would be diagnostic when evaluating individuals such as a 75-year-old smoking male with modest asbestos exposure and interstitial lung disease. To be clinically useful in individual cases, standard CT films, akin to ILO standard films, would need to be available that demonstrate the features of coarse versus fine interstitial fibrosis. (Copley SJ, Wells AU, Sivakumaran P et al. Asbestosis and idiopathic pulmonary fibrosis: Comparison of thin-section CT features. *Radiology* 2003;229(3):731–6.)

Carrillo and others from Toronto, Ontario, Canada, published a study indicating that low-dose CT is useful in detecting parenchymal abnormalities in asbestos-exposed workers as well as pleural plaques. Unfortunately, the study provides no information on the type, duration, and quantity of asbestos exposure to allow any dose–response assessment or ability to discern whether the parenchymal abnormalities observed were due to asbestos or a variety of other causes. (Carrillo MC, Alturkistany S, Roberts H et al. Low-dose computed tomography (LDCT) in workers previously exposed to asbestos: Detection of parenchymal lung disease. *J Comput Assist Tomogr* 2013;37:626–30.)

German and Dutch investigators noted in their chest x-ray and CT scan survey of power industry workers that parenchymal changes found on chest x-ray and CT and diffuse pleural thickening on chest x-ray were both associated with smoking. Finnish investigators carefully quantitated the effects of smoking in asbestos-exposed workers and found that smoking increased all emphysema signs and contributed to bronchial wall thickening. Smoking was negatively associated with curvilinear and septal lines as well as with parenchymal bands. In persons who had smoked <10 pack-years, smoking was positively related to para-septal emphysema and to bronchial wall thickening and negatively related to septal lines, subpleural nodules, and honeycombing. Smoking was related to several abnormal CT scans, even among those with relatively small exposures. (Eisenhawer C, Felten MK, Tamm M et al. Radiological surveillance of formerly asbestos-exposed power industry workers: Rates and risk factors of benign changes on chest X-ray and MDCT. *J Occup Med Toxicol* 2014;9:18; Vehmas T, Kivisaari L, Huuskonen MS, Jaakkola MS. Effects of tobacco smoking on findings in chest computed tomography among asbestos-exposed workers. *Eur Respir J* 2003;21(5):866–71; Geyer SJ. Asbestos, asbestosis, smoking, and lung cancer: Study bias and confounding issues that complicate the interpretation of the results. *Am J Respir Crit Care Med* 2014;189(1):115–6; Churg A, Hall R, Bilawich A. Respiratory bronchiolitis with fibrosis-interstitial lung disease: A new form of smoking-induced interstitial lung disease. *Arch Pathol Lab Med* 2015;139(4):437–40.)

The clinical/radiological diagnosis of interstitial lung disease is still imperfect. The sensitivity and positive predictive value for a HRCT diagnosis of idiopathic fibrosing alveolitis (IPF)/chronic fibrosing alveolitis (CFA) were 71% each, while specificity and negative predictive value were 67% each. For the ATS/ERS criteria, sensitivity, specificity, positive predictive value, and negative predictive value were 71%, 75%, 77%, and 69%, respectively. The inter-observer variability values, expressed as a kappa coefficient, for HRCT and the ATS/ERS criteria were 0.59 and 0.53, respectively. Both HRCT and the ATS/ERS clinical criteria may lead to misdiagnosis of patients with interstitial lung disease. (Peckham RM, Shorr AF, Helman

DL Jr. Potential limitations of clinical criteria for the diagnosis of idiopathic pulmonary fibrosis/cryptogenic fibrosing alveolitis. *Respiration* 2004;71(2):165–9.)

Tiwari conducted an agreement analysis between HRCT and chest x-ray and found that there was a poor agreement between HRCT and chest x-rays (kappa = 0.34) in diagnosing interstitial lung disease. (Tiwari RR. Agreement between chest radiography and high-resolution computed tomography in diagnosing dust-related interstitial lung fibrosis. *Toxicol Ind Health* 2015;31(3):235–8; Ren H, Lee DR, Hruban RH et al. Pleural plaques do not predict asbestosis: A high-resolution computed tomography and pathology study. *Mod Pathol* 1991;4:201–9; Hillerdal G, Malmberg P, Hemmingsson A. Asbestos-related lesions of the pleura: Parietal plaques compared to diffuse thickening studied with chest roentgenography, computed tomography, lung function, and gas exchange. *Am J Ind Med* 1990;18(6):627–3.)

The gold standard for the diagnosis of asbestosis is pathology, via lung biopsy or autopsy, with elevation of asbestos body or lung fiber counts, since the history of asbestos exposure is often unreliable. The pulmonary fibrosis of asbestosis is interstitial and has a bilateral basal peri-bronchial fibrosis with subpleural distribution, often with honeycombing, similar to that seen in IPF, which is the principal differential diagnosis. However, there are differences between the two diseases, apart from the presence or absence of increased asbestos bodies or fibers. First, the interstitial fibrosis of asbestosis is accompanied by very little inflammation, which, although not marked, is better developed in IPF. Second, in keeping with the slow tempo of the disease, the fibroblastic foci that characterize IPF are infrequent in asbestosis. Third, asbestosis is almost always accompanied by mild fibrosis of the visceral pleura, a feature that is rare in IPF. (Roggli VL, Gibbs AR, Attanoos R et al. Pathology of asbestosis—An update of the diagnostic criteria: Report of the asbestosis committee of the College of American Pathologists and Pulmonary Pathology Society. *Arch Pathol Lab Med* 2010;134(3):462–80.)

Asbestosis is one of many forms of diffuse interstitial pulmonary fibrosis. Its histologic diagnosis rests on the pattern of diffuse lung fibrosis and the presence of elevated numbers of asbestos bodies by light microscopy in lung biopsies. Roggli and Sanders reviewed pathological lung sections from 234 patients with lung cancer referred mostly for forensic analysis of fiber counts to their laboratory. Only 6.5% had pleural plaques without histological asbestosis. (Roggli VL, Sanders LL. Asbestos content of lung tissue and carcinoma of the lung: A clinicopathologic correlation and mineral fiber analysis of 234 cases. *Ann Occup Hyg* 2000;44:109–17.) Roggli and Sanders concluded:

The pulmonary concentration of asbestos fibers in 234 cases of primary carcinoma of the lung was determined by means of a tissue digestion technique. Asbestos body counts were performed in 229 cases and fiber analysis by scanning electron microscopy in 221 cases. Asbestos content was recorded as total asbestos fibers, commercial amphibole fibers, noncommercial amphibole fibers, and chrysotile fibers 5 mm or greater in length per gram of wet lung tissue. The study group included 70 patients with asbestosis

(Group I), 44 patients with parietal pleural plaques but without asbestosis (Group II), and 120 patients with neither (Group III). The median asbestos body content of Group I was more than 35 times greater than Group II and more than 300 times greater than Group III. The total asbestos fiber count for Group I was nearly 20 times greater than Group II and more than 50 times greater than Group III. The difference was due almost entirely to commercial amphiboles.

In 2008, Roggli reviewed his laboratory experience in correlating asbestos body and fiber counts and disease. Asbestos content was measured in lung tissue samples from 819 individuals using light microscopy (to measure asbestos body concentrations) and scanning electron microscopy (to measure types and concentrations of mineral fibers). Cases were divided chronologically according to those occurring in the first half (group 1) versus those occurring in the second half (group 2). The study included 419 cases of malignant mesothelioma, 206 cases of asbestosis, and 340 cases of lung cancer. The median asbestos body count (in asbestos bodies per gram) decreased from group 1 to group 2 for each disease: malignant mesothelioma, 480–350; asbestosis, 24,700–19,200; and lung cancer, 1600–174 (reference range: 0–20). A similar trend was observed for fiber counts by scanning electron microscopy. Amosite was the most frequently detected asbestos fiber type and decreased in frequency of detection and median concentration from group 1 to group 2. Crocidolite showed an increased detection frequency from group 1 to group 2 across all three disease categories. The decrease in asbestos body and amosite concentrations over time is consistent with the banning of asbestos from insulation products in 1972. The source for the increased detection of crocidolite was not identified and needs further investigation. (Roggli VL, Vollmer RT. Twenty-five years of fiber analysis: What have we learned? *Hum Pathol* 2008;39(3):307–15.)

A follow-up study was published in 2010, which correlated the number of asbestos fibers found in lungs with asbestosis and IPF, and a quantitative degree of fibrosis was analyzed. The fibrosis scores of the asbestosis cases correlated best with the number of uncoated commercial amphibole fibers. (Schneider F, Sporn TA, Roggli VL. Asbestos fiber content of lungs with diffuse interstitial fibrosis: An analytical scanning electron microscopic analysis of 249 cases. *Arch Pathol Lab Med* 2010;134(3):457–61.)

Finally, the clinical course for IPF is usually rapidly progressive over a course of 2–5 years prior to death. Asbestosis usually progresses very slowly over 10–15+ years or does not progress at all in the currently surviving exposed population. The very heavily exposed population such as those seen in the asbestos textile industry in the early twentieth century developed rapidly advancing pulmonary fibrosis, but those with historically high exposures have expired, leaving a small remaining population with milder disease. This is consistent with the lower level of interstitial inflammation when compared to IPF. (Świątkowska B, Sobala W, Szubert Z. Progression of small, irregular opacities in chest radiographs of former asbestos workers. *Int J Occup Med Environ Health* 2012;25:481–91; Isidro MI, Abu SK, Alday E et al. Guidelines on asbestos-related pleuropulmonary disease. *Arch Bronconeumol* 2005;41(3):153–68. Spanish, English translation available online.)

I am always suspicious for an alternate diagnosis to asbestosis, if, in retrospect, I do not find radiologic evidence of chronic interstitial fibrosis going back several years. (Bar-Shai A, Tiran B, Topilsky M, Greif J, Fomin I, Schwarz Y. Continued progression of asbestos-related respiratory disease after more than 15 years of non-exposure. *Isr Med Assoc J* 2012;14(9):560–5.) New onset of rapidly progressive interstitial fibrosis suggests an alternative diagnosis to asbestosis. (Roggli VL, Gibbs AR, Attanoos R et al. Pathology of asbestosis—An update of the diagnostic criteria: Report of the Asbestosis Committee of the College of American Pathologists and Pulmonary Pathology Society. *Arch Pathol Lab Med* 2010;134(3):462–80; Raghu G, Collard H, Egan JJ et al. An official ATS/ERS/JRS/ALAT statement: Idiopathic pulmonary fibrosis: Evidence-based guidelines for diagnosis and management. *Am J Respir Crit Care Med* 2011;183:788–824.)

Some claim that work history of asbestos exposure establishes the likelihood of asbestos-related lung disease. Van Cleemput and coworkers comment: "Why do we not agree that the past work history should be the gold standard for past asbestos exposure? The history is rarely, if ever, an accurate reflection of the level of exposure, particularly if this is obtained by questioning the patient." The authors concluded that people sometimes totally ignore that they have ever been exposed to asbestos, either at work or elsewhere; in addition, when they do know that they have worked with asbestos-containing materials, clinical experience demonstrates that a substantial asbestos exposure may remain "occult," even after extensive questioning. Often patients claim—or fear—that they have been exposed to huge quantities of asbestos, although their exposure has only been trivial. While a detailed occupational history is essential in the diagnosis of asbestos-related lung disease; I do not think that it can ever be the best indicator, or even a gold standard. Quantitative assessments of fiber burden in lung tissue, and to some extent also in BAL, are generally more accurate indicators, although not perfect, but are useful for assessing remote exposures to asbestos. If there is no gold standard for evaluating past exposure to asbestos, then we are left with having to use combined approaches, including fiber analysis, exposures associated with job title, industrial hygiene measurements, and the occupational history. Small-to-moderate pleural plaques do not correlate well with the estimated cumulative exposure to asbestos as discussed in Chapter 8. (Van Cleemput J, De Raeve H, Verschakelen J, Nemery B. The gold standard for past asbestos exposure. *Am J Respir Crit Care Med* 2002;165:134.)

A surrogate for actual lung fiber analysis has been BAL with measurement of asbestos bodies. In individuals with a history of asbestos exposure, the presence of asbestos bodies in BAL cells is associated with higher prevalence of parenchymal abnormalities, respiratory symptoms, and reduced pulmonary function. Sebastien has demonstrated that asbestos bodies in sputum in vermiculite-exposed workers in Libby, Montana, is a better indicator of chest x-ray abnormality than measurements of cumulative exposure. (Vathesatogkit P, Harkin TJ, Addrizzo-Harris DJ, Bodkin M, Crane M, Rom WN. Clinical correlation of asbestos bodies in BAL fluid. *Chest* 2004;126(3):966–71; Rivolta G, Prandi E, Sogliani M, Picchi O. Significance of bronchoalveolar lavage in demonstrating previous exposure to asbestos. *Med Lav* 2001;92(3):166–72; Sebastien P,

Armstrong B, Monchaux G, Bignon J. Asbestos bodies in bronchoalveolar lavage fluid and in lung parenchyma. *Am Rev Respir Dis* 1988;137(1):75–8.)

Andrew Churg suggested in 1983 (which was later confirmed by Warnock and Isenberg) that the discovery of one asbestos body per square centimeter of a fibrotic lung section is sufficient for histological diagnosis of asbestosis. This is roughly equivalent to 1000 asbestos bodies per cubic centimeter of lung. (Churg A. Current issues in the pathologic and mineralogic diagnosis of asbestos-induced disease. *Chest* 1983;84(3):275–80; Warnock ML, Isenberg W. Asbestos burden and the pathology of lung cancer. 1986. *Chest* 2009;136(5 Suppl.):e30.) The general population has many asbestos bodies in their normal lungs due to environmental exposure and the finding of an occasional asbestos body is not sufficient evidence of significant asbestos exposure. (Thompson JG, Kaschula ROC, MacDonald RR. Asbestos as a modern urban hazard. *S Afr Med J* 1963;37:77–81; Churg A. Asbestos fibers and pleural plaques in a general autopsy population. *Am J Pathol* 1982;109(1):88–96.) Roggli and the Asbestos Committee require two or more asbestos bodies per square centimeter of 5-μm thick lung pathologic sections. This is roughly equivalent to 2000 asbestos bodies per cubic centimeter of lung. (Roggli VL, Gibbs AR, Attanoos R et al. Pathology of asbestosis—An update of the diagnostic criteria: Report of the Asbestosis Committee of the College of American Pathologists and Pulmonary Pathology Society. *Arch Pathol Lab Med* 2010;134(3):462–80.)

The problem with the asbestos body standard for the diagnosis of asbestosis is it fails to recognize that asbestosis is a dose-related disease, meaning that the higher the asbestos body count, the greater the likelihood of a cause-and-effect relationship between the asbestos body count and asbestosis. The median asbestos body count (in asbestos bodies per gram) in a previously quoted study by Roggli was 19,200–24,700 asbestos bodies per gram. This is quite different from 1000–2000 asbestos bodies per gram suggested as the asbestosis standard! (Roggli VL, Vollmer RT. Twenty-five years of fiber analysis: What have we learned? *Hum Pathol* 2008;39(3):307–15.)

The finding of an occasional asbestos body alerts the pathologist to the possibility of asbestosis only. The finding of two or more asbestos bodies in a square centimeter of a microscopic field of lung tissue is suggestive of sufficient, albeit minimal asbestos content in the lung tissue to produce asbestosis, but higher concentrations of asbestos bodies are usually found. Whenever a diagnosis of asbestosis is in question, the reasonable approach is to take a larger sample of lung from several different areas and measure the asbestos body count or fiber count from these areas in order to quantitate asbestos exposure. Often, asbestos body counts are lower in areas of fibrosis and asbestos body counts in the upper lobes may be higher. Low and intermediate levels of asbestos fibers are difficult to interpret because cigarette smoking enhances fiber retention and may cause a nonspecific form of mild pulmonary fibrosis. Lung distortion from emphysema may also enhance fiber retention.

The definition of asbestosis by the Committee of the College of American Pathologists and Pulmonary Pathology Society is a medical–legal definition. The finding of elevated numbers of asbestos bodies does not exclude other causes of interstitial fibrosis as major contributing factors or the major cause of the interstitial lung disease. Most experts recognize that many of the elderly asbestos-exposed workers we see today who have elevated asbestos fiber counts from prior exposures many decades ago, are more likely to have IPF or some other cause of interstitial lung disease in a setting of prior asbestos exposure, particularly if the lung fibrosis is of recent onset and rapidly progressive. Medico-legally, these workers with elevated asbestos bodies would likely meet the pathologic criteria of asbestosis. It is important for the clinician, radiologist, and pathologist to consider other cases of interstitial fibrosis that might be treatable, such as hypersensitivity pneumonitis. Unfortunately, many of these cases of late-onset progressive pulmonary fibrosis never get evaluated for other causes of pulmonary fibrosis once a history of heavy asbestos exposure is found or pleural plaques are evident radiologically in the presence of bilateral lower-lobe pulmonary fibrosis.

American researchers performed a study of 53,454 current or ex-smokers with a history of smoking at least 30 pack-years to compare the sensitivity of low-dose CT scanning with chest x-ray screening. They demonstrated that low-dose CT scanning of current and ex-smokers can find lung cancers at an early stage before they could be visible on chest x-ray. Lung cancer was discovered in 1.1% of the CT-scanned group compared with 0.7% of the chest x-ray-screened group. The limitation of CT scanning for the detection of lung cancer is related to the cost of the frequently found false positives, small scars, and benign nodules that may result in unnecessary surgery for a benign condition. (The National Lung Screening Trial. Results of initial low-dose computed tomographic screening for lung cancer. *N Engl J Med* 2013;368:1980–91; Ollier M Jr, Chamoux A, Naughton G, Pereira B, Dutheil F. Chest computed tomography screening for lung cancer in asbestos occupational exposure: A systematic review and meta-analysis. *Chest* 2014;145(6):1339–46.) CT scanning not only discovers early small lung cancers, but also detects many other abnormalities, such as focal lung scarring, which could be confused with an asbestos-related condition.

Italian investigators have been using HRCT to find early lung cancers in heavy smokers. They noted that some of the patients had previously undiagnosed interstitial lung disease. The usual interstitial pattern and the other chronic interstitial pattern were identified in two (0.3%) out of 692 and 26 (3.8%) out of 692 patients, respectively; 109 (15.7%) out of 692 patients showed CT abnormalities consistent with smoking-related respiratory bronchiolitis, while an indeterminate CT pattern was reported in 21 out of 692 (3%) patients. Age, male sex, and current smoking status were factors associated with the presence of chronic and usual interstitial fibrotic patterns. This research study is very important in that it identifies the prevalence of interstitial lung disease in a smoking population. In summary, approximately 3%–4% of an older smoking population will have non-specific fibrotic changes on routine HRCT examination possibly consistent with asbestosis, even though they may have never been exposed to asbestos. "Thin-section CT features of ILD, probably representing smoking-related ILD, are not uncommon in a lung cancer screening population and should not be overlooked." (Sverzellati N, Guerci L, Randi G et al. Interstitial lung diseases in a lung cancer screening trial. *Eur Respir J* 2011;38(2):392–400; Sverzellati N. Highlights of HRCT imaging in IPF. *Respir Res* 2013;14(Suppl. 1):S3; Caminati A, Cavazza A, Sverzellati N, Harari S. An integrated approach in the diagnosis of smoking-related interstitial lung disease. *Eur Respir Rev* 2012;21(125):207–17.)

German pathologists in 2012 evaluated 88 cases of interstitial fibrosis or fibrosing alveolitis and found 63 patients (72%) were diagnosed as idiopathic interstitial pneumonias (IPF) according to ATS/ERS criteria. Furthermore, ten (11%) cases of hypersensitivity pneumonitis, seven (8%) Langerhans cell histiocytosis, and eight (9%) interstitial pneumonias of other known causes or associations were detected without finding significant cases of asbestosis. (Theegarten D, Müller HM, Bonella F, Wohlschlaeger J, Costabel U. Diagnostic approach to interstitial pneumonias in a single centre: Report on 88 cases. *Diagn Pathol* 2012;7:160; Oikonomou A, Prassopoulos P. Mimics in chest disease: Interstitial opacities. *Insights Imaging* 2013;4(1):9–27; Noble PW, Barkauskas CE, Jiang D. Pulmonary fibrosis: Patterns and perpetrators. *J Clin Invest* 2012;122(8):2756–62; Schneider F, Gruden J, Tazelaar HD, Leslie KO. Pleuropulmonary pathology in patients with rheumatic disease. *Arch Pathol Lab Med* 2012;136(10):1242–52; Vassallo R, Ryu JH. Smoking-related interstitial lung diseases. *Clin Chest Med* 2012;33(1):1.)

Asbestosis remains a rare disease, even in asbestos-exposed workers with sufficient latency for the detection of asbestosis. Laurent and French coworkers evaluated 5511 participants in an asbestos postsurvey study between October 2003 and December 2005. 4106 workers were between 60 and 74 years of age and 197 were over the age of 75 years. Most were ex-smokers (59.5%), 7.2% were still smoking and 25.6% were nonsmokers. Approximately 85% had a duration of asbestos exposure of 20–40+ years. The authors found a very low rate of asbestosis by their HRCT criteria of 0.896% and of honeycombing of 0.18% in their study population. (Laurent F, Paris C, Ferretti GR et al. Inter-reader agreement in HRCT detection of pleural plaques and asbestosis in participants with previous occupational exposure to asbestos. *Occup Environ Med* 2014;71(12):865–70.) Asbestosis remains a difficult diagnosis in an adult population aged >75 years in which 69% of the normal population have interstitial abnormalities. These discrete parenchymal abnormalities slowly increase with age. (Copely SJ, Wells AU, Hawtin KE et al. Lung morphology in the elderly: Comparative CT study of subjects over the age 75 years versus those under 55 years old. *Radiology* 2009;251:566–73; Hansell DM. The thin section CT of the lungs: The hinterland of normal. *Radiology* 2010;256:695–711.) Previous studies by Gordon Gamsu have shown that CT findings of asbestosis are neither perfectly sensitive nor specific. (Gamsu G, Salmon CJ, Warnock ML. CT quantification of interstitial fibrosis in patients with asbestosis. *Am J Roentgenol* 1995;164:63–8.)

The diagnosis of asbestosis remains a clinical diagnosis. The clinician must integrate the radiologic, pathologic, serologic, smoking history, and environmental exposure data with all of the other clinical information, such as family history, drug exposures, other medical illnesses such as collagen vascular disease, gastroesphageal reflux disease (GERD), and personal habits such as bird or pigeon exposure and household mold exposure. (Colby T. Pulmonary pathology: LC22-1 diagnosis of idiopathic pulmonary fibrosis (IPF): Histologic and HRCT diagnosis. *Pathology* 2014;46(Suppl. 2):S36.)

6

The association of lung cancer and asbestosis

Early studies of asbestos workers in asbestos textile manufacturing noted the association between lung cancer and asbestosis, but it took many years before scientists concluded that asbestosis caused lung cancer. These early studies did not mention any smoking history. Dr. Lynch and Dr. Smith of the University of South Carolina were the first to publish a case report of a patient with asbestosis and carcinoma of the lung in 1935. They noted the association but did not feel that a definite causal relationship was proven. (Lynch KJ, Smith WA. Pulmonary asbestosis III. Carcinoma of the lung in asbestos-silicosis. *Am J Cancer* 1935;24:56–64.) At the same time, Gloyne also reported two cases of carcinoma of the lung associated with asbestosis (Gloyne SR. Two cases of squamous carcinoma of the lung occurring in asbestosis. *Tubercle* 1935;17:5–10), as did Egbert and Geiger. Other cases began to filter in through the 1930s, and in 1938, Nordmann described another case of asbestosis associated with lung cancer, and he felt the data of the association between asbestosis and lung cancer were strong. (Nordmann M. Der Berufskrebs der Asbestarbeiter Eingegangen am 18. *Marz* 1938:288–30; Nordmann M, Sorge A. Lungenkrebs durch Asbestaub im Tierversuch *Z Krebsforch* 1941;51:168–82.)

Holleb and Angrist in 1942 felt that lung cancer was related to asbestosis. (Holleb HB, Angrist A. Bronchogenic carcinoma associated with pulmonary asbestosis. *Am J Pathol* 1942;18:123–31.) Homburger, a pathologist at Yale Medical School, reviewed the literature in 1943 and found 19 cases of asbestosis associated with lung cancer reported in the literature, including three of his own cases, but felt that there was no reliable answer as to whether pulmonary asbestosis was associated with lung cancer. (Homburger F. Coincidence of primary carcinoma of the lungs and pulmonary asbestosis. *Am J Pathol* 1943;19(5):797–807.)

Other reports in the literature were summarized in 1943 by HW Wedler in Heidelberg, Germany, who felt that after reviewing the world's literature on asbestos exposure and lung cancer, there were enough cases reported of lung cancer in patients with asbestosis plus his own cases to prove an association. He found 14 cases of lung cancer out of 92 postmortem examinations of lungs with asbestosis. He felt that the incidence of lung cancer of 16% was much too high and also noted that latency for lung cancer was correlated with the length and intensity of exposure to asbestos. (*Dtsch Arch Klin Med* 1943;191:189–209.) This was also summarized in the *Bulletin of Hygiene* in May 1944. His stature as a German pathologist was strong, and shortly thereafter, the German government in 1943 made lung cancer associated with asbestosis a recognizable, compensable, work-related condition.

In the meantime, there were numerous other case reports of patients with lung cancer in asbestos workers in the world literature, both in the United States and elsewhere. In 1948, Lynch and Cannon reviewed 40 cases of asbestosis, three of which had lung cancers. The authors considered that lung cancer was possibly inducible by severe asbestosis and should remain uncertain until proven by further investigation. (*Dis Chest* 1948;14:874–89.) H Wyers reviewed the literature on asbestosis and noted 17 patients with lung cancer out of 115 autopsies (14.8%). (*Postgrad Med J* 1949;26:631–8.)

It is important to point out at this juncture that the German government had a very strong bias in the favor of an environmental cause of all cancers. It was around 1940 that the German government mandated that soldiers and others stop smoking because they felt there were adequate data to prove an association between lung cancer and cigarette smoking. Other investigators felt the evidence was insufficient, and it was not until 1964 that the Surgeon General issued a report in the United States of the health hazards of cigarette smoking in relation to lung cancer. Thus, the Germans were 24 years ahead of the United States in making that association, and as we will see later, they were many years ahead of the United States in making the association between asbestos exposure and lung cancer. Unfortunately, the demonization of Germany by other Western nations during and after World War II resulted in xenophobia and rejection of advances in German medicine that lasted for decades. (Procter R. *The Nazi War on Cancer.* Princeton University Press, 1999, pp. 111–3; Lifton RJ. *The Nazi Doctors.* Basic Books, 1986; Harrington JM. Re: Attitudes and opinions regarding asbestos and cancer, 1934–1965. *Am J Ind Med* 1993;23:505–6; Burdorf L, Swuste PHJJ, Heederik D. A history of awareness of asbestos disease and the control of occupational asbestos exposures in The Netherlands. *Am J Ind Med* 1991;20:547–55; Corn M, Corn JK. Re: Historical reasons for attitudes and opinions regarding asbestos and cancer, 1934–1965. *Am J Ind Med* 1993;23:513–5; Langard S. Attitudes and opinions regarding asbestos and cancer 1934–1965. *Am J Ind Med* 1992;22:267–9; Criaghead JE. Re: Changing attitudes and opinions regarding asbestos and cancer 1934–1965. *Am J Ind Med* 1992;22:271–3.)

Meanwhile, further research was done in 1947. Merewether studied a group of asbestos workers in Great Britain and found 31 cases of lung cancer (13.2%) out of 235 cases of asbestosis. This was reported in his annual report of the Chief Inspector of the Factories of the year 1947 and published in January 1949. (*Annual Report of the Chief Inspector of Factories for the Year 1947.* London: His Majesty's Stationary Office, 1949.) He noted a much higher incidence of lung cancer in patients with asbestosis who had been working as textile workers in asbestos plants as compared to workers who had had silicosis. Gloyne reviewed 1205 cases of pneumoconiosis autopsies and noted an increased incidence of lung cancer in his asbestosis necropsies. (Gloyne SR. Pneumoconiosis: A histological survey of necropsy material in 1205 cases. *Lancet* 1951;1:810–4.) However, in spite of these data, Merewether and Gloyne did not feel the evidence of the association between asbestos exposure and lung cancer was proven. Merewether mentioned his reservations on the association between asbestosis and lung cancer in a paper given at the Second Conference on Industrial Hygiene in Zagreb, Yugoslavia, in September 1953.

Perhaps one of the most outspoken advocates for the relationship between asbestosis and lung cancer was the prolific writer Dr. Wilhelm C Hueper, a German-trained physician who emigrated to the United States before World War II and later became Chief of the Environmental Cancer Section of the National Cancer Institute. Hueper articulated his views in many medical articles. (Hueper W. *Occupational Tumors and Allied Diseases*; Hueper W. Environmental lung cancer. *Ind Med Surg* 1951;20:50–62; Hueper W. Lung cancer and the tobacco smoking habit. *Ind Med Surg* 1954;23(1):13–9; Hueper W. Recent developments in environmental cancer. *AMA Arch Pathol* 1954;58:360–99; Hueper W. Silicosis, asbestosis, and cancer of the lung editorial. *Am J Clin Pathol* 1955;25:1388; Hueper WC. A quest into the environmental causes of cancer of the lung. *Public Health Monogr* 1955;36:1–54.) Dr. Hueper was a cigarette smoker and in a 1959 paper opined that studies in experimental animals that cigarette smoke caused cancer were inconclusive. He stated, "Human observations are in agreement with this interpretation of experimental evidence. If tobacco tar would be a potent carcinogen, one would expect that intimate contact of the skin of the fingers often deeply stained by it and the mucosa of the lip and mouth bathed in the tarry fluid exuding from the tip would exhibit cancerous lesions to an unusually high degree, since such reactions are not uncommon in individuals exposed to coal tar. The facts are that there is not a single case of cancer of the fingers in chain smokers and that there is no positive statistical association between cigarette smoking and lip and oral cancer, such relations have been claimed for cigar and pipe smoking." (Hueper WC. Environmental cancer. In: F Homberger (Ed.), *Pathophysiology of Cancer*, 1959, pp. 919–70.)

There are many problems with Hueper's approach to the medical literature, which I believe was not fair or balanced. He completely ignored the great strides made by Doll, Wynder, and others proving that cigarette smoking causes lung cancer. Wynder and coworkers had produced cancer from cigarette tar in 1953. (Wynder El, Graham EA, Croninger AB. Experimental production of carcinoma with cigarette tar. *Cancer Res* 1953;13:855–64.) Hueper made much noise but few listened. It is helpful to gain perspective by reviewing another commentary on lung cancer and smoking by a world expert on the subject and an author of the early research that demonstrated the relationship between smoking and lung cancer. Ernst Wynder and Dr. Evarts Graham submitted a paper on 684 proven cases of lung cancer and their relationship to cigarette smoking. (Wynder El, Graham EA. Tobacco smoking as a possible etiologic factor in bronchogenic cancer. *JAMA* 1950;143:329–36.) In 1997, Dr. Wynder provided a great review and commentary on the early research on the relationship of cigarette smoking and cancer. (Wynder EL. Tobacco as a cause of lung cancer: Some reflections. *Am J Epidemiol* 1997;146:687–94.)

In 1958, an important paper was published by Braun and Truan that claimed that there was no increased risk of lung cancer in their large Canadian asbestos miner worker cohort of 5958 workers. (Braun DC, Truan TD. An epidemiologic study of lung cancer in asbestos miners. *AMA Arch Ind Health* 1958;17:634–53.) Approximately 66% were aged 20–44 years and 30% had less than 10 years of employment and 70% had less than 20 years of employment. This created a large selection bias that minimized the ability of this study to capture the true incidence of lung cancer, since relatively few of these workers would have had sufficient time and exposure to develop lung cancer. Their data in retrospect were very tenuous at best. There is no evidence that any data were manipulated by this industry-sponsored study. Subsequent studies of many of the same workers by McDonald and others later found an increased incidence of lung cancer in a more mature population of many of the same workers. (McDonald JC, Liddell FDK, Gibbs GW et al. Dust exposure and mortality in chrysotile mining 1910–1975. *Br J Ind Med* 1980;37:11–24.) Many felt reassured by this large 1958 study, in spite of its many deficiencies, as elucidated by Thomas F Mancuso in 1965. (Mancuso T. Comments at biological effects of asbestos. *Ann NY Acad Sci* 1965;132:589–94.)

Other scientists were reassured by the paper by Bohlig and Jacob in 1956, who reported their experiences with asbestos workers in Dresden, Germany, where they found no increases in lung cancer. A later report in 1965 by the same authors did find an increased incidence of lung cancer associated with asbestosis. (Bohlig H, Jacob G. Neue Gesichtpunke Uber den Lungenkrebs der Asbestarbeiter. *Deutsche Med Wehnschr* 1956;81:231; Jacob G, Anspach M. Pulmonary neoplasia among Dresden asbestos workers. *Ann NY Acad Sci* 1965;132:536–47.)

It was Sir Richard Doll who was the first British researcher to study asbestos textile workers in a specific plant in Great Britain, where a combination of crocidolite and chrysotile asbestos had been used, and noted a tenfold increased risk of lung cancer in those former workers who had asbestosis. There were two cases of pleural tumors, presumably mesotheliomas, which were ignored, since no association between asbestos exposure and mesothelioma had been made in the general scientific community in 1955. (Doll R. Mortality from lung cancer in asbestos workers. *Br J Ind Med* 1955;12:81–6.) Ironically, this study was not controlled for cigarette smoking by the very author of the classic paper in 1954 about cigarette smoking and cancer in British physicians. A review of the world's literature by Doll in 1953 does not mention asbestos as a lung carcinogen. (Doll R. Bronchial carcinoma: Incidence and aetiology. *Br Med J* 1953;2:521–7.) Generally, experts felt that this study suggested that employment in a specific plant in Great Britain, where there were very heavy exposures to crocidolite amphibole asbestos prior to 1933, was associated with an increased incidence of lung cancer associated with asbestosis. The author mentions that it was thought that after the exposure levels were reduced on January 1, 1933 by regulation, further cases of significant asbestosis and asbestos-related lung cancer would not develop. Knox analyzed the same group of workers that were studied by Doll, and his data were published in the *Annals of the New York Academy of Sciences* in 1965. Knox's paper was summarized in an editorial *The Lancet* on March 5, 1966 as follows:

A follow-up of this same factory after 1933 now shows that vigorous action taken then and later to reduce dust levels has been largely successful in eliminating the hazard, though a further period of observation is necessary before complete success can be claimed.

It was the seminal work of Irving Selikoff, who studied a large population of United States and Canadian asbestos insulators, in which the magnitude of the risk of lung cancer in these workers became apparent. (Selikoff IJ, Churg J, Hammond EC. Asbestos exposure and neoplasia. *JAMA* 1964;188:22–6.) The increased incidence of lung cancer and asbestosis was very much related to latency. There was no significant increase in lung cancer prior to 15 years after exposure in these asbestos insulation workers, and most of the increased risk was observed 25–35 years after the first exposure. The increased incidence of lung cancer tracked well with the increased incidence of asbestosis. (Selikoff IJ, Seidman H. Asbestos-associated deaths among insulation workers in the United States and Canada, 1967–1987. *Ann NY Acad Sci* 1991;643:1–14.)

Prior to Selikoff's study on asbestos insulators, the scientific community remained skeptical about the relationship between asbestosis and lung cancer. Cordova et al. from Seattle stated in 1962, "There now exists considerable data to suspect the contention that pulmonary asbestosis has a definite role in the development of neoplastic change in the respiratory system. None of the agents studied have been clearly implicated except uranium." (Cordova JF, Tesluk H, Knutson KP. Asbestosis and carcinoma of the lung. *Cancer* 1962;15:1181–7.)

The U.S. Department of Health, Education, and Welfare published a reference text in 1964 on recognizing occupational diseases. This reference book for physicians and industrial hygienists discussed the Doll epidemiology study on lung cancer that had been issued 6 years earlier in 1955, and noted that following the publication of that study, there was some skepticism about the validity of Doll's conclusions. Specifically, the guide stated, "Conflicting opinions and differences in reports make it difficult to confirm or deny conclusively a causal relationship between asbestosis and cancer of the lung or extrapulmonary tissue. However, there is increasing evidence to suggest that such a relationship exists." (Gafafer WM. *Occupational Diseases. A Guide to their Recognition*. Washington, DC: U.S. Government Printing Office, 1964, p. 52).

Much more work had to be done before the world would be convinced of the adverse health effects from asbestos. Drs. Selikoff, Churg, and Hammond noted in their article, "Nevertheless, some investigators have held that while these observations might be suggestive, they do not establish an increased incidence of carcinoma of the lung in pulmonary asbestosis, and further the association was unproved." (Selikoff IJ, Churg J, Hammond EC. Asbestos exposure and neoplasia. *JAMA* 1964;188:22–6.) Basically, it was unproven until the seminal studies of Dr. Selikoff and the reports of others at the New York Academy of Sciences.

Dr. Selikoff goes on to summarize the literature and explain about the lack of interest in the study of Dr. Doll in Great Britain on the association between lung cancer and asbestosis. Selikoff went on to publish an article in *The Environment* in 1969;11:2–7, where on page 1 he states,

> Thus Kenneth Lynch reported a death from lung cancer in association with asbestosis in 1935, and several similar reports of this association between these two uncommon diseases followed. For the most part, however, these reports were categorized as biological curiosities. Even the careful studies of Richard Doll reported in 1955 failed to disturb our calm, perhaps because of the reticence with which the statistician summarized his findings. Listing 18 deaths due to lung cancer and 105 consecutive postmortem examinations at one asbestos works in England, he concluded, "...lung cancer was a specific industrial hazard of certain asbestos workers..." Even those who accepted Doll's conclusions—and there were some who did not – could point to a problem with a rather narrow spectrum. A single neoplasm (lung cancer) was (past tense) a specific industrial hazard (no hint that it could be more than this) of certain asbestos workers (the heavily exposed individuals in this factory).

In 1968, Dr. Selikoff published further studies on the asbestos workers that he and Dr. Hammond followed, and his conclusion was that cigarette smoking was present in all those individuals who developed lung cancer. If individuals, who were asbestos workers, could avoid cigarette smoking, they would not develop lung cancer, as noted in his publication in the *JAMA* in 1968. (Selikoff I, Hammond EC, Churg J. Asbestos exposure, smoking and neoplasia. *JAMA* 1968;204:1104–9.)

The issue of who was responsible for the lag in the identification of the health risk from exposure has gone to physicians, industry, and labor unions, and this issue was summarized by Dr. Selikoff in *Industrial Medicine* 1970;39:21–25. In this article, Dr. Selikoff states:

> It is too easy to indulge in what may be called the demonological theory of industrial hygiene history. One version would place the responsibility for early identification of risk and its correction upon industry and then indict it for trading human health for profits. Similarly, the other side of the counterfeit coin puts the blame on organized labor for having been more interested in premium pay for hazardous work than in eliminating known hazards. Both conclusions are too convenient and are essentially erroneous. It is much nearer the truth to say that both industry and labor shared in ignorance and neglect of the problem. Science and medicine are also at fault here for inadequate attention to environmental and occupational health. In retrospect, however, it is possible to see why the recognition was so long in coming. We know now that it

may take 20 to 30 or more years from onset of exposure before the effects of this particular hazard begins to manifest themselves in the morbidity and mortality of the workers.

The initial epidemiologic studies by Selikoff suggested that asbestos was a cocarcinogen rather than a primary complete carcinogen in that it appeared that only smokers developed lung cancer. (Selikoff IL, Hammond EC, Churg J. Asbestos exposure, smoking, and neoplasia. *JAMA* 1968;204:106–12.) Further studies indicated that asbestos was a complete carcinogen and could produce lung cancer in nonsmokers with asbestosis. (Hammond EC, Selikoff IJ, Seidman H. Asbestos exposure, cigarette smoking and death rates. *Ann NY Acad Sci* 1979;330:473–90.)

Crocidolite asbestos was used in the manufacture of cigarette filters between 1951 and 1957. The contribution to the risk of mesothelioma in smokers of KOOL cigarettes is unclear. Talcott studied a cohort of 33 men who worked in a Massachusetts factory that manufactured KOOL cigarette filters containing crocidolite fibers from 1951 to 1957. Twenty-eight of the men had died, as compared with the 8.3 deaths expected. This increased mortality was attributable to asbestos-associated diseases. Fifteen deaths were caused by cancer, as compared with the 1.8 expected (relative risk: 8.2; 95% confidence interval: 4.6–13.4), including eight from lung cancer, five from malignant mesothelioma, and two from other types of cancer. There were seven deaths from nonmalignant respiratory disease, as compared with the 0.5 expected (relative risk: 14.7; 95% confidence interval: 5.9–30.3), of which five were due primarily to asbestosis. In contrast, the mortality rates from cardiovascular diseases and all other causes were not increased. Four of the five living workers had pulmonary asbestosis; three of them had recently diagnosed cancers, including two additional lung cancers. The authors concluded that the extremely high morbidity and mortality rates in these workers were caused by intense exposure to crocidolite asbestos fibers. (Talcott JA, Thurber WA, Kantor AF et al. Asbestos-associated diseases in a cohort of cigarette-filter workers. *N Engl J Med* 1989;321(18):1220–3.)

Originally, based on a report by Whitwell et al., physicians believed that asbestos-related lung cancers developed in areas of lung fibrosis or usually in the lower lobes in patients with asbestosis, the thought being that asbestosis causes lung inflammation that, in turn, causes scar cancers or adenocarcinomas due to chronic inflammation. The normal ratio of nonasbestosis-caused lung cancer of the upper lobe to the lower lobe was 2 to 1 and thought to be reversed in asbestosis. (Whitwell F, Newhouse ML, Bennett DR. A study of the histological cell types of lung cancer in workers suffering from asbestosis in the United Kingdom. *Br J Ind Med* 1974;31(4):298–303.) Several later studies have confirmed that this hypothesis was not true, and that the distribution of lung cancers between the upper and lower lobes was not different than that found in the general population of nonasbestos-exposed smokers as to tumor type and tumor site being predominately in the upper lobes in individuals with asbestosis. (Karjalainen A, Anttila S, Heikkilä L et al. Lobe of origin of lung cancer among asbestos-exposed patients with or without diffuse interstitial fibrosis. *Scand J Work Environ Health*

1993;19(2):102–7; Churg A. Lung cancer cell type and asbestos exposure. *JAMA* 1985;253(20):2984–5; Mossman BT, Craighead JE. Mechanisms of asbestos associated bronchogenic cancer. In: K Antman, J Aisner (Eds.), *Asbestos-Related Malignancy*. Orlando: Grune & Stratton, 1987, pp. 137–150.)

ASBESTOS AND ANIMAL STUDIES

Our understanding of cancer pathogenesis has traditionally been based on animal studies. The lack of animal confirmation of asbestos exposure and production of cancer was always a problem for scientists and delayed the recognition of the carcinogenic potential of asbestos. Dr. LeRoy Gardner at the Saranac Laboratory in New York State did early studies in 1931 on animals but did not initially find any relationship between asbestos exposure and lung cancer. Nordmann and Sorge in Germany reported an association between asbestosis and lung cancer in a small study published in a German medical journal in 1941. Later studies were submitted to the Johns Manville Corporation in 1943 by Dr. Gardner, which were possibly suggestive of a relationship between asbestos exposure and lung cancer in animals. Some pundits have suggested that Dr. Gardner was refused further financing because of pressure by asbestos industry advocates. There is no foundation for this speculation. No larger studies were performed as requested by Dr. Gardner. However, mice have been shown to be largely unsuitable for asbestos cancer research because of the high incidence of spontaneous tumors in mice. Arthur Vorwald continued to work at the Saranac Laboratories, and in 1951, concluded that long fibers greater 20 μm in length were primarily responsible for asbestosis. He also concluded that the irritant and not chemical properties of asbestos dust were responsible for the fibrotic reaction of asbestosis, but reached no conclusion about asbestos exposure and lung cancer.

Schepers, Duran, and Delahant carried on the work of Gardner and Vorwald at the Saranac Research Laboratory with a mixture of calcium silicate mixed with approximately 15% chrysotile asbestos. They used guinea pigs, rats, and hamsters, exposing these animals to high concentrations of the mixture of 100–125 million particles of asbestos dust per cubic feet (mppcf) for 8 hours a day for up to 36 months. The animals developed terminal peri-bronchiolar focal fibrosis, chronic bronchitis, bronchiectasia, and epithelialization of atelectatic alveoli, but no lung cancers or mesotheliomas were found. (Schepers GWH, Durkan TM, Delahant AB. Effect of inhaled commercial hydrous calcium silicate dust on animal tissues. *AMA Arch Ind Health* 1955;12:348–60.)

Lynch did a larger study in mice in 1957 and the study was again uninterruptable because of the high incidence of spontaneous cancers in both the study and control groups. The study by Lynch in 1957 was similar to Leroy Gardner's animal studies in 1943, and exculpates Dr. Gardner from any false claim that he held back any information from his earlier animal studies on asbestos exposure and lung cancer. Cancers in mice are largely spontaneous adenomas, which are not thought to be malignant and occur randomly in mice. (Lynch KM, McIver FA, Cain JR. Pulmonary tumors in mice exposed to asbestos dust. *Arch Ind Health* 1957;15:207–14.)

It was not until 1967 that Gross et al. reported an association between asbestos exposure and lung cancer in white rats. (Gross P, DeTreville R, Tolker E et al. Experimental asbestosis. *Arch Environ Health* 1967;15:343–55.) Davis in 1979 concluded that mice were not suitable for studying the fiber effects of asbestos. Various investigators have exposed guinea pigs, rabbits, cats, dogs, monkeys, and other species to asbestos, and have found that the rat appears to be the best model for research on the carcinogenicity of asbestos. Animal models have not been able to demonstrate lung cancers without asbestosis. (Davis JM. The use of animal models for studies on asbestos bioeffects. *Ann NY Acad Sci* 1979;330:795–8.)

The first report of pleural mesotheliomas in animals was by JC Wagner in the journal *Nature* in 1962, who inoculated asbestos dust into the pleural cavity of rats. (Wagner JC. Experimental production of mesothelial tumours of the pleura by implantation of dusts in laboratory animals. *Nature* 1962;196:180–1.) Previous inhalation studies in animals had been unsuccessful in producing mesotheliomas. Earlier reports of dust exposure by inhalation in 1965 showed the production of lung fibrosis but no mesotheliomas. However, when Wagner switched to pathogen-free healthy rats with a much longer life expectancy, mesotheliomas could be produced in greater quantities and consistencies. Inhalation studies of asbestos fiber exposure in rats were not successful in producing mesotheliomas until 1973. Wagner also used intratracheal administration to produce malignancies, but the technique was never standardized, making it difficult to analyze comparative studies from other researchers. Later, German scientists used the intraperitoneal model of asbestos injection into the abdominal cavity of rats, popularized by Pott. (Pott F, Roller M, Rippe RM et al. Tumors by the intraperitoneal and intrapleural routes and their significance for the classification of mineral fibers. In: *Mechanisms of Fiber Carcinogeneisis*. New York: Plenum Press, 1991, pp. 547–65.) This method of Pott in producing mesotheliomas from all asbestos fiber types is very sensitive but controversial, since the intraperitoneal methodology does not always correlate with the traditional intrapleural or inhalational studies. The test is so sensitive that Pott required a tumor response of 10% and even the saline control occasionally produced positive results. (Bernstein D, Dunnigan J, Hesterberg T et al. Health risk of chrysotile revisited. *Crit Rev Toxicol* 2013;43(2):154–83.) Furthermore, the dose of asbestos fibers used in these experiments in animals was many magnitudes greater than that found in human exposures. This type of experimental asbestos bolus dose overwhelms the normal physiologic defenses of the experimental animal, allowing for a much higher dose of fibers to remain in the pleural or peritoneal space. Unfortunately, because asbestos fibers are so small, it has not been possible to perform experimental studies with small doses of asbestos that would produce dose–response information. The very high doses of asbestos fibers used in animal studies makes extrapolation from chronic animal inhalation studies difficult for comparing with human epidemiologic studies. Animals such as the rat and guinea pig have very short life expectancies and different lung anatomies, which produces bias in inhalation studies, particularly with chrysotile asbestos because of its high solubility, rapid dissolution, and low bio-persistence in humans. No chronic inhalation studies using chrysotile asbestos with fiber selection techniques have ever been performed. (Hesterberg TW, Hart GA, Chevalier J et al. The importance of fiber biopersistence and lung dose in determining the chronic inhalation effects of X607, RCF1, and chrysotile asbestos in rats. *Toxicol Appl Pharmacol* 1998;153(1):68–82; Mossman BT, Lippmann M, Hesterberg TW et al. Pulmonary endpoints (lung carcinomas and asbestosis) following inhalation exposure to asbestos. *Toxicol Environ Health B Crit Rev* 2011;14(1–4):76–121.)

Geoffrey Berry, an international expert on asbestos, stated in 1999 related to animal studies that

The health effects of inhaled fibers are related to the intensity and duration of exposure and occur many years after the exposure. In particular, the incidence of mesothelioma after exposure to asbestos is proportional to the intensity of exposure (fibers per milliliter of air) and the duration of exposure, and to the time that has elapsed since the exposure. The incidence increases with time since exposure to a power of between 3 and 4. The disease process resulting from exposure to fibers in the air is presumably related to the dose of fibers in the lungs, which depends on the exposure level and duration, and also on the size characteristics of the fibers influencing their inhalation and retention in the lungs. Models incorporating these characteristics have been found to be satisfactory in explaining the incidence of mesothelioma over time after exposure to asbestos. Most of the epidemiological modeling has been for occupational exposure to one of the amphibole asbestos types (crocidolite or amosite), for which heavy exposure produces a high incidence of mesothelioma. Occupational exposure to chrysotile asbestos has resulted in a much lower incidence of mesothelioma. Crocidolite asbestos is much more biopersistent than chrysotile asbestos in the sense that after retention in the lungs it is eliminated only slowly (half-time of several years). If fibers are eliminated then the dose in the lungs declines following exposure, and this may influence the disease process. This concept is more important for synthetic mineral fibers, such as glass wool, which are used as a substitute for asbestos. These fibers are much less biopersistent than asbestos, with half-times of weeks or even days. Biopersistence is related to the dissolution of fibers. This is a physical-chemical process that may be expected to proceed at about the same rate in rats and humans. The predicted effect of biopersistence of fibers has been explored using the basic mesothelioma incidence model generalized to include a term representing exponential elimination over time. The influence of solubility of fibers on the mesothelioma rate is 17 times higher in humans than in rats. This is because rats are aging and developing cancer at a much quicker rate than humans, and hence the influence of dissolution is less. Thus, the predicted mesothelioma incidence in humans is highly dependent on the rate of elimination across the range covering asbestos and the more durable synthetic fibers, but in rats a similar dependence occurs at a 17 times higher rate of elimination corresponding to the less durable synthetic fibers. The possible carcinogenic effects of fibers are often determined from animal experiments, but these results suggest that the extrapolation from rats to humans is highly dependent on the biopersistence of fibers, in the situation where the elimination is through dissolution of fibers at a rate independent of species and the speed of the cancer process is species dependent. This implies that relatively soluble fibers that do not produce disease in rat experiments are even less likely to produce disease in humans. (Berry G. Models for mesothelioma incidence following exposure to fibers in terms of timing and duration of exposure and the biopersistence of the fibers. *Inhal Toxicol* 1999;11(2):111–30.)

PATHOPHYSIOLOGY

Early studies of asbestosis cases reported increased numbers of adenocarcinomas in the lower lobes, which were thought to be scar carcinomas. The distribution of histologic cell types of lung cancer related to asbestos exposure appears to be the same histologically as lung cancer caused by cigarette smoking, radiation, or chemical carcinogens. (Churg A. Lung cancer cell type and asbestos exposure *JAMA* 1985;253:2984–85; Mollo F, Piglatto G, Bellis D et al. Asbestos exposure and histologic cell types of lung cancer in surgical and autopsy series. *Int J Cancer* 1990;46:576–80.)

The latency period for lung cancer is generally 20–30 years. Lung cancer begins in the lung parenchyma and invades locally, often blocking airways and eroding into blood vessels, leading to hemoptysis. Metastatic spread also occurs throughout the lung and to other parts of the body, especially to the spine or brain.

The reasons that combined exposure to asbestos and cigarette smoking greatly increase the risk for lung cancer are not clear. Smoking itself is the most common cause of lung cancer. Cigarette smoke also inhibits ciliary function in the lung epithelium, inhibiting clearance of asbestos from the lung and possibly increasing the risk of lung cancer from asbestos.

In the period during and after World War II, when many U.S. workers had their heaviest asbestos exposures, the prevalence of cigarette smoking among blue-collar workers was about 80%. Since lung cancer caused by asbestos and lung cancer from cigarette smoking look the same histologically, attribution of the cause of lung cancer is often a contentious issue in litigation in the United States. In Germany and the United Kingdom, lung cancer is legally attributed to asbestos if asbestosis is also present.

The German physicians were the first to establish a relationship between lung cancer and asbestosis in the early 1940s. The world scientific community did not generally accept this association between asbestosis and lung cancer until a retrospective cohort epidemiologic study was published by Dr. Doll in 1955 about the observations made in an asbestos textile factory in England, where they found a tenfold increased risk of lung cancer in those with asbestosis. His conclusion was that further cases of asbestosis and lung cancer were unlikely to appear in those individuals that began work after the safety regulations of 1933 were instituted to reduce exposure to asbestos. Based on these other studies, it was generally thought by the scientific community that if you could protect workers from asbestosis, you would protect them from lung cancer. This was the basis of the British occupational hygiene standard for asbestos in 1968.

The recognition by the general medical community that all forms of asbestos exposure with asbestosis may cause lung cancer occurred after the publication of the seminal work of Selikoff in 1965, 1968, and 1972. Studies by Wagner in South Africa and others in Great Britain in the 1960s suggested that exposure to crocidolite asbestos was strongly and almost exclusively associated with the development of mesotheliomas. Amosite was also incriminated as a cause of mesotheliomas in 1972. (Selikoff I, Hammond E, Churg J. Carcinogenicity of amosite asbestos. *Arch Environ Health* 1972;25:183–86; Seidman H, Selikoff IJ, Gelb SK. Mortality experience of amosite asbestos factory workers: Dose–response relationships 5–40 years after onset of short-term exposure. *Am J Ind Med* 1986;10:479–514.) It is now generally recognized that the majority of mesotheliomas are due to amphibole exposures. All forms of asbestos cause lung cancer, but amphibole asbestos is much more carcinogenic than chrysotile asbestos.

Determining the mechanisms of asbestos-related carcinogenesis has been the source of extensive research over the last 30 years. The role of different mechanisms of asbestos-related cell injury and tumor initiation is still unresolved. Asbestos fibers may effect tumor formation either through indirect mechanisms (e.g., formation of active oxygen species or growth factors) or by the fibers causing direct interference with cell division.

Asbestos is unique among the carcinogens in that most mutagens are genotoxic and cause abnormalities or evidence of DNA damage when assayed by the Ames test. Asbestos is not mutagenic in the Ames test, but is genotoxic when using a sensitive human–hamster hybrid cell. It is now recognized that asbestos fibers cause point mutations and large deletions of chromosomes in normal cells. Recent studies using high-resolution time-lapse microscopy have demonstrated that long asbestos fibers interfere with chromosome distribution during cell division, causing genomic changes such as chromosomal deletions, translocations, and aneuploidy. These genomic changes lead to cell transformation and neoplastic progression. These types of chromosomal changes have been found in asbestos-related mesotheliomas and lung cancers. (Mossman BT, Shukla A, Heintz NH et al. New insights into understanding the mechanisms, pathogenesis, and management of malignant mesotheliomas. *Am J Pathol* 2013;182(4):1065–77.)

Asbestos as a carcinogen has been associated with lengthy latency periods from initial exposure to the development of cancer. Asbestos, like a variety of other carcinogens, causes genetic changes in the cell that occur over a long period of time. A series of oncogenic mutations must occur before the actual tumor develops. The greater number of mutations required, or the length of time required to produce these mutations, explains the long latency period from exposure to asbestos to the development of an asbestos-related neoplasm. The long latency time from first exposure to development of asbestos-related malignancy was the cause of early underestimations of the risk of asbestos exposure and later development of malignancy (see Figure 6.1). (Richardson DB, Cole SR, Chu H et al. Lagging exposure information in cumulative exposure–response analysis. *Am J Epidemiol* 2011;174:1416–22.)

Asbestos fibers are taken up by inflammatory cells such as pulmonary macrophages in the lung, and these inflammatory cells in turn release cytokines as well as active oxygen species, which in turn produce DNA alterations. The chronic production of transforming growth factor, insulin-like growth factor II, and other cytokines such as platelet-derived growth factor, are responsible for recruitment of inflammatory cells. Mesothelial cells may produce these cytokines by an autocrine loop, which in turn perpetuates the inflammatory response. Asbestos-induced cell proliferation in both epithelial cells and mesothelial cells via growth factors is important to tumor cell initiation, promotion, and progression. This may be a secondary effect of active oxygen species generation, or there may other effects of cytokines themselves on mutagenesis and genetic changes in cells. This is an area of current research. The pro-inflammatory molecule HMGB-1 seems to be the master switch that starts the inflammatory process. Genetic predisposition and viral infections such as simian virus 40 as well as radiation are important co-factors. (Carbone M, Bevan Hl, Dodson RF et al. Malignant mesothelioma: Facts, myths and hypotheses. *J Cell Physiol* 2012;227:44–58.)

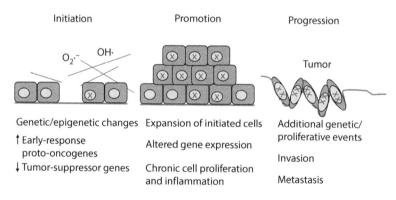

Figure 6.1 Multistage carcinogenesis. The latency period of mesotheliomas is protracted (an average of >40 years since initial exposures to amphibole asbestos) and consists of three phases. Initiation may involve chromosomal (genetic) changes yet to be defined or, more likely, epigenetic changes, most likely perpetuated by reactive oxygen species and inflammation. Increases in expression of early-response proto-oncogenes of the Fos/Jun family and decreases in several tumor-suppressor genes have been observed in some mesotheliomas. Promotion is characterized by expansion of initiated cells through proliferation and inflammation, and progression may entail additional genetic and proliferative events. These three phases of tumor development are integral to the formation of a variety of tumor types. (Courtesy of Brooke Mossman, PhD. With permission.)

Asbestos is primarily a cytotoxin, meaning that it causes changes in the genetic make-up of a cell via chronic inflammation. Another purported mechanism of cell and genome damage is thought to be related to the propensity of long asbestos fibers to invoke a chronic inflammatory reaction, which in turn evokes the recruitment of cell-damaging cytokines and inflammatory products. A variety of investigators have noted that active oxygen species are produced when asbestos is placed in a medium with cultured lymphocytes. This is the third method of asbestos-related cell damage. The critical target molecule for reactive oxygen species is DNA. A variety of anti-toxic enzymes such as superoxide dismutase inhibit asbestos-related cytotoxicity. Free iron catalyzes the formation of the highly toxic hydroxyl radical (OH) from superoxide anion (O_2^-) and hydrogen peroxide (H_2O_2) through the Haber–Weiss reaction. Only minute quantities of free iron are necessary for catalytic enhancement of this reaction. Iron chelation inhibits the formation of free radicals in cell culture, and indicates that iron seems to be a critical and necessary cofactor in asbestos-induced cytotoxicity, liquid preoccupation, and DNA breakage. (Mossman BT, Shukla A, Heintz NH et al. New insights into understanding the mechanisms, pathogenesis, and management of malignant mesotheliomas. *Am J Pathol* 2013;182(4):1065–77.)

Morimoto and Japanese coworkers studied the use of nanoparticles in producing inflammation and the effects of inflammation on potential carcinogenesis. Pulmonary inflammation, especially persistent inflammation, has been found to play a key role in respiratory disorders induced by nanoparticles in animal models.

In inhalation studies and instillation studies of nanomaterials, persistent inflammation is composed of neutrophils and alveolar macrophages, and its pathogenesis is related to chemokines such as the cytokine-induced neutrophil chemoattractant (CINC) family and macrophage inflammatory protein-1α and oxidant stress-related genes such as heme oxygenase-1. DNA damages occur chemically or physically by nanomaterials. Chemical and physical damage are associated with point mutation by free radicals and double strand brake, respectively. The failure of DNA repair and accumulation of mutations might occur when inflammation is prolonged, and finally normal cells could become malignant. These free radicals can not only damage cells but also induce signaling molecules containing immunoreaction. Nanoparticles and asbestos also induce the production of free radicals. (Morimoto Y, Izumi H, Kuroda E. Significance of persistent inflammation in respiratory disorders induced by nanoparticles. *J Immunol Res* 2014;2014:962871.)

Chrysotile asbestos contains relatively little iron, approximately 2%–3% in the average sample, whereas crocidolite asbestos, which is generally considered the most carcinogenic form of asbestos, has up to 36% iron by weight. It has been reported that individuals that consume excessive amounts of iron have an increased risk of cancer. Iron appears to be toxic and when asbestos fibers are phagocytized there may be abnormal release of iron not controlled by the proteins involved in normal iron metabolism. Asbestos-related pulmonary toxicity appears to be initiated by reactive oxygen species generated from mobilized iron via the Haber–Weiss reaction, as mentioned above. Epidermal growth factor is a trans-membrane protein that is involved in cell injury from both inhibition of apoptosis and increased cell proliferation. The administration of the antioxidant enzyme catalase to rats during inhalation of asbestos fibers can ameliorate inflammation, lung damage, and pulmonary fibrosis or asbestosis in part related to inactivation of epidermal growth factor. It seems plausible that asbestos fiber iron content relates to its carcinogenicity. In fact, the evidence that asbestos-related cytotoxicity is inhibited by anti-toxin enzymes and iron chelation by desferrioxamine, indicates a strong biological contribution of active oxygen species, and the secondary role of iron content in asbestos fibers in its toxic effects, which may have future clinical implications. (Baldys A, Aust A. Role of iron in inactivation of epidermal growth factor after asbestos treatment of human lung and pleural target cells. *Am J Respir Cell Mol Biol* 2005;32:436–42.)

The majority of studies on asbestos-related cytotoxicity have been done with models of human or animal mesothelial cells in culture. Bronchial epithelial cells seem to be more resistant to the genotoxic and cytotoxic effects of asbestos. This correlates with clinical epidemiologic studies, which have shown a relatively low incidence of asbestos-related lung cancers in heavily exposed nonsmokers with asbestosis. Asbestos acts primarily as a cocarcinogen and promoter, and while cigarette smoke is the primary cocarcinogen with asbestos, there is very little information as to the role of other cocarcinogens in the workplace in the induction of asbestos-related lung cancers. It is quite likely that a variety of other carcinogens, such as radon, may play an important role in the induction of asbestos-related lung cancers.

The dose required for the production of an asbestos-related lung cancer must be high enough to produce asbestosis since asbestos-related lung cancers are not seen in most clinical studies unless there is coexistent asbestosis. This is also true of animal models. Animal inhalation studies demonstrate that the threshold dose of asbestos for causing lung cancer is related to the dose of asbestos necessary to produce asbestosis. (Ilgren EB, Browne K. Asbestos-related mesothelioma: Evidence for a threshold in animals and humans. *Regul Toxicol Pharmacol* 1991;13:116–32; Ilgren EB, Browne K. Background incidence of mesothelioma: Animal and human evidence. *Regul Toxicol Pharmacol* 1991;13:133–49.) Thus, there seems to be a threshold dose for lung cancer and that threshold dose is the dose above which asbestosis is likely to develop. A variety of clinical pathological studies have confirmed that the risk of lung cancer is only elevated when asbestosis is present.

Murphy and others studied shipyard workers and reported in 1971 that asbestosis was not evident until an estimated exposure was 60 mppcf/years of total dust (not asbestos dust), which is roughly equivalent to a total dust exposure of 360 fibers/cc/years, if 1 mppcf = 6 fibers/cc. (Murphy RL, Ferris BG, Burgess WA, Worcester J, Gaensler EA. Effects of low concentrations of asbestos— Clinical, radiologic, and epidemiologic observations in shipyard pipe covers and controls. *N Engl J Med* 1971;285:1271–8.) Wells also began to see asbestosis at the same level. (Wells J. Biological effects of asbestos: Section V human exposure to asbestos: Dust controls and standards: Discussion. *Ann NY Acad Sci* 1965;132:335–6.) Fulton reported 17% prevalence of asbestosis after an exposure to 27–75 mppcf/years or 162–450 fibers/cc/years. (Fulton WB, Dooley A et al. *Asbestosis. Part II, III, Bulletin 42*. Harrisburg: Pennsylvania Department of Labor and Industry, 1935.)

In summary, reactive oxygen species are generated by long thin asbestos fiber–cell interactions, which in turn activate a host of kinases, transcription factors, and cytokines that up-regulate and down-regulate a variety of genes involved in inflammation, fibrosis, and malignant transformation. (Mossman BT, Lippmann M, Hesterberg TW et al. Pulmonary endpoints (lung carcinomas and asbestosis) following inhalation exposure to asbestos. *Toxicol Environ Health B Crit Rev* 2011;14(1–4):76–121.)

THE HELSINKI CRITERIA

In 1997, a group of self-selected experts, many of whom were plaintiffs' litigation experts, met in Helsinki, Finland, to discuss two major issues. There were 19 participants from eight countries covering seven to nine disciplines. Their first opinion was on the attribution of lung cancer to asbestos exposure and the second opinion was related to mesothelioma causation from both chrysotile and amphibole asbestos and the minimum dose of asbestos required for mesothelioma causation. (Anon. Asbestos, asbestosis, and cancer: The Helsinki criteria for diagnosis and attribution. *Scand J Work Environ Health* 1997;23(4):311–6.) The Helsinki statement created significant controversy since the selected expert panel did not include any conservative or defense-oriented litigation experts or reflect their opinions. The views of this group did not reflect or represent the opinions of the general scientific community as a whole. The Helsinki criteria were revaluated in 2014 with new recommendations. (Wolff H, Vehmas T, Oksa P, Rantanen J, Vainio H. Asbestos, asbestosis, and cancer, the Helsinki criteria for diagnosis and attribution 2014: Recommendations. *Scand J Work Environ Health* 2015;41(1):5–15.)

In 2009, using the Delphi technique, the American College of Physicians Committee on Asbestos attempted to obtain a global representation of scientific opinion by surveying those scientists who have published papers regarding asbestos health effects. (Gibbs A, Attanoos RL, Churg A et al. The "Helsinki criteria" for attribution of lung cancer to asbestos exposure: How robust are the criteria? *Arch Pathol Lab Med* 2007;131(2):181–3; Banks DE, Shi R, McLarty J et al. American College of Chest Physicians consensus statement on the respiratory health effects of asbestos: Results of a Delphi study. *Chest* 2009;135:1619–27. Available at http://www.sh.lsuhsc.edu/medicine/delphi.)

The Australian Dust Diseases Board met in November 2001 to provide an evaluation of the exposure criteria and lung fiber burden associated with the Helsinki criteria and its applicability to Australia. The problems elucidated by the Australian Dust Diseases Board included the following in their executive summary:

1. The attribution value of 25 fibers/cc-years cumulative exposure leading to a doubling of lung cancer risk appears to be derived from some of the data from epidemiological studies conducted in the U.S. textile industries. A value of 100–200 fiber/cc-years appears to be more applicable.
2. The basis of evaluation of cumulative exposure using the 90th percentile exposure data that are used in Germany and by Helsinki recommendations results in an overestimate of exposure levels.
3. The value of 1 million amphibole fibers (>5 μm) per gram of dry lung tissue was not particularly useful in application to Australian conditions. This criterion is based on a single study by Karjalainen in Finland. This small study with low statistical power lacks the scientific basis for generalization for a criteria statement. (Karjalainen A, Anttila S, Vanhala E, Vainio H. Asbestos exposure and the risk of lung cancer in a general urban population. *Scand J Work Environ Health* 1994;20(4):243–50.)
4. An occupational history of 1 year of heavy exposure to asbestos is required as a minimal standard (manufacture of asbestos products, asbestos spraying, and insulation work with asbestos materials) or 5–10 years of moderate exposure (construction or shipbuilding). The problem with this criterion is that estimates of exposure from German accident insurance measurements of exposure used in this criterion are not consistent with epidemiologic studies. Worker estimates of exposure are not reliable.

The Helsinki criterion for the attribution of asbestos exposure to the causation of lung cancer is a cumulative exposure to asbestos of 25 fibers/mL-years (1 fiber/cc for 1 year = 1 fiber/mL-year). The expert panel felt that an exposure of 25 fiber/mL-years was sufficient to double the risk of lung cancer, or a history of 1 year of heavy exposure to asbestos, such as asbestos manufacturing, asbestos spraying, or insulation work, or 5–10 years of moderate exposure, such as in construction and shipbuilding. This cumulative exposure is equivalent to 5000–15,000 asbestos bodies per gram of dry lung tissue or 500–1500 asbestos bodies per gram of wet lung tissue, a lung fiber count of $>2 \times 10^3$ amphibole fibers of 5 μm or longer per gram of dry lung tissue. A level of 100 asbestos bodies per gram of wet lung tissue was thought to be sufficient to indicate occupational exposure. No distinction was made based on fiber type, size, or length. Chrysotile was considered to be just as carcinogenic as crocidolite! No distinction was made between the source of chrysotile exposure and risk. This means that chrysotile exposure from wallboard or brake dust is considered to be just as risky as exposure to long chrysotile fibers from a textile mill. There are no data to support this conclusion.

Any proposal that suggests risk estimates from asbestos exposure that does not take into account fiber type, fiber size, fiber length, and source of exposure is not consistent with current scientific knowledge of fiber toxicology and asbestos epidemiological studies that are discussed elsewise in this book. The Helsinki criteria are based on speculation that lung fiber counts and industrial hygiene estimates of exposure are reasonable surrogates of an asbestos exposure adequate to produce asbestosis. There is a very large variation between individuals in the susceptibility to asbestosis from asbestos exposure. In spite of heavy exposure, the vast majority of asbestos insulation workers do not develop asbestosis or lung cancer. Irving Selikoff and coworkers studied the deaths from a cohort of 17,800 asbestos insulation workers from January 1, 1967 to December 31, 1976 and observed 2271 deaths in this heavily exposed cohort with 1659 deaths expected, of which only 168 were due to asbestosis and 486 were due to lung cancer. Asbestosis must be present to be the causative agent for asbestos-related lung cancer, as was demonstrated by a later study of these insulators by Kipen et al., who found that 100% of these insulators with lung cancer had asbestosis. (Selikoff IJ, Hammond EC, Seidman H. Mortality experience of insulation workers in the United States and Canada 1943–1976. *Ann NY Acad Sci* 1979;330:91–116; Kipen H, Lilis R, Suzuki Y et al. Pulmonary fibrosis in asbestos insulation workers with lung cancer: A radiologic and histopathological evaluation. *Br J Ind Med* 1987;44:96–100; Henderson DW, Rödelsperger K, Woitowitz HJ et al. After Helsinki: A multidisciplinary review of the relationship between asbestos exposure and lung cancer, with emphasis on studies published during 1997–2004. *Pathology* 2004;36(6):517–50; Roggli VL, Hammar SP, Maddox JC et al. Re: The "Helsinki criteria" for attribution of lung cancer to asbestos exposure: How robust are the criteria? *Arch Pathol Lab Med* 2008;132(9):1386–7; Helsinki Criteria—Critique. In: JE Craighead, AR Gibbs. *Asbestos and its Diseases*, Oxford University Press, 2008, pp. 181–3.)

The London Pneumoconiosis Panel in 1987 reviewed 155 cases of asbestosis and found that 39% of the 59 deaths of these asbestosis cases died of lung cancer and 10% died of mesothelioma according to death certificates. Actually, lung cancer was present in 44% of the cases after careful review. The authors reviewed the chest x-rays and noted no increased mortality of those with 0 to 0/1 films. If the profusion score was >1/0, indicating clinical asbestosis, the mortality was increased for lung cancer. These data were similar to those from Liddell's study of Canadian miners and millers who also found that an International Labor Office (ILO) profusion score of >1/0 was associated with increased mortality and lung cancer. Most but not all of the Canadian cases had evidence of asbestosis, but there was often a long lag between their last chest x-ray and the diagnosis of lung cancer, which would explain why not all of their asbestos workers with lung cancer had evidence of radiologic asbestosis. (Coutts II, Gilson JC, Kerr JH et al. Mortality in cases of asbestosis diagnosed by a pneumoconiosis panel. *Thorax* 1987;42:111–6; Liddell FDS, McDonald JC. Radiological findings as predictors of mortality in Quebec asbestos workers. *Br J Ind Med* 1980;37:257–67.) This evidence is consistent with the results of a later prospective mortality study by Hughes and Weill. (Hughes JM, Weill H. Asbestosis related lung cancer: Results of a prospective mortality study. *Br J Ind Med* 1991;48:229–33.)

While some experts, such as the Helsinki group, contend that asbestos exposure of an amount that possibly was sufficient to cause asbestosis is a sufficient surrogate for actual subclinical pathological or radiological asbestosis, the data are lacking to support this hypothesis. This is scientific speculation or wishful thinking, but not science. A review of 34 asbestos cohort studies by Weiss revealed a direct correlation between the degree of asbestosis and lung cancer. The data in the medical literature indicate that asbestosis is a better predictor of excess lung cancer risk than estimates of asbestos exposure. (Weiss W. Asbestosis: A marker for the increased risk of lung cancer among workers exposed to asbestos. *Chest* 1999;115:536–49.)

All experts agree that some cases of pathologic asbestosis may be subclinical or not present on chest x-ray or high-resolution computerized tomography (HRCT) scanning. However, there are no data on quantifying the relative risk of lung cancer from subclinical asbestosis corrected for cigarette smoking. The only data available is the correlation of radiologic asbestosis, not subclinical asbestosis, with the incidence of lung cancer corrected for smoking. The presumption by some has been that subclinical asbestosis should also increase the risk of lung cancer, but subclinical asbestosis is often burnt-out disease with low levels of inflammation. Most experts agree that it is the intensity of inflammation and not the degree of fibrosis that is the critical factor in carcinogenesis.

Kevin Browne reviewed eight published cohort studies in which there was quantitation of asbestos exposure correlated with risk of lung cancer. He concluded that a threshold exposure is required to develop lung cancer. This is biologically plausible because of the ability of lung molecular repair mechanisms to suppress oncogenic development. The biologic defense mechanisms have to be overwhelmed before malignancy can develop. (Browne K. A threshold for asbestos related lung cancer. *Br J Ind Med* 1986;43:556–8; Browne K. Letter to the editor: The quantitative risks of mesothelioma and lung cancer in relation to asbestos exposure. *Ann Occup Hyg* 2001;45(4):327–438.)

Various epidemiologic studies have primarily demonstrated increased risk with radiologically identifiable x-ray changes of ILO 1/0 or greater. Oksa and coworkers reported that 11 out of 24 patients with progressive asbestosis developed lung cancer, but only five out of 54 patients with stable asbestosis developed lung cancer. (Oksa P, Klokars M, Karjalainien A et al. Progression of asbestosis predicts lung cancer. *Chest* 1998;113:1517–21.) It is well recognized that chronic inflammation results in the production of growth-promoting and angiogenic cytokines and changes in apoptosis, as well as the production of cytotoxic reactive oxygen species. (Kamp DW. Asbestos-induced lung disease: An update. *Transl Res* 2009;153:143–52; Mossman BT, Churg A. Mechanisms in the pathogenesis of asbestosis and silicosis. *Am J Respir Crit Care Med* 1998;157:1666–80.)

In response to these papers, the Helsinki group and other authors have demonstrated in retrospective pathological studies lung cancer patients' elevated levels of asbestos in lung tissue samples in some of these patients without asbestosis. These authors have concluded that high levels of asbestos exposure may not always be associated with pathological asbestosis, and therefore heavy exposures without asbestosis can be a cause of asbestos-related lung cancer. The problem with these studies is that often the cigarette smoking exposure history is either not available on a first-hand basis or is absent, creating tremendous bias. Cigarette smoking increases lung fiber burden, parenchymal opacities, and upgrades lung inflammatory defenses and can produce interstitial changes. (Caminati A, Cavazza A,

Sverzellati N et al. An integrated approach in the diagnosis of smoking-related interstitial lung disease. *Eur Respir Rev* 2012;21(125):207–17.) The inference that elevated lung tissue levels of asbestos, without asbestosis, causes asbestosis cannot be supported by epidemiological data that control for smoking and other confounders. (Dave SK, Ghodasara NB, Moharao N et al. The relationship of exposure to asbestos and smoking habit with pulmonary function tests and chest radiograph. *Ind J Pub Health* 1997;41:16–34; Pearle J. Smoking and duration of asbestos exposure in the production of functional and roentgenographic abnormalities in shipyard workers. *J Occup Med* 1982;24(1):37–40.)

A critical assessment of the epidemiological evidence on the relationships between asbestos exposure, asbestosis, and lung cancer was published in 2005 by three of the best epidemiologists in the field of occupational lung disease. (Hessel PA, Gamble JF, McDonald JC. Asbestos, asbestosis, and lung cancer: A critical assessment of the epidemiological evidence. *Thorax* 2005;60:433–6.) These experts concluded that the epidemiological evidence could not settle this issue of causation. This is similar to the view expressed in the American College of Chest Physicians Delphi study, published in 2009. (Banks DE, Shi R, McLarty J et al. American College of Chest Physicians consensus statement on the respiratory health effects of asbestos: Results of a Delphi study. *Chest* 2009;135:1619–27. Available at http://www.sh.lsuhsc.edu/medicine/delphi.)

Every individual over the age of 50 years has had significant enough asbestos exposure to produce some asbestos bodies in the lung. The issue is not whether someone has had asbestos exposure, but rather how much exposure. Patient histories are very difficult to interpret in that lay people are not experts in identifying significantly high asbestos exposures that would be considered injurious. The job title by itself is not very useful in estimating exposure to asbestos in a specific individual. Some experts testify that, to a reasonable medical certainty, specific irrefutable evidence of heavy asbestos exposure equivalent to the exposure that will cause asbestosis must be present to establish a cause-and-effect relationship between the exposure and the lung cancer. That type of testimony is speculation in that there is no epidemiologic evidence that heavy exposure without asbestosis increases the risk of lung cancer. This evidence of high exposure requires that asbestosis is present on pathological sections and, less reliably, HRCT or chest x-rays. Plaintiff testimonials of exposures, without additional clinical evidence of heavy exposure with asbestosis, are not sufficient scientific evidence to establish causation of lung cancer. There is no relationship between cigarette smoking and mesothelioma. Again, a history of asbestos exposure is not sufficient evidence for attributability of asbestos exposure as the cause of lung cancer. The only reliable marker of attribution for lung cancer is radiologic asbestosis with diffuse pulmonary interstitial fibrosis with a suitable increase in asbestos bodies. In most cases, cigarette smoking is the primary cause of lung cancer if the individual with lung cancer has been a smoker.

A recent study of the Mount Sinai asbestos worker cohort claimed to demonstrate an increased risk of lung cancer in those with asbestos exposure without asbestosis on chest x-ray. (Markowitz SB, Levin SM, Miller A et al. Asbestos, asbestosis, smoking and lung cancer: New findings from the North American insulator cohort. *Am J Respir Crit Care Med* 2013;188(1):90–6.) The authors have concluded that this large study demonstrated that asbestos exposure without asbestosis can cause lung cancer. An editorial comment by John Balmes reviewed the Markowitz data and also concluded that asbestos exposure alone, without radiologic demonstration of asbestosis, is capable of causing lung cancer. (Balmes J. Asbestos and lung cancer: What we know. *Am J Respir Dis Crit Care Med* 2013;188:8–9.)

Robert Ross from the Baylor College of Medicine reevaluated the data of Markowitz et al. and came to a different conclusion from the authors. Ross concluded that the data supported the prevailing concept that the risk of lung cancer from asbestos exposure is due to asbestosis and not asbestos exposure alone. (Ross R. Asbestosis, not asbestos exposure, is the primary risk factor for lung cancer. *Am J Respir Crit Care Med* 2014;189:114–5.) Stanley Geyer also raised some methodological issues with this paper. (Geyer S. Asbestos, asbestosis, smoking, and lung cancer: Study bias and confounding issues that complicate the interpretation of the results. *Am J Respir Crit Care Med* 2014;189:115–6.) The authors responded to Drs. Geyer and Ross in defense of their paper and I will leave it to the reader to decide whether their defense was adequate. (Markowitz S, Morabela A, Miller A. Reply to letters to the editor. *Am J Respir Crit Care Med* 2014;189:116–7.)

The limitations of the Markowitz study are that previous studies of the same population by Kipen and others from the same institution have shown that chest x-rays are not a sensitive instrument for detecting asbestosis. (Kipen H, Lilis R, Suzuki Y et al. Pulmonary fibrosis in asbestos insulation workers with lung cancer: A radiologic and histopathological evaluation. *Br J Ind Med* 1987;44:96–100.) Of the 138 cases of lung cancer in insulation workers, all of whom had asbestosis pathologically, only 82% had radiologically detectable small irregular opacities (ILO >1/0). The authors concluded in their abstract summary: "Thus a negative chest radiograph does not exclude the presence of interstitial fibrosis (asbestosis) in a substantial proportion of insulation workers previously exposed to asbestos who develop lung cancer." Some experts have implied that the Kipen study confirms that 18% of asbestos workers may not have radiologic evidence of asbestosis even though it is present pathologically. William Weiss pointed out that 23.6% of these asbestos-exposed workers would have likely developed lung cancer from cigarette smoking without asbestosis. Therefore, it is highly likely that those workers with lung cancer and no radiologic asbestosis developed their lung cancer from cigarette smoking. (Weiss W. Pulmonary fibrosis in asbestos insulation workers with lung cancer. *Br J Ind Med* 1989;46;430.) The poor sensitivity of the chest x-ray in establishing the diagnosis of parenchymal fibrosis was again confirmed by Miller et al. in 2013 and discussed below.

The same authors originally from Dr. Selikoff's laboratory at Mount Sinai Hospital in New York City evaluated the different sensitivity and specificity of computed tomography (CT) scans versus chest x-rays. They compared low-dose scans and x-ray films in 2760 nuclear workers potentially exposed to asbestos in order to assess their ability to detect interstitial lung disease (ILD) and pleural thickening (PT). Of the 2760 workers, 271 showed circumscribed PT on CT scans and 73 showed this on x-ray films, 54 (74%) of which were confirmed on CT scans; 76 showed ILD on CT scans and 15 showed this on x-ray film, 10 (67%) of which were confirmed on CT scans. Their conclusion was that CT scans detected three to five times more cases. The authors claimed that the majority of differences were minor. No mention was made of the difficulty of interpreting CT scans in smokers, the obese, or those of older age. An international classification system for interpreting HRCT scans is available (International Classification of Occupational and Environmental Respiratory Diseases [ICOERD]) but not used. Any study that uses HRCT scans to screen workers without the use of a standardized reference system of interpretation is of little value. (Hering KG, Hofmann-Preiß K, Kraus T. Update: Standardized CT/HRCT classification of occupational and environmental thoracic diseases in Germany. *Radiologe* 2014;54(4):363–84.) The international system of classification (ICOERD) is more sensitive and specific for interstitial lung abnormalities. (Vehmas T, Oksa P. Chest HRCT signs predict deaths in long-term follow-up among asbestos exposed workers. *Eur J Radiol* 2014;83(10):1983–7.)

This paper is important in that it establishes the low sensitivity of chest x-rays in discovering ILD in 13.2% of their study population and pleural disease of 19.7% of those verified on CT, resulting in a positive predictive value of 66.7% for interstitial disease and 74.0% for pleural disease as compared to CT scans. In short, only ten of the 76 CT scan-diagnosed cases of ILD and 54 of the 274 CT scan-diagnosed PT cases that were detected by chest x-ray were confirmed by CT. The study further demonstrated the poor correlation between chest x-rays and CT scans in estimating lung ILO profusion scores. (Miller A, Widman SA, Miller JA et al. Comparison of x-ray films and low-dose computed tomographic scans: Demonstration of asbestos-related changes in 2760 nuclear weapons workers screened for lung cancer. *J Occup Environ Med* 2013;55:741–45.) Another limitation of this study is due to the fact that only 74% of the chest x-rays were read and only a small percentage of workers had both a CT scan and a chest x-ray. Diffuse PT was not included because the authors stated "most such cases were unilateral, often attributable to thoracic or cardiac surgery." Only circumscribed pleural plaques were counted in their study. Their criteria for the diagnosis of asbestosis was interlobular septal thickening and honeycombing of both lower lobes or one lower lobe in addition to another lobe. Their definition of asbestosis is not consistent with the classical definition of asbestosis as being rather symmetrical, bilateral, lower-lobe interlobular septal thickening or honeycombing. No exposure measurements of individual subjects were available. No autopsy data were available for determining the true sensitivity of CT scanning in the detection of asbestos-related disease. No age-matched control population was available. The diagnosis of lung cancer can be difficult, particularly if the tumor is poorly differentiated, which further complicates some epidemiological studies. (Thunnissen E, Noguchi M, Aisner S et al. Reproducibility of histopathological diagnosis in poorly differentiated NSCLC: An international multiobserver study. *J Thorac Oncol* 2014;9(9):1354–62.)

There is an additional bias in this study by Miller et al. related to the accuracy of smoking histories, since the workers were all referred for medical–legal evaluation because of issues related to exposure, symptoms, or possible asbestos-related disease. Therefore, many of these more "heavily exposed" workers from different occupations have had a variety of exposures to other carcinogens, confounding the data analysis of the major cause of their lung cancer, or they had inaccurate smoking histories.

There have been varying opinions expressed by experts on exposure assessment and fiber type in relation to causation of lung cancer from asbestos exposure. The risk of lung cancer associated with chrysotile exposure compared with amphibole asbestos is highly contested. Asbestos–lung cancer risk relationships are highly heterogeneous and different experts have had great differences in distinguishing which epidemiologic studies best represent exposure assessment–lung cancer risk relationships, as well as differences in evaluating risk differences according to fiber type. Hodgson and Darnton estimated that the potency differential between chrysotile and amphibole asbestos for lung cancer was between 1:10 and 1:50. The risk for mesothelioma according to fiber type was 1:100:500 for chrysotile, amosite and crocidolite asbestos. Later, Berman and Crump estimated that chrysotile asbestos was less potent in the cause of lung cancer than amphibole asbestos by a factor of between 6 and 60 when considering fiber dimensions. Longer, thinner fibers are more carcinogenic than shorter fibers, as shown in the animal models by Stanton et al., Davis and Jones, and Lippmann. (Stanton MF, Kayard M, Tegris A et al. Relation of particle dimension to carcinogenicity in amphibole asbestos and other fibrous minerals. *J Natl Cancer Inst* 1981;67:965–75; Davis JM, Jones AD. Comparisons of the pathogenicity of long and short fibers of chrysotile asbestos in rats. *Br J Exp Pathol* 1988;69:717–37; Lippmann M. Effects of fiber characteristics on lung deposition, retention, and disease. *Environ Health Perspect* 1990;88:311–7.) This means that the lung cancer risk in Quebec asbestos workers with primarily shorter, thicker fiber exposure is not comparable to South Carolina textile workers who have longer, thinner fiber exposure. (Hodgson JT, Darnton A. The quantitative risks of mesothelioma and lung cancer in relation to asbestos exposure. *Ann Occup Hyg* 2000;44(8):565–601; Berman DW, Crump KS. A meta-analysis of asbestos-related cancer risk that addresses fiber size and mineral type. *Crit Rev Toxicol* 2008;38(Suppl. 1):49–73 and 38(Suppl. 1):1–47.)

Dutch researchers performed a meta-analysis of selective epidemiologic studies on the relationship between asbestos exposure and lung cancer. The authors claimed that studies with higher-quality asbestos exposure assessment yield higher meta-estimates of lung cancer risk per unit of exposure. The rebuttal from other experts was that the main finding of the original meta-analysis was less robust than claimed, and should be interpreted cautiously. (Lenters V, Burdorf A, Vermeulen R et al. Quality of evidence must guide risk assessment of asbestos. *Ann Occup Hyg* 2013;57(5):667–9.)

The question of why some chrysotile asbestos exposures (i.e., those of South Carolina textile plants) seem to be more carcinogenic than others is related to the old problem of comparing apples with oranges. Short, wider asbestos fiber exposure data, as in Quebec miners and millers, cannot be extrapolated to compare risk with a cohort exposed to more carcinogenic long, thin fibers, as in South

Carolina textile workers. Estimates of risk are determined not only by fiber type and exposure, but also by fiber length and diameter, which requires transmission electron microscopy in order to perform a more accurate analysis of respiratory exposure. Long, thin fibers are more fibrogenic than shorter, wider fibers, and therefore are more likely to cause asbestosis and asbestos-related lung cancer.

Järvholm and Aström studied Swedish workers exposed to asbestos and used the incidence of mesothelioma as a marker of exposure. There were in total 2835 cases of lung cancer. Workers with heavy exposure to asbestos had an increased risk of lung cancer (relative risk: 1.74; 95% confidence interval: 1.25–2.41) before exposure ended and a similar risk to those with low exposure 20 years after the exposure had ceased (relative risk: 0.94; 95% confidence interval: 0.77–1.15). They concluded that workers with heavy exposure to asbestos have a similar risk of lung cancer as persons with low or no exposure 20 years after the exposure has ended. The fact that there was no change in risk for lung cancer with increased asbestos exposure demonstrates that there was *no dose response* in their cohort. This is consistent with animal and many epidemiologic studies demonstrating that the *threshold dose* of asbestos necessary to produce clinical asbestosis does not significantly increase the risk of lung cancer unless clinical asbestosis is present. (Järvholm B, Aström E. The risk of lung cancer after cessation of asbestos exposure in construction workers using pleural malignant mesothelioma as a marker of exposure. *J Occup Environ Med* 2014;56(12):1297–301.)

In summary, *clinical asbestosis* is the necessary, certain link between asbestos exposure and causation of lung cancer, since there is no other reliable biological, molecular, or clinical marker between exposure and causation of lung cancer other than asbestosis. (Cagle PT. Criteria for attributing lung cancer to asbestos exposure. *Am J Clin Pathol* 2002;117:9–15; Jones R. Asbestos exposures and thoracic neoplasms. *Semin Roentgen* 1992;27:94–101; Hughes JM. Epidemiology of lung cancer in relation to asbestos exposure. In: D Liddell, K Miller (Eds.), *Mineral Fibers and Health.* Boca Raton: CRC Press, 1991, pp. 135–45; Edelman DA. Does asbestosis increase the risk of lung cancer? *Int Arch Occup Environ Health* 1990;62:345–9; Browne K. Is asbestos or asbestosis the cause of the increased risk of lung cancer in asbestos workers? *Br J Ind Med* 1986;43:145–9; Weiss W. Asbestosis: A marker for the increased risk of lung cancer among workers exposed to asbestos. *Chest* 1999;115:536–49; Hessel PA, Gamble JF, McDonald JC. Asbestos, asbestosis, and lung cancer: A critical assessment of the epidemiological evidence. *Thorax* 2005;60:433–6.)

7

The effect of smoking and lung cancer

Lung cancer is the leading cause of death in both men and women in the United States, and much of the world. Sir Richard Doll did a mortality study of British physicians in relation to their smoking habits, which was published in the *British Medical Journal* in 1950, 1954, and again in 1956, demonstrating a clear association between cigarette smoking and the causation of lung cancer. At the same time, Drs. Wynder and Graham reported the increased risk of lung cancer associated with cigarette smoking in the *Journal of the American Medical Association* in 1950. (Wynder El, Graham EA. Tobacco smoking as a possible etiologic factor in bronchogenic cancer. *JAMA* 1950;143:329-36; Doll R, Hill AB. The mortality of doctors in relation to their smoking habits: A preliminary report. 1954. *Br Med J* 2004;328(7455):1529-33; Doll R, Hill AB. Mortality in relation to smoking: Ten years observations of British doctors. *Br Med J* 1964;1(5395):1399-410.) It was not until 1964 that the Surgeon General of the United States presented a comprehensive review of the health effects of cigarette smoking as a cause of lung cancer based on 29 retrospective and seven prospective studies. (*Smoking and Health: Report of the Advisory Committee to the Surgeon General of the Public Health Service.* Public Health Services Publication No. 1103, 1964.) In 1986, the International Agency for Research on Cancer Working Group found that there was sufficient evidence that tobacco smoking was carcinogenic in humans, and concluded that cigarette smoking caused cancers, not only of the lung, but also of the lower urinary tract, including the renal pelvis and bladder, and the upper gastrointestinal tract including the oral cavity, pharynx, larynx, esophagus, and pancreas. (International Agency for Research on Cancer. *Tobacco smoking, IARC Monographs on the Evaluation of Carcinogenic Risks in Humans.* Lyon, France: International Agency for Research, 1986.)

Perhaps the best review on the early historical studies on the relationship between smoking and cancer was published at the end of the career of a very distinguished physician, Dr. Ernst Wynder, who participated personally with and knew many of the great epidemiologists who published the early studies on the relationship between smoking and lung cancer. (Wynder E. The past, present and future of the prevention of lung cancer. *Cancer Epidemiol Biomarkers Prev* 1998;7:735–48.)

The number of people smoking in Western nations has slowly decreased but the hazard remains. The incidence of lung cancer in women is now the same as men, thought to be largely due to a change in smoking habits in women. Most people are unaware that smokers lose at least one decade in life expectancy as compared with those who never smoked. The risk for lung cancer falls with the passage of time, but the effects on cardiovascular disease, stroke, and other diseases remain. The increased risk of death is not only due to lung cancer, but also due to an increased risk of chronic obstructive pulmonary disease, ischemic heart disease, other cancers, and stroke. (Jha P, Ramsundarahettige C, Landsman V et al. Twenty first century hazards of smoking and benefits of cessation in the United States. *N Engl J Med* 2013;368:341–50; Thun MJ, Carter BD, Feskanich D et al. 50-year trends in smoking-related mortality in the United States. *N Engl J Med* 2013;368:351–64; Wynder EL. Tobacco as a cause of lung cancer: Some reflections. *Am J Epidemiol* 1997;146:687–94.)

The risk of lung cancer is increased fourfold in former cigarette smokers. Those who have smoked more than 25 cigarettes a day have a risk of lung cancer that is 24.5 times greater than nonsmokers, and the risk continues to increase linearly with the number of cigarettes smoked, based on another study by Dr. Doll, published in the *British Medical Journal* in 1994, with a follow-up study of British doctors published in the same journal in the year 2004. This means that if you triple the number of cigarettes smoked, per day, you triple the risk of developing lung cancer. However, the duration of smoking is more important than the intensity, and it is estimated that tripling the duration of cigarette smoking increases the risk of lung cancer 100-fold, according to the American Cancer Society in 2006. In summary, both the number of cigarettes smoked and the duration of cigarette smoking have separate distinct effects on the risk of developing lung cancer. The duration of cigarette smoking is a greater risk factor than the number of cigarettes smoked, according to the U.S. Surgeon General's study on the relationship between smoking and lung cancer. (Reducing the health consequences of smoking: 25 years of progress. *A Report of the Surgeon General 1989*, DHHS Publication No. (CDC) 89-8411, 1989; Smoking and health in America. *A Report of the Surgeon General in collaboration with the Pan-American Health Organization 1992*, DHHS Publication No. (CDC) 92–8419.)

It was hoped that lowering the amount of nicotine, tobacco, and cigarette smoke would reduce the risk of lung cancer. However, the data have shown that there has been no significant risk reduction from smoking the newer low-tar cigarettes as compared to the previous higher-tar cigarettes. Also, menthol cigarettes, such as Kool increase the systemic exposure to various carcinogens, and increasing the risk of lung cancer. African–American men and women are much more likely to smoke menthol cigarettes, and it is thought that this explains the increased risk of lung cancer amongst African–American men and women.

Several studies have shown an increased incidence of lung cancer, or broncho-genic carcinoma, in groups of workers with moderate-to-heavy asbestos exposure and asbestosis. All fiber types are associated with this disease, but crocidolite is most toxic, followed by amosite and chrysotile. About 222,520 new cases of lung cancer occurred in the United States in 2010, with 157,300 deaths. Less than 5% of these cases were attributed, at least partially—and I believe incorrectly—to asbestos exposure, while cigarette smoking accounted for at least 90%. A dose–response relationship appeared to only exist for high cumulative asbestos exposures, which must have been heavy enough to cause asbestosis, even though this does not hold true at lower doses.

Cigarette smokers who have also had heavy cumulative exposure to asbestos have a combined lung cancer risk that is greater than expected for each exposure alone. Selikoff's study of insulators with 20 years of heavy asbestos exposure in 1979 found that, when compared to nonsmokers with no asbestos exposures, the relative risks for lung cancer in the heavily asbestos-exposed workers were 5.0 for nonsmokers, and 50.0 for cigarette smokers. This is called a synergistic effect since the effect is multiplicative rather than additive. This study was compared to other studies of nonasbestos-exposed persons for whom the relative risk for lung cancer was 11.0 for cigarette smokers compared to nonsmokers.

The earlier studies by Selikoff had noted an increased risk of lung cancer only in smokers with exposure to asbestos. Nonsmokers were not thought to be at risk for lung cancer based on epidemiologic studies through 1974. (Selikoff IJ, Hammond EC. Multiple risk factors in environmental cancer. *Proceedings of Conference: Persons at High Risk of Cancer: An Approach to Cancer Etiology and Control*, December 10–12, 1974; *Environ Cancer* 1975;467–83.) In 1972, Berry and others studied the smoking habits of 1780 asbestos workers and noted no significant excess risk of lung cancer in workers, whether smokers or nonsmokers, with low-to-moderate asbestos exposure. Smoking workers who were heavily exposed to asbestos had a highly significant increased risk of lung cancer. (Berry G, Neuhouse ML, Turok M. Combined effect of asbestos exposure and smoking on mortality from lung cancer in factory workers. *Lancet* 1972;2:476–79.) A later study of asbestos factory workers exposed to amosite asbestos also found an increased risk of lung cancer only in current smokers exposed to high levels of asbestos. (Acheson ED, Gardner MJ, Winter PD, Bennett C. Cancer in a factory using amosite asbestos. *J Epidemiol* 1984;13:3–10.)

Previous theories maintained that very low cumulative exposures to asbestos presented a real, although small, risk for developing lung cancer. However, there is now a significant amount of evidence that lung cancer from asbestos exposure only occurs after very large cumulative asbestos exposures. Warnock and Isenberg wrote in 1986 that "There is a consensus that a diagnosis of asbestos-related cancer requires the presence of asbestosis as proof of substantial asbestos burden." (Warnock ML, Isenberg BS. Asbestos burden and the pathology of lung cancer. *Chest* 1986;89:20–6.) Several studies suggest that lung cancer due to asbestos exposure only occurs in the presence of asbestosis, suggesting that this may be a type of scar cancer. Patients with nonasbestos-related idiopathic interstitial pulmonary fibrosis have a definite increase incidence of lung cancer. The scientific literature indicates that chronic inflammation and lung scarring from a variety of sources may produce lung cancer without any asbestos exposure. The common denominator for the production of lung cancer is chronic inflammation with pulmonary fibrosis from any cause. (Vancheri C. Common pathways in idiopathic pulmonary fibrosis and cancer. *Eur Respir Rev* 2013;22(129):265–72; Archontogeorgis K, Steiropoulos P, Tzouvelekis A et al. Lung cancer and interstitial lung diseases: A systematic review. *Pulm Med* 2012;2012:315918; Raghu G, Nyberg F, Morgan G. The epidemiology of interstitial lung disease and its association with lung cancer. *Br J Cancer* 2004;91(2):S3–S10.)

In 1995, Wilkinson and colleagues raised the question again as to whether the risk of lung cancer is increased in asbestos-exposed individuals in the absence of small opacities on chest x-ray. (Wilkinson P, Hansell DM, Janssens J et al. Is lung cancer associated with asbestos exposure when there are no small opacities on the chest radiograph? *Lancet* 1995;345:1074.) This paper was very controversial and resulted in a vigorous response by other experts who felt that there were major methodological problems with the research design, producing a false impression that asbestos-related lung cancer risk was elevated in some individuals with "normal chest x-rays," implying that no radiological evidence of asbestosis was necessary to increase the risk of lung cancer from asbestos exposure. (Asbestos: A risk to far, Letters to the Editor, *Lancet* 1995;346:304–306.) The authors retreated and responded to their critics by stating, "No single study can provide certain proof of cause and effect, and account must be taken of biologic plausibility."

The threshold dose (i.e., cumulative asbestos exposure) needed to develop lung cancer from asbestos exposure appears to be the same as that needed to develop asbestosis or interstitial lung fibrosis. Cumulative asbestos exposures of 25–100 fiber years for amphibole asbestos, and 250–500 fiber years for chrysotile exposure, are needed to develop lung cancer (this would require 250 years of exposure at the current Occupational Safety and Health Administration permissible exposure limit of 0.1 fibers/cc). Persons with cumulative exposures below this level may not be at any real increased risk for lung cancer. The threshold dose and latency for cancer is complicated by the impact of the intensity of exposure. (Jones HB, Grendon A. Environmental factors in the origin of cancer and estimation of the possible hazard to man. *Food Cosmet Toxicol* 1975;18:251–68.) The issues of the relationship between cigarette smoking and health effects is further complicated by significant bias. Significant differences in smoking habits, such as smoking to the end of the cigarette, deeper inhalation, and the use of nonfiltered cigarettes, as well as social class and occupational group, affect the risk for an adverse health effect. (Axelson O. Confounding from smoking in occupational epidemiology. *Br J Ind Med* 1989;46:505–7; Jarholm B, Thringer G. Epidemiological studies of lung cancer: Influence of smoking habits. *Eur J Respir Dis* 1980;61(Suppl. 107):125–9.)

Once a diagnosis of a lung cancer is made, the human response of many individuals is *shame followed by blame* because of the guilt from cigarette smoking. Patients tend to minimize their smoking history once they have developed a serious smoking-related health condition. Some accept responsibility for their smoking-related condition, while others may blame other causes such as asbestos exposure for their lung cancer. It is difficult to obtain an accurate smoking and asbestos exposure history in retrospect after the diagnosis of lung cancer has been given to a patient. The excellent clinician recognizes that the reality of the emotional response to any diagnosis of a serious medical condition may include some degree of denial, or unwillingness to accept responsibility for smoking, or adverse health habits such as obesity, diet, drugs, or alcohol consumption, etc.

More recently, the issue has been whether asbestos is a complete carcinogen, since most lung cancers occurred in asbestos-exposed individuals who have been smokers. Tobacco smoke is clearly the most important factor associated with the development of lung cancer, accounting for 80%–90% of all cases. Asbestos is another significant inhaled carcinogen, contributing to the development of about 5%–7% of all lung cancers. (LaDou J. The asbestos cancer epidemic. *Environ Health Perspect* 2004;112:285–90.) The efficacy of asbestos exposure as a complete lung carcinogen, independent of tobacco smoke, has not been demonstrated conclusively in humans, since lung cancers of asbestos-exposed individuals frequently occur in smokers and ex-smokers. The majority of asbestos-related lung cancers may result from the combined effects of asbestos and carcinogens in tobacco smoke, with the possibility of a synergistic relationship. Many studies on asbestos-related lung carcinogenesis have analyzed the genotoxic effects of asbestos; asbestos fibers induce DNA damage, chromosome aberrations, mitotic disturbances, and gene mutations (Figure 6.1). In addition, asbestos fibers can stimulate a range of other effects including cell proliferation, chronic inflammation, enhanced gene expression (such as c-fos and c-jun overexpression), and transformation. P53 is important in lung cancers but does not seem to be affected in mesotheliomas. The complete mechanism of asbestos-induced lung carcinogenesis still remains unclear. (Inamura K, Ninomiya H, Nomura K et al. Combined effects of asbestos and cigarette smoke on the development of lung adenocarcinoma: Different carcinogens may cause different genomic changes. *Oncol Rep* 2014;32(2):475–82; Jaurand MC. Mechanisms of fiber-induced genotoxicity. *Environ Health Perspect* 1997;105(Suppl. 5):1073–84; Husgafvel-Pursiainen K, Karjalainen A, Kannio A et al. Lung cancer and past occupational exposure to asbestos. Role of *p53* and *K-ras* mutations. *Am J Respir Cell Mol Biol* 1999;20:667–74; Luanpitpong S, Wang L, Stueckle TA et al. Caveolin-1 regulates lung cancer stem-like cell induction and p53 inactivation in carbon nanotube-driven tumorigenesis. *Oncotarget* 2014;5(11):3541–54.) The good news is that molecular cell biological research has resulted in elucidating various oncogenic pathways that now can be interrupted by drugs. Now that oncogenic drivers have been identified, genomic testing has become very useful for guiding treatment in the majority of patients with lung adenocarcinomas. (Kris MG, Johnson BE, Berry LD et al. Using multiplexed assays of oncogenic drivers in lung cancers to select targeted drugs. *JAMA* 2014;311(19):1998–2006.)

Tobacco exposure is the major cause of lung cancer. Lung cancer in never-smokers accounts for 10%–25% of all lung cancer cases. Arsenic, asbestos, and radon are three prominent nontobacco carcinogens strongly associated with lung cancer. Exposure to these agents can lead to genetic and epigenetic alterations in tumor genomes, impacting genes and pathways involved in lung cancer development. Unfortunately, most of the medical literature has focused on the interaction of tobacco smoke and asbestos, and the additional roles of other causes of lung cancer have not been well studied in asbestos-exposed cohorts. (Hubaux R, Becker-Santos DD, Enfield KS et al. Arsenic, asbestos and radon: Emerging players in lung tumorigenesis. *Environ Health* 2012;11:89.)

8

Asbestos-related pleural disease

Pleural plaques are well-circumscribed discrete elevated gray–white fibrohyaline thickenings involving the parietal pleural surface of the chest wall or diaphragm, without any associated pleural effusion or adhesions. These plaques vary in size and most commonly occupy the posterior gutter of the chest cavity and the diaphragm. They often have a "holly leaf" appearance due to irregular borders. The plaques are covered by a layer of mesothelial cells, which protect the surface of the plaque from impairing lung function or normal lung movement in the chest cavity. They may calcify and enlarge over time. Plaques are asymptomatic unless complicated by diffuse pleural thickening and usually go undetected during the lifetime of an individual. (Smith DD. Asbestos-related pleural disease: Questions in need of answer. *Clin Pulm Med* 1994;1:289–300.) Most pleural plaques found at autopsy are not seen radiologically by standard PA chest x-ray because they lay predominately in the para-spinal areas of the posterior chest and diaphragm. (Meurman L. Asbestos bodies in pleural plaques in the Finnish series of cases. *Acta Pathol Scand* 1966;181:8.) Hourihane et al. found that 85% of pleural plaques found at autopsy are invisible by chest x-ray. Svener noted in 1986 not only false-negative findings but also false-positive correlations with chest x-rays and pleural plaques. In less than half the pleural plaque cases was this diagnosis suggested from the roentgenological examination. On the other hand, the two interpreting radiologists found 13 and 14 cases, respectively, with positive or uncertain findings in the 33 control cases with no pleural plaques found at autopsy. There was no correlation between plaque area and plaque thickness ($r = 0.037$), but plaque thickness influenced the accuracy of roentgenological diagnosis significantly. In this series, no oblique views were obtained, and the x-rays were of mixed quality. (Hourihane DOB, Lessof L, Richardson PC. Hyaline and calcified pleural plaques as an index of exposure to asbestos: A study of 100 cases with consideration of epidemiology. *BMJ* 1966;1:1069–74; Hillerdal G, Lindgren A. Pleural plaques: Correlation of autopsy findings to radiographic findings and occupational history. *Eur J Respir Dis* 1980;61:315–9; Svener KB, Borgersen AM,

Haaversen O, Holton K. Parietal pleural plaques: A comparison between autopsy and X-ray findings. *Eur J Respir Dis* 1986;69:10–5.)

The problem of the poor correlation between chest x-ray findings and autopsy studies has been further complicated by significant inter-observer variation in interpreting chest x-rays of asbestos-exposed workers. The degree of inter-observer variability has made the results of many chest x-ray studies, including those that use International Labor Office (ILO) B-Readers, questionable. Rossiter, in 100 test films among 12 chosen test readers, measured the between-observer variability for the prevalence of pleural abnormality, and found that the chest x-ray findings varied from under 20% to more than 50%. The use of ILO-certified B-Readers reduces the variability slightly, but the concordance between readers is still disappointing. (Rossiter CE. Initial repeatability studies of the UICC/Cincinnati classification of the radiographic appearances of the pneumoconiosis. *Br J Ind Med* 1972;29:407–19; Ducatman AM. Variability in interpretation of radiographs for asbestosis abnormalities: Problems and solutions. *Ann NY Acad Sci* 1991;643:108–20.) The inter-observer variability, as well as the poor correlation with autopsy findings, make the radiological observation of pleural plaques a poor instrument for epidemiological studies, because of its lack of statistical precision. This raises serious reservations as to the conclusion of the more than 500 published articles correlating chest x-ray-detected pleural plaques, and risk for lung cancer, mesothelioma, and reduced lung function.

Pleural plaques usually take 20 or more years from date of first exposure to become visible on chest x-ray. Only those plaques that are tangential to the x-ray beam are usually seen on survey chest x-rays. The more common posterior plaques are not usually seen by chest x-ray unless they are calcified. Plaques tend to calcify 30 or more years after exposure and then become more visible on a survey chest x-ray. They may enlarge slowly over the lifetime of an individual without causing any symptoms or impairment. The plaques may become confluent without compromising lung function. When plaques are bilateral and symmetrical, the most common cause is amphibole asbestos exposure. A combination of bilateral posterior–lateral plaques, or bilateral diaphragmatic pleural involvement, is consistent with asbestos exposure. No treatments are necessary for benign pleural plaques and the frequency or necessity for follow-up should be based on the type and intensity of exposure, as well as the latency time related to prior asbestos exposure. (Cugell DW, Kamp DW. Asbestos and the pleura: A review. *Chest* 2004;125:1103–17; Peacock C, Copley SJ, Hansell DM. Asbestos-related pleural disease. *Clin Radiol* 2000;55:422–32.)

Previous studies based on chest radiographs have reported an unexplained left-sided predominance of pleural plaques. In a study by Gallego, a comparison of summed surfaces and location of plaques calculated from computed tomography (CT) studies was performed. Thoracic CT scans from 40 adults with asbestos exposure and pleural plaques were analyzed. The results showed a lack of significant predominance for any hemithorax. (Gallego JC. Absence of left-sided predominance in asbestos-related pleural plaques: A CT study. *Chest* 1998;113(4):1034–6.)

Plaques may be unilateral and related to chest wall scarring from a variety of other causes such as chest trauma, thoracic/cardiovascular surgery, tuberculosis, hemothorax, pneumonia/empyema, rib fractures, chest or breast radiation, or infection. Chest x-rays are frequently false positive or false negative. Rib companion shadows, fat, intercostal vessels, and muscles can appear as plaques. Mineral fibers, other than asbestos, can also cause pleural effusions, rounded atelectasis, bilateral pleural plaques, and diffuse pleural disease. Plaques are also related to genetic susceptibility and may be seen in many different occupational and environmental exposures:

- Kaolinosis
- Talc mining
- Vermiculite
- Ophiolite
- Environmental exposures in Greece, New Caledonia, Turkey, Corsica, Italy, Finland, and Balkan areas of Europe
- Silica
- Wollastonite
- Liparitosis
- Erionite
- Carbon nanotubes
- Anthophylite
- Antigorite
- Balangeroite
- Fluoro-edenite
- Pulmonary alveolar microlithiasis
- Nephite jade
- Australian gold mine workers
- Refractory ceramic fibers
- Silicon carbide
- Metsovo lung
- Taconite mining
- Refractory ceramic fibers

(Chaudhary BA, Kanes GJ, Pool WH. Pleural thickening in mild kaolinosis. *South Med J* 1997;90(11):1106–9; Fitzgerald EF, Stark AD, Vianna N, Hwang SA. Exposure to asbestiform minerals and radiographic chest abnormalities in a talc mining region of upstate New York. *Arch Environ Health* 1991;46(3):151–4; Antao VC, Larson TC, Horton DK. Libby vermiculite exposure and risk of developing asbestos-related lung and pleural diseases. *Curr Opin Pulm Med* 2012;18(2):161–7; Bayram M, Dongel I, Bakan ND et al. High risk of malignant mesothelioma and pleural plaques in subjects born close to ophiolites. *Chest* 2013;143(1):164–71; Sahin U, Ozturk O, Songur N, Bircan A, Akkaya A. Observations on environmental asbestos exposure in a high risk area. *Respirology* 2009;14(4):579–82; Baris YI, Saracci R, Siminoto L et al. Malignant mesothelioma in two villages in central Turkey. *Lancet* 1981;1:984–7; Bignon J, Peto J, Saracci R. *Non-Occupational Exposure to*

Mineral Fibers. Lyon, France: IARC Scientific Publications, 1989; Kukkonen MK, Hämäläinen S, Kaleva S et al. Genetic susceptibility to asbestos-related fibrotic pleuropulmonary changes. *Eur Respir J* 2011;38(3):672–8; Mazziotti S, Gaeta M, Costa C et al. Computed tomography features of liparitosis: A pneumoconiosis due to amorphous silica. *Eur Respir J* 2004;23(2):208–11; Arakawa H, Honma K, Saito Y et al. Pleural disease in silicosis: Pleural thickening, effusion, and invagination. *Radiology* 2005;236:685–93; Patel A, Choudhury S. Pleural tuberculosis presented as multiple pleural masses: An atypical presentation. *Lung India* 2013;30(1):54–6; Rous V, Studený J. Aetiology of pleural plaques. *Thorax* 1970;25(3):270–84; Maxim LD, Niebo R, Utell MJ et al. Wollastonite toxicity: An update. *Inhal Toxicol* 2014;26(2):95–112; Donaldson K, Poland CA, Murphy FA, MacFarlane M. Pulmonary toxicity of carbon nanotubes and asbestos—Similarities and differences. *Adv Drug Deliv Rev* 2013;65(15):2078–86; Turci F, Tomatis M, Comagnoni R, Fubini B. Role of associated mineral fibers in chrysotile asbestos health effects: The case of balangeroite. *Ann Occup Hyg* 2009;53:491–97; Turci F, Tomatis M, Comagnoni R, Fubini B. Role of associated mineral fibers in chrysotile asbestos health effects: The case of balangeroite. *Ann Occup Hyg* 2009;53:491–7; Biggeri A, Pasetto R, Belli S et al. Mortality from chronic obstructive pulmonary disease and pleural mesothelioma in an area contaminated by natural fiber (fluoro-edenite). *Scand J Work Environ Health* 2004;30:249–52; Baumann F, Maurizot P, Mangeas M et al. Pleural mesothelioma in New Caledonia: Associations with environmental risk factors. *Environ Health Perspect* 2011;119:695–700; Yang HY, Shie RH, Chen PC. Pulmonary fibrosis in workers exposed to non-asbestiform tremolite asbestos minerals. *Epidemiology* 2012;23:1–7; Lee YC, De Klerk NH, Musk AW. Asbestos-related pleural disease in Western Australian gold-miners. *Med J Aust* 1999;170(6):263–5; Lockey J, Lemasters G, Rice C et al. Refractory ceramic fiber exposure and pleural plaques. *Am J Respir Crit Care Med* 1996;154(5):1405–10; Scancarello G, Romeo R, Sartorelli E. Respiratory disease as a result of talc inhalation. *J Occup Environ Med* 1996;38(6):610–4; Durand P, Bégin R, Samson L et al. Silicon carbide pneumoconiosis: A radiographic assessment. *Am J Ind Med* 1991;20(1):37–47; Constantopoulos SH, Goudevenos JA, Saratzis N et al. Metsovo lung: Pleural calcification and restrictive lung function in northwestern Greece. Environmental exposure to mineral fiber as etiology. *Environ Res* 1985;38(2):319–31; Mandel J, Lambert C, Alexander B, MacLehose R, Ramachandran G. A study of radiographic abnormalities in Minnesota taconite workers. *Occup Environ Med* 2014;71(Suppl. 1):A41.)

Exposure to environmental anthophylite asbestos is common in Finland, Bulgaria, and Japan. Karjalainen and coinvestigators found the prevalence of pleural plaques in their autopsy population of 288 Finnish urban men was 58%. Approximately 38% of these plaques occurred in non-occupationally exposed men. Plaques had been previously reported in 52% of urban dwellers and 32% of those living in the countryside in Finland. The risk for plaques correlated with intensity of exposure and exposure to crocidolite/amosite as well as anthophylite. (Karjalainen A, Karhunen PJ, Lalu K et al. Pleural plaques and exposure to mineral fibres in a male urban necropsy population. *Occup Environ Med* 1994;51(7):456–60.)

The identification of diffuse pleural changes suggests an intermediate exposure between the very low exposure necessary to cause pleural plaques, and the heavy exposure necessary to cause asbestosis. Very low levels of amphibole exposure (<1 fiber/cc-year) may be sufficient to produce pleural plaques. A study by Larson and colleagues found that 46% of individuals exposed to vermiculite in Libby, Montana, had pleural thickening at a median exposure of 3.6 fibers/cc-year. (Larson TC, Antao VC, Bove FJ, Cusack C. Association between cumulative fiber exposure and respiratory outcomes among Libby vermiculite workers. *J Occup Environ Med* 2012;54(1):56–63; Christensen KY, Bateson TF, Kopylev L. Low levels of exposure to Libby amphibole asbestos and localized pleural thickening. *J Occup Environ Med* 2013;55:1350–5.)

Pleural plaques occur in the general population of the United States and the prevalence by x-ray diagnosis varies from 0.2% to 6.4% in the National Health and Nutrition Examination II Study (NHANES II). The prevalence estimates in NHANES II in the age group of 35–74 years are 6.4% (±0.9%) among males, 1.7% (±0.6%) among females, and 3.9% (±0.6%) overall. These prevalence values are approximately twice those estimated from NHANES I data (1971–1975). (Rogan WJ, Ragan NB, Dinse GE. X-ray evidence of increased asbestos exposure in the US population from NHANES I and NHANES II, 1973–1978. National Health Examination Survey. *Cancer Causes Control* 2000;11(5):441–9.)

A survey of 1212 patients in a Veteran's hospital found a 2.3% incidence of pleural plaques, and only 18% had knowledge of asbestos exposure. (Miller JA, Zurlo JV. Asbestos plaques in a typical Veteran's hospital population. *Am J Ind Med* 1996;30(6):726–9.)

A US Navy study was part of a programmatic review of the Asbestos Medical Surveillance Program database, which included 233,353 radiographic examinations from 1990 to 1999. The initial review focused on incidental findings recorded by B-Readers for 23,460 radiographs. Pleural thickening was found in 2.35% of chest x-rays. (Muller JG, Bohnker BK, Philippi AF, Litow FK, Rudolph G, Hernandez JE. Trends in pleural radiographic findings in the Navy Asbestos Medical Surveillance Program (1990–1999). *Mil Med* 2005;170(5):375–80.) Chest x-ray diagnosis of pleural plaques lacks the precision to be useful based on the poor correlation between autopsy findings. (Meurman L. Asbestos bodies and pleural plaques in a Finnish series of autopsy cases. *Acta Pathol Microbiol Scand* 1966;Suppl. 181:1+.)

Exposure to chrysotile asbestos in asbestos miners and millers was evaluated by Graham Gibbs in 1979, and after surveying 15,689 chest x-rays, he found a very low incidence of calcified pleural plaques (1.3%), noting only 206 cases. This incidence is lower than that found in the general population and suggests the low sensitivity of survey chest x-rays as well as the low incidence of calcified pleural plaques associated with chrysotile exposure. (Gibbs GW. Etiology of pleural calcification: A study of Quebec chrysotile asbestos miners and millers. *Arch Environ Health* 1979;34:76–83.) Martha Warnock and colleagues studied the correlation of asbestos fiber types and pleural plaques found at autopsy and measured the lung fiber counts. Pleural plaques were associated with a higher mean concentration of amphibole (crocidolite and amosite), but not chrysotile.

(Warnock ML, Prescott BT, Kuwahara TJ. Numbers and types of asbestos fibers in subjects with pleural plaques. *Am J Pathol* 1982;109:37–46.) Warnock's data were confirmed by Andrew Churg. (Churg A. Asbestos fibers in pleural plaques in a general autopsy population. *Am J Pathol* 1982;109:88–96.)

Subpleural fat is easily confused with asbestos-related diffuse pleural disease, or pleural plaques. In 1984, Sargent and colleagues estimated that as many as 20%–40% of findings of apparent pleural thickening are due to pleural fat. In obese patients, chest x-rays present too many false positives to be reliable indicators of asbestos-related pleural disease, without confirmation by chest CT. Ultrasound has been unable to identify pleural plaques or distinguish between subpleural fat and diffuse pleural thickening. (Sargent EN, Boswell WD, Ralls WP, Markowitz A. Subpleural fat pads in patients exposed to asbestos: Distinction from non-calcified pleural plaques. *Diagn Radiol* 1984;152:273–7; Larson TC, Franzblau A, Lewin M, Goodman AB, Antao VC. Impact of body mass index on the detection of radiographic localized pleural thickening. *Acad Radiol* 2014;21(1):3–10.) Muscle shadows can also be confused with pleural thickening (Figures 8.1 and 8.2). (Collins JD, Brown RK, Batra P. Asbestosis and the serratus anterior muscle. *J Natl Med Assoc* 1983;75(3):296–300; Gilmartin D. The serratus anterior muscle on chest radiographs. *Radiology* 1979;131:629–35.)

Some radiologists use the term "pleural asbestosis" when discovering pleural plaques or asbestos-related diffuse pleural disease on a chest x-ray. The failure to distinguish between asbestos-related diffuse parenchymal fibrosis and asbestos-related benign diffuse pleural disease, results an unnecessary concern and agitation for families and physicians. There is no such thing as "pleural asbestosis" and the term should not be used. Asbestos-related pleural plaques are a benign condition related to amphibole asbestos exposure or to amphibole-contaminated chrysotile asbestos. (Smith DD. What is asbestosis? *Chest* 1990;98:963–4; Smith DD. When should you suspect asbestos-related pulmonary disease? *J Respir Dis*

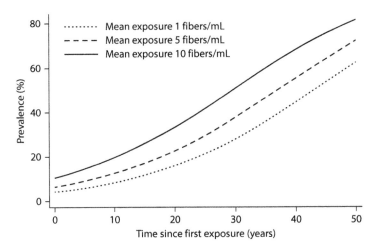

Figure 8.1 Prevalence and latency of pleural plaques since time of first exposure. (Adapted from Paris C et al. *Environ Health* 2008;7:30.)

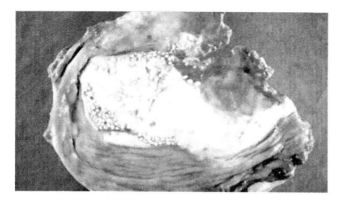

Figure 8.2 A diaphragmatic pleural plaque. (Adapted from Leslie KO, Wick MR. *Practical Pulmonary Pathology.* Philadelphia: Elsevier, 2005.)

2005;11:499–510.) Many pleural plaques are not radiologically detectable on chest x-rays. The percentage of pleural plaques found postmortem and detected premortem by chest x-ray has ranged from 8% to 40%. Plaques were not an uncommon finding in the attorney referral population studied by Victor Roggli and colleagues, being found in 39% of routine post-mortem examinations. (Roggli VL, Oury TD, Sporn TA. *Pathology of Asbestos Associated Diseases.* New York: Springer-Verlag, 2004.) The study population evaluated by Roggli and co-workers was a largely forensic population of patients referred by both defense and plaintiff attorneys because of probable asbestos-related disease, which explains the high number of patients with pleural plaques.

Various amphibole mineral fibers are associated with pleural reactions to these fibers. The most common reaction to mineral fibers is pleural plaques. Plaques suggest amphibole mineral fiber exposure, but the shape, size, or location remains the same regardless of the type—asbestos versus asbestiform—of amphibole mineral fiber exposure.

Pleural plaques are seen less frequently in Quebec chrysotile workers. The question has been whether workers exposed to pure chrysotile—uncontaminated by amphibole—can produce pleural plaques. In the Canabrava mine in the state of Gola, Central Region of Brazil, the asbestos mine appears not to have significant amphibole contamination, but chest x-ray surveys, not confirmed by CT, have demonstrated abnormalities thought to be due to pleural plaques. (Bagatin E, Neder JA, Nery LE et al. Non-malignant consequences of decreasing asbestos exposure in the Brazil chrysotile mines and mills. *Occup Environ Med* 2005;62(6):381–9; Oliveira MCB, Frazzoo EB, Valorelli JV et al. Technological characteristics of serpentines in the Cana Brava Mine, Go, Brazil. *Proc Int Symp Mine Planning Equip.* Rotterdam: A.A. Balkema, 1997, pp. 77–80.)

Asbestos-related bilateral pleural plaques, either small or large, are a signature of asbestos exposure only when other causes of pleural disease are excluded. Only 10%–15% of pleural plaques found at autopsy are visualized on a chest x-ray and conversely only 50% of plaques seen on chest x-ray can be confirmed at autopsy. Historical epidemiology studies have relied on chest x-rays, which lack the sensitivity and specificity to accurately diagnose pleural plaques! (Meurman L. Asbestos bodies and pleural plaques in a Finnish series of autopsy cases. *Acta Pathol Microbiol Scand* 1966; Suppl. 181:7–107; Hourihane DOB, Lessof L, Richardson PC. Hyaline and calcified pleural plaques as an index of exposure to asbestos: A study of 100 cases with consideration of epidemiology. *BMJ* 1966;1:1069–74; Hillerdal G, Lindgren A. Pleural plaques: Correlation of autopsy findings to radiographic findings and occupational history. *Eur J Respir Dis* 1980;61:315–9; Hillerdal G. Pleural plaques and risk of bronchial carcinoma and mesothelioma: A prospective study. *Chest* 1994;105:144–50; Churg A. Asbestos fibers and pleural plaques in a general autopsy population. *Am J Pathol* 1982;109:88–96; Karjalainen A, Karhunen PJ, Lalu K et al. Pleural plaques and exposure to mineral fibres in a male urban necropsy population. *Occup Environ Med* 1994;51:456–60.)

Many pleural plaques are from unknown causes, in that autopsy studies have found no evidence of elevated asbestos body counts in up to 50% of patients. (Churg A. Asbestos fibers in pleural plaques in a general autopsy population. *Am J Pathol* 1982;109:88–96; Clarke CC, Mowet FS, Kelsh MA, Roberts MA. Pleural plaques: A review of diagnostic issues and possible non-asbestos factors. *Arch Environ Occup Health* 2006;61:183–92.) Pleural plaques are more common in males. Andrion and coworkers found hyaline pleural plaques were searched for in 1019 consecutive autopsies performed on adults in the heavily industrialized area of Turin, Italy. Pleural lesions were found in 173/706 (24.5%) of males and 22/313 (7%) of females (p < 0.001). (Andrion A, Colombo A, Dacorsi M, Mollo F. Pleural plaques at autopsy in Turin: A study on 1019 adult subjects. *Eur J Respir Dis* 1982;63:107–12.)

Previous studies have provided conflicting results about the role of intensity and duration of exposure on amphibole mineral fibers in the production of asbestos-related pleural disease. Italian investigators have assessed the relationship between the risk of benign asbestos-related diseases, and different aspects of asbestos exposure, in previous asbestos workers who underwent low-dose CT. They studied 772 formally exposed asbestos workers and found 14 (1.8%) cases of asbestosis, 187 (24.2%) cases of pleural plaques, and 50 (6.5%) cases of diffuse pleural thickening. The significant risk factors for pleural changes were cumulative exposure for asbestosis (p for trend = 0.004), time since first exposure (p for trend <0.001), peak exposure (p for trend <0.001) for pleural plaques, and time since first exposure for diffuse pleural disease (p for trend = 0.024). They concluded that parenchymal asbestosis and pleural plaques are associated with different aspects of asbestos exposure. Diffuse pleural thickening appears to be less specific for asbestos exposure. (Mastrangelo G, Ballarin MN, Bellini E et al. Asbestos exposure and benign asbestos diseases in 772 formerly exposed workers: Dose–response relationships. *Am J Ind Med* 2009;52(8):596–602.)

A large French study concluded that time since first exposure (p < 0.0001) and either cumulative or mean exposure (p < 0.0001) showed independent associations with both pleural plaques and asbestosis prevalence and pleural plaques incidence. Modelling incidence of pleural plaques showed a 0.8%–2.4%

yearly increase for a mean exposure of 1 fiber/mL. The major limitation of this study is that exposures were estimated and not directly measured. It is likely that the intensity and duration of exposures were underestimated. (Paris C, Martin A, Letourneux M, Wild P. Modelling prevalence and incidence of fibrosis and pleural plaques in asbestos-exposed populations for screening and follow-up: A cross-sectional study. *Environ Health* 2008;7:30.) These results are consistent with those of Finkelstein and Vingilis. (Finkelstein MM, Vingilis JJ. Radiographic abnormalities among asbestos cement workers: An exposure response study. *Am Rev Respir Dis* 1984;129:17–22.)

A major concern has been whether pleural plaques by themselves, uncomplicated by diffuse pleural disease, pleural effusions, or asbestosis, may cause impairment of lung function or disability. Experts have been divided on this issue; some claim that uncomplicated pleural plaques may cause some reduction in lung function. (Schwartz DA, Davis CS, Merchant JA et al. Longitudinal changes in lung function among asbestos-exposed workers. *Am J Respir Crit Care Med* 1994;150(5 Pt 1):1243–9.) The issue relates to the failure to distinguish diffuse pleural disease from pleural plaques. There is no argument among experts that diffuse pleural disease may cause a restrictive type of lung function impairment. Epidemiological studies that do not distinguish pleural plaques from diffuse pleural disease are uninterpretable when efforts attempt to establish whether pleural plaques cause lung function impairment. High-resolution CT (HRCT) is necessary for distinguishing pleural plaques from diffuse pleural thickening. (Schwartz DA, Fuortes LJ, Galvin JR et al. Asbestos-induced pleural fibrosis and impaired lung function. *Am Rev Respir Dis* 1990;141(2):321–6.)

Teresa McCloud, Professor of Chest Radiology at Harvard Medical School, and coworkers from Boston, did the best study published for distinguishing the frequency and functional impact of pleural plaques versus diffuse pleural disease. Two types of pleural reaction have been described in association with asbestos exposure: pleural plaques and diffuse pleural thickening. The study was undertaken to determine the prevalence and causes of diffuse thickening in asbestos-exposed persons.

Serial chest radiographs in 1373 exposed individuals and 717 controls were interpreted according to the ILO scheme by two B readers. Diffuse pleural thickening was defined as a smooth, non-interrupted pleural density extending over at least one-fourth of the chest wall, with or without costophrenic angle obliteration. Among the exposed group, plaques and diffuse thickening occurred with almost equal frequency, 16.5% and 13.5%, respectively. Of the 185 cases with diffuse thickening, the radiographic appearance was most often due to the residual of a benign asbestos effusion (31.3%) or confluent plaques (25.4%). The most commonly held explanation of diffuse thickening, an extension of pulmonary fibrosis to the visceral and parietal pleura, was actually infrequent (10.2%). Among the group with diffuse thickening without asbestosis, the forced vital capacity and single-breath diffusing capacity were significantly lower than those of comparable normal persons and those with confluent plaques. (McLoud TC, Woods BO, Carrington CB, Epler GR, Gaensler EA. Diffuse pleural thickening in an asbestos-exposed population: Prevalence and causes. *AJR Am J Roentgenol* 1985;144(1):9–18.)

Ernst, Bourbeau, and Becklake, from Quebec, investigated the association between pleural disease and lung function impairment, and noted that pleural plaques are not associated with impairment unless there is accompanying parenchymal disease or blunting of the costophrenic angle, which confirmed the earlier study of McCloud and others. (Ernst P, Bourbeau J, Becklake MR. Pleural abnormality as a cause of impairment and disability. *Ann NY Acad Sci*, 1991;643:157–61.)

Ruth Lilis and others examined 2907 active and retired asbestos insulators and found that the presence of parenchymal changes only, or of pleural changes only, as factors contributing to dyspnea, did not reach the level of statistical significance in the regression analysis. (Lilis R, Miller A, Godbold J, Chan E, Selikoff IJ. Radiographic abnormalities in asbestos insulators: Effects of duration from onset of exposure and smoking. Relationships of dyspnea with parenchymal and pleural fibrosis. *Am J Ind Med* 1991;20(1):1–15.)

Israeli scientists have followed a cohort of very heavily exposed power plant workers and claim that some of these workers had deterioration of pulmonary function correlated with progression of pleural plaques. They did not address the issue of whether there was diffuse pleural disease present, which would explain any detrimental loss of lung function. Diffuse pleural disease certainly was likely to be present in a cohort with a death rate of 14% from asbestosis. (Bar-Shai A, Tiran B, Topilsky M et al. Continued progression of asbestos-related respiratory disease after more than 15 years of non-exposure. *Isr Med Assoc J* 2012;14:560–5.)

A recent French study evaluated the functional effects of isolated pleural plaques.

The study population consisted of 2743 subjects presenting with no parenchymal interstitial abnormalities on the high-resolution CT (HRCT) scan. All functional parameters studied were within normal limits for subjects presenting with isolated pleural plaques and for those presenting with no pleuropulmonary abnormalities. However, isolated parietal and/or diaphragmatic pleural plaques were associated with a significant decrease in total lung capacity (TLC) (98.1% predicted in subjects with pleural plaques vs. 101.2% in subjects free of plaques, p = 0.0494), forced vital capacity (FVC) (96.6% vs. 100.4%, p < 0.001) and forced expiratory volume in 1 s (FEV(1)) (97.9% vs. 101.9%, p = 0.0032). In contrast, no significant relationship was observed between pleural plaques and FEV1/FVC ratio, forced expiratory flow at 25–75% FVC and residual volume. A significant correlation was found between the extent of pleural plaques and the reduction in FVC and TLC, whereas plaque thickness was not related to functional impairment. The results show a relationship between isolated parietal and/or diaphragmatic pleural plaques and a trend towards a restrictive pattern, although the observed decrease in FVC and TLC is unlikely to be of real clinical relevance for the majority of subjects in this series. (Clin B, Paris C, Ameille J et al. Do asbestos-related pleural plaques on HRCT scans cause restrictive impairment in the absence of pulmonary fibrosis? *Thorax* 2011;66(11):985–91.)

The Beta Carotene and Retinol Efficacy Trial (CARET) study of 4060 asbestos-exposed workers for chemoprevention of lung cancer, followed for 9–17 years, evaluated the relationship between chest x-ray and lung function testing and asbestos exposure and smoking. Of the asbestos-exposed men, 1839 were eligible for inclusion in the heavy smoking arm (80% exposed in shipbuilding). The authors concluded that men with more than 40 years of exposure in high-risk trades had a fivefold higher risk for lung cancer than men with 5–10 years of exposure after adjusting for smoking and other risk factors. Those workers with 0–10 years in a high-risk trade had a risk of 1 as compared to 5.17 for those with the highest exposure. Only those with an ILO profusion rating of 1/0 to 1/2 had an increased risk of lung cancer when controlled for smoking. The authors claimed that there was an increased lung cancer risk without clear-cut fibrosis on chest x-ray. However, their data do not justify that claim. In fact, the data confirm that the risk of lung cancer occurs only in the presence of asbestosis.

The authors also conclude that the presence of pleural plaques doubled the risk of lung cancer in ILO-negative chest x-rays. There are major criticisms of this study since the chest x-rays were not read by National Institute for Occupational Safety and Health (NIOSH)-certified B-Readers or confirmed by HRCT, and therefore the results are unsubstantiated. All experts agree that chest x-rays are a very imprecise assessment of asbestos-related disease. (Ross RM. The clinical diagnosis of asbestosis in this century requires more than a chest radiograph. *Chest* 2003;124:120–8.) Later studies have used HRCT to develop a more accurate and specific assessment of asbestos-related abnormalities, and have not been able to confirm the conclusions of the CARET study. These authors of CARET also concluded that obstructive airways disease was a strong independent predictor of lung cancer, but ignored the data that indicated that chronic obstructive pulmonary disease (COPD) is a strong independent predictor of lung cancer in individuals without any exposure to asbestos. (Cullen MR, Barnett MJ, Balmes JR et al. Predictors of lung cancer among asbestos-exposed men in the β-Carotene and Retinol Efficacy Trial. *Am J Epidemiol* 2005;161:260–70.)

Numerous epidemiological studies have consistently linked the presence of COPD to the development of lung cancer, independently of cigarette smoking dosage or asbestos exposure. The mechanistic explanation for the increased risk of lung cancer in COPD remains poorly understood. The data do not support any role of asbestos exposure as a cause of COPD or COPD-related lung cancer. Asbestos-related pleural disease is not related to COPD. (Houghton AM. Mechanistic links between COPD and lung cancer. *Nat Rev Cancer*

2013;13(4):233–45; Roca M, Roca IC, Mihăescu T. Lung cancer—A comorbidity in chronic obstructive pulmonary disease. *Rev Med Chir Soc Med Nat Iasi* 2012;116(4):1055–62; Smith DD. Letter to the editor: Does asbestos exposure cause obstructive airways disease. *Chest* 2004;126:1000; Jones RN, Glindmeyer HW, Weil H. Review of the Kilburn and Warshaw *Chest* article—Airways obstruction from asbestos exposure. *Chest* 1995;107:1727–29.)

Subsequent studies, using more accurate and specific HRCT, by Ameille and others found that, among asbestos-exposed individuals, those having radiographic evidence of pleural plaques are at increased risk for lung cancer and pleural mesothelioma, compared to the general population. "However, there is no evidence that pleural plaque confers an increased risk of lung cancer or pleural mesothelioma within a population of individuals having the same cumulative asbestos exposure." (Ameille J, Brochard P, Letourneux M, Paris C, Pairon JC. Asbestos-related cancer risk in patients with asbestosis or pleural plaques. *Rev Mal Respir* 2011;28(6):e11–7.) Earlier studies by the same French authors using HRCT demonstrated both time–response and dose–response relationships for pleural plaques, while only dose–response relationships were demonstrated for asbestosis. (Paris C, Thierry S, Brochard P et al. Pleural plaques and asbestosis: Dose– and time–response relationships based on HRCT data. *Eur Respir J* 2009;34(1):72–9.)

A more recent French study by Pairon et al. came to a different conclusion. The study was conducted in the 5287 male subjects for whom chest CT scan data were available. Annual determination of the number of subjects eligible for free medical care because of pleural mesothelioma was carried out. Diagnosis certification was obtained from the French mesothelioma panel of pathologists. Survival regression based on the Cox model was used to estimate the risk of pleural mesothelioma associated with pleural plaques, with age as the main time variable and time-varying exposure variables, namely duration of exposure, time since first exposure, and cumulative exposure index to asbestos. All statistical tests were two-sided. A total of 17 incident cases of pleural mesothelioma were diagnosed. A statistically significant association was observed between mesothelioma and pleural plaques (unadjusted hazard ratio [HR]: 8.9, 95% confidence interval [CI]: 3.0–26.5; adjusted HR: 6.8, 95% CI: 2.2–21.4 after adjustment for time since first exposure and cumulative exposure index to asbestos). Their conclusion was that the presence of pleural plaques might be an independent risk factor for pleural mesothelioma. The problem with this study is that no comparison to individuals with the same asbestos exposure and latency period without plaques for risk of mesothelioma was conducted. Pleural plaques are a surrogate of asbestos exposure, and some plaques may not be visible on CT scanning. The risk of mesothelioma is due to the intensity, fiber type, size, and duration of asbestos exposure to amphibole asbestos, not pleural plaques. (Pairon JC, Laurent F, Rinaldo M et al. Pleural plaques and the risk of pleural mesothelioma. *J Natl Cancer Inst* 2013;105(4):293–30; Harber P, Mohsenifar Z, Oren A, Lew M. Pleural plaques and asbestos-associated malignancy. *J Occup Med* 1987;29(8):641–4; Ren H, Lee DR, Hruban RH et al. Pleural plaques do not predict asbestosis: A high-resolution computed tomography and pathology study. *Mod Pathol* 1991;4:201–9;

Hillerdal G, Malmberg P, Hemmingsson A. Asbestos-related lesions of the pleura: Parietal plaques compared to diffuse thickening studied with chest roentgenography, computed tomography, lung function, and gas exchange. *Am J Ind Med* 1990;18(6):627–3.)

Reid and others from Western Australia found those with pleural plaques shown by chest x-ray had an increase in abdominal (peritoneal) mesothelioma risk, but there was no increase in risk of pleural mesothelioma in those with pleural plaques. Specifically, after adjusting for age, time since first exposure, and cumulative exposure to asbestos, Reid found a nonsignificant adjusted odds ratio of development of pleural mesothelioma of 1.12 (95% CI: 0.61–2.07). (Reid A, de Klerk N, Ambrosini G et al. The additional risk of malignant mesothelioma in former workers and residents of Wittenoom with benign pleural disease or asbestosis. *Occup Environ Med* 2005;62(10):665–9.)

Many studies may suffer from the uncertainty in the estimated exposure level or a *recall bias*. Reid's study included residents. Residents in the crocidolite mining area of Western Australia who had no disease may still overestimate their exposure levels because of their concerns about past asbestos exposure and subsequent development of mesothelioma. Pairon's study may also suffer from the recall bias from the workers who had plaques. If they already knew they had plaques before the questions were asked about the exposure levels, they may be overestimated. This will lead to a high hazard ratio.

Albert Miller and coworkers reported pulmonary function results from a screening study population of union workers evaluated for asbestos-related disease, performed in a mobile clinic between 1997 and 2004. There was no clear information as to fiber type of asbestos, intensity of exposure, duration of exposure, asbestos product information, or work practice at time of exposure. The only information given was the number of years exposed. The group included plumbers, pipefitters, boilermakers, machinists, laborers, insulators, carpenters, electricians, and oil and chemical workers. No information was given about the numbers in each occupational group and the results of pulmonary function testing for that group. The authors concluded that both diffusing capacity and vital capacity were negatively correlated with profusion score over the full spectrum of radiographic severity. ILO profusion scores 0/1 (conventionally classified as normal) and 1/0 (conventionally classified as abnormal) were associated with similar diffusing capacity and vital capacity values. The highest profusion scores were associated with a greater proportionate decrease in diffusing capacity than in FVC. Both tests showed an effect of pleural fibrosis. The authors mentioned that one of the limitations of the study was that studying workers for medical–legal evaluation may select more impaired workers and that CT scans offer greater sensitivity and specificity than chest x-rays for evaluating pleural and parenchymal lung disease. The limitations of this study make any conclusions uninterpretable. (Miller A, Warshaw R, Nezamis J. Diffusing capacity and forced vital capacity in 5003 asbestos-exposed workers: Relationships to interstitial fibrosis (ILO profusion score) and pleural thickening. *Am J Ind Med* 2013;22:1–11.)

Dutch investigators investigated the size of pleural plaques and the relationship to asbestos exposure and disordered lung function. There was no correlation with the size of the pleural plaques, asbestos exposure, and lung function. (Van Cleemput J, De Raeve H, Verschakelen JA et al. Surface of localized pleural plaques quantitated by computed tomography scanning: No relation with cumulative asbestos exposure and no effect on lung function. *Am J Respir Crit Care Med* 2001;163:705–10.)

I personally have evaluated over 1000 patients with asbestos-related pleural disease and I have never found an example of significant impairment of lung function associated with isolated pleural plaques, without diffuse pleural disease or asbestosis. Asbestos-related diffuse pleural disease is the cause of significant impairment of lung function in many patients with pleural plaques and absent interstitial disease. It frequently is present simultaneously in patients with pleural plaques. (Smith DD. Asbestos-related pleural disease: Questions in need of answer. *Clin Pulm Med* 1994;1:289–300.)

Clark and co-investigators evaluated lung function in Libby, Montana, vermiculite miners with pleural plaques diagnosed by HRCT. Nearly 90% of miners (n = 149) had evidence of pleural plaques on HRCT. No significant differences in spirometry results, lung volumes, or diffusion of lung for carbon monoxide (DLCO) were found between miners with pleural plaques alone and miners with normal HRCT studies. Miners with both interstitial fibrosis and the presence of pleural plaques had a significantly decreased total lung capacity in comparison to miners with normal HRCT studies (p = 0.03). Age, cumulative smoking history, and body mass index (BMI) were significant covariates that contributed to abnormal lung function. The results of HRCT and complete pulmonary function test (PFT) performed between January 2000 and August 2012 were obtained from medical records of 166 Libby, Montana, vermiculite miners. Multivariate regression analyses with Tukey multivariate adjustment was used to assess statistical associations between the presence of pleural plaques and lung function. Adjustments were made for age, BMI, smoking history, duration of employment, and years since last occupational asbestos exposure. Nearly 90% of miners (n = 149) had evidence of pleural plaques on HRCT. *No significant differences in spirometry results, lung volumes, or DLCO were found between miners with pleural plaques alone and miners with normal HRCT studies.* Miners with both interstitial fibrosis and the presence of pleural plaques had a significantly decreased total lung capacity in comparison to miners with normal HRCT studies (p = 0.03). Age, cumulative smoking history, and BMI were significant covariates that contributed to abnormal lung function. (Clark KA, Flynn JJ 3rd, Goodman JE et al. Pleural plaques and their effect on lung function in Libby vermiculite mine. *Chest* 2014;146(3):786–94.) This was a well done study that again concludes that isolated pleural plaques do not impair lung function.

Larson et al. noted that no significant differences were found with regard to measures of exposure in Libby, Montana, vermiculite workers, between workers with, and those without, progression of their pleural disease. (Larson TC, Meyer CA, Kapil V et al. Workers with Libby amphibole exposure: Retrospective identification and progression of radiographic changes. *Radiology* 2010;255(3):924–33.)

Another important issue has been conflicting claims as to the association of pleural plaques and an increased risk of lung cancer or mesothelioma. The controversy was largely related to the imprecision of using chest x-rays to evaluate asbestos-related pleural disease. HRCT has proven to be more sensitive and specific in the assessment of asbestos-related pleural and parenchymal disease. (Peacock C, Copley SJ, Hansell DM. Asbestos-related benign pleural disease. *Clin Radiol* 2000;55(6):422–32; Neri S, Antonelli A, Falaschi F, Boraschi P, Baschieri L. Findings from high resolution computed tomography of the lung and pleura of symptom free workers exposed to amosite who had normal chest radiographs and pulmonary function tests. *Occup Environ Med* 1994;51:239–43; Ren H, Lee DR, Hruban RH et al. Pleural plaques do not predict asbestosis: High-resolution computed tomography and pathology study. *Mod Pathol* 1991;4(2):201–9; Smith DD. Plaques, cancer, and confusion. *Chest* 1994;105(1):8–9; Solomon A. Radiological features of asbestos-related visceral pleural changes. *Am J Ind Med* 1991;19:339–55; Janower ML, Berlin L. "B" readers' radiographic interpretations in asbestos litigation: Is something rotten in the courtroom? *Acad Radiol* 2004;11(8):841–2.)

It is the intensity, fiber type, fiber size, and duration of asbestos exposure that determine risk of any asbestos-related malignancy, not pleural plaques. If you make the distinction in individuals, without adequately correcting for asbestos exposure, then pleural plaques, confirmed by HRCT, may confer an increased risk for mesothelioma since pleural plaques are only a surrogate for asbestos exposure. Amphibole asbestos exposure is the cause of mesothelioma, not pleural plaques. (Smith DD. Plaques, cancer, and confusion. *Chest* 1994;105(1):8–9.) This was confirmed by a French study among asbestos-exposed individuals, with those having radiographic evidence of pleural plaques being at increased risk for lung cancer and pleural mesothelioma, compared to the general population. However, there is no evidence that pleural plaques confer an increased risk of lung cancer or pleural mesothelioma within a population of individuals having the same cumulative asbestos exposure. (Ameille J, Brochard P, Letourneux M, Paris C, Pairon JC. Asbestos-related cancer risk in patients with asbestosis or pleural plaques. *Rev Mal Respir* 2011;28(6):e11–7.)

Diffuse pleural thickening, or diffuse pleural fibrosis, involves primarily the visceral pleura and the fusion with the parietal pleura, which may impair lung function. It is usually asymptomatic but may be associated with episodes of pleurisy. It is thought to be the result of a previous pleural effusion from any cause. Diffuse pleural disease may be associated with parenchymal bands, crow's feet, rounded atelectasis, and mild focal subpleural parenchymal fibrosis. (Solomon A, Webster I. The visceral pleura in asbestosis. *Environ Res* 1976;11(1):128–34; Stephens M, Gibbs AR, Pooley FD, Wagner JC. Asbestos-induced diffuse pleural fibrosis: Pathology and mineralogy. *Thorax* 1987;42:583.) A prior history of an asbestos-related pleural effusion is common. Focal rales can be present over some areas of pleural fibrosis. Diffuse pleural disease can progress episodically and decrements in lung function may occur in a stair-step fashion, rather than the linear fashion that would be typical of asbestosis. Because the pleural reaction is on the surface of the lung, there can be sub-pleural interlobular thickening and curvilinear lines, as well as parenchymal bands developing that can cause confusion with asbestosis. These pleural/parenchymal reactions are generally focal and just adjacent to the pleural reaction. Asbestosis is a generalized disease associated

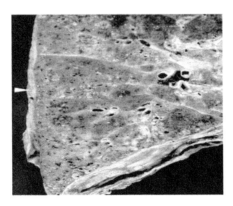

Figure 8.3 Diffuse pleural thickening. (Adapted from Leslie KO, Wick MR. *Practical Pulmonary Pathology*. Philadelphia: Elsevier, 2005.)

with bilateral, largely symmetrical changes of interstitial fibrosis, which differentiates it from asbestos-related inflammatory pleural disease, which tends to be focal and unilateral (Figure 8.3). (Gevenois PA, de Maertelaer V, Madani A, Winant C, Sergent G, De Vuyst P. Asbestosis, pleural plaques and diffuse pleural thickening: Three distinct benign responses to asbestos exposure. *Eur Respir J* 1998;11(5):1021–7; Yates DH, Browne K, Stidolf PN, Neville E. Asbestos-related bilateral diffuse pleural thickening: Natural history of radiographic and lung function abnormalities. *Am J Respir Crit Care Med* 1996;153:301–6; Smith KA, Sykes LJ, McGavin CR. "Diffuse pleural fibrosis—An unreliable indicator of heavy asbestos exposure?" *Scand J Work Environ Health* 2003;29(1):60–3.)

Jeebun and Stenton studied 75 patients with asbestos-related diffuse pleural disease from 1992 to 2007. They defined diffuse pleural fibrosis to be present if there was obliteration of the costophrenic angle in continuity with at least 3 mm of pleural thickening, in accordance with the International Labor Organization 2000 classification. The median latency for development of diffuse pleural fibrosis from first asbestos exposure was 34 years. A total of 73% of patients had unilateral disease at presentation, and 24% of these were observed to develop contralateral disease after a median of 2 years. Unilateral pleural disease was most common on the right. A total of 40% of patients presented with pleural effusions preceding the development of diffuse pleural thickening. The median latency for development of pleural effusions from onset of exposures was 38 years. A total of 80% of the pleural effusions were unilateral. Once established, pleural thickening was reported to have remained stable in 91% on the ipsilateral side. (Jeebun V, Stenton SC. The presentation and natural history of asbestos-induced diffuse pleural thickening. *Occup Med (Lond)* 2012;62(4):266–8.)

There are many causes of diffuse pleural scarring, which makes diffuse pleural disease less specific for asbestos-related changes. Tuberculosis, with or without pneumothorax treatment, hemothorax, empyema, chest trauma, collagen vascular disease, rheumatoid arthritis, retroperitoneal fibrosis, postpericardotomy syndrome (Dressler's syndrome), various other mineral dust exposures, and other causes of an inflammatory reactions in the pleural space can all cause x-ray or

HRCT changes that are indistinguishable from asbestos-related pleural disease. Unilateral diffuse pleural disease, with or without pleural calcification, is commonly seen from a variety of causes and should not be considered to be related to asbestos exposure if the contralateral lung and pleura are normal. Pleural calcification may occur from any cause of diffuse pleural disease. Small left-sided pleural effusions following cardiac surgery are common, and a common cause of left-sided pleural scarring, and may be followed by rounded atelectasis. Mild restrictive lung function impairment is common in patients with diffuse pleural thickening and can occur from any cause of diffuse pleural thickening, but severe impairment is very uncommon. The diagnosis is further complicated by the occasional simultaneous presence of asbestosis in heavily exposed workers.

Pleural plaques need to be distinguished from diffuse pleural disease. Diffuse pleural disease generally suggests a higher asbestos exposure and consequently a greater risk for mesothelioma than pleural plaques alone. It may be associated with a short or long latency of 40–50 years. (Pairon JC, Laurent F, Rinaldo M et al. Pleural plaques and the risk of pleural mesothelioma. *J Natl Cancer Inst* 2013;105(4):293–301.) For more detail, please consult my editorial in *Chest*. (Smith DD. Plaques, cancer, and confusion. *Chest* 1994;105:8–9; Smith DD. Diagnosis and initial management of nonmalignant diseases related to asbestos. *Am J Respir Crit Care Med* 2005;171:665–6; Smith DD. Asbestos-related pleural disease: Questions in need of answers. *Clin Pulm Med* 1994;1:289–300; Ameille J, Brochard P, Letourneux M, Paris C, Pairon JC. Asbestos-related cancer risk in patients with asbestosis or pleural plaques. *Rev Mal Respir* 2011;28(6):e11–7; Miles SE, Sandrini A, Johnson AR, Yates DH. Clinical consequences of asbestos-related diffuse pleural thickening: A review. *Am J Ind Med* 2009;52(8):596–602; Jeebun V, Stenton SC. The presentation and natural history of asbestos-induced diffuse pleural thickening. *Occup Med (Lond)* 2012;62(4):266–8; McLoud TC, Woods BO, Carrington CB, Epler GR, Gaensler EA. Diffuse pleural thickening in an asbestos-exposed population: Prevalence and causes. *Am J Roentgenol* 1985;144:9–18; Weiss W. Asbestos-related pleural plaques and lung cancer. *Chest* 1993;103:1854–9.)

Not all studies agree that workers with asbestos-related diffuse pleural disease have had heavier exposures to asbestos. Smith and coworkers measured the asbestos burden for 192 naval dockyard workers (96 with diffuse pleural fibrosis and 96 with plaques) by calculating the exposure ratings from the trade and the years spent in that trade. In 53 cases, the diffuse pleural fibrosis was bilateral. The mean exposure ratings for diffuse pleural fibrosis do not differ from those for pleural plaques, although the ratings are significantly higher for men with bilateral diffuse pleural fibrosis than for those with unilateral diffuse pleural fibrosis. The authors concluded that diffuse pleural fibrosis cannot be used as a reliable marker of heavy asbestos exposure. (Smith KA, Sykes LJ, McGavin CR. Diffuse pleural fibrosis—An unreliable indicator of heavy asbestos exposure? *Scand J Work Environ Health* 2003;29(1):60–3.)

Some radiologists incorrectly confuse these pleural/parenchymal changes of asbestos-related diffuse pleural disease such as crow's feet, parenchymal bands, ground glass changes, and changes from rounded atelectasis with asbestosis. I have called these changes *pseudo-asbestosis* as opposed to true bilateral lower-lobe symmetrical parenchymal fibrosis from asbestosis. HRCT is usually adequate for distinguishing diffuse parenchymal disease (asbestosis) from the inflammatory pleural-based focal changes of diffuse pleural disease. In rare cases, an autopsy or exploratory thoracotomy is necessary to determine the complete diagnosis. (Smith DD. Asbestos-related pleural disease: Questions in need of answers. *Clin Pulm Med* 1994;1:289–300.)

Diffuse pleural disease from any cause may cause impaired lung function. An Australian group studied the functional effects of diffuse pleural disease and/or rounded atelectasis in 25 patients with abnormal lung function on the 6-minute walk test (6MWT). They concluded that the 6MWT was useful in predicting the health quality of life. (Dale MT, McKeough ZJ, Munoz PA et al. Functional exercise capacity and health-related quality of life in people with asbestos related pleural disease: An observational study. *BMC Pulm Med.* 2013;13:1; Miller A. Asbestos-related bilateral diffuse pleural thickening: Natural history of radiographic and lung function abnormalities. *Am J Respir Crit Care Med* 1996;154(6 Pt 1):1919–20; Kee ST, Gamsu G, Blanc P. Causes of pulmonary impairment in asbestos-exposed individuals with diffuse pleural thickening. *Am J Respir Crit Care Med* 1996;154(3 Pt 1):789–93; Cotes JE, King B. Relationship of lung function to radiographic reading (ILO) in patients with asbestos related lung disease. *Thorax* 1988;43(10):777–83; McGavin CR, Sheers G. Diffuse pleural thickening in asbestos workers: Disability and lung function abnormalities. *Thorax* 1984;39(8):604–7; Lumley KP. Physiological changes in asbestos pleural disease. *Inhaled Part* 1975;4(Pt 2):781–8; Fujimoto N, Kato K, Usami I et al. Asbestos-related diffuse pleural thickening. *Respiration* 2014;88(4):277–84.)

Investigators from Thessaloniki, Greece, studied 266 out of the total 317 employees who had worked in an asbestos cement factory during the period 1968–2004, with chest x-ray, HRCT, and lung function tests. Abnormal HRCT findings were found in 75 subjects (67%) and were related to age, occupational exposure duration, and spirometric data. The presence of parenchymal or visceral pleural lesions (exclusively or as the predominant abnormality) was accompanied by lower total lung capacity and diffusion capacity. HRCT was much more sensitive than chest x-ray for occupational chrysotile exposure. Lung function impairment was related to parenchymal but not to pleural HRCT abnormalities. (Spyratos D, Chloros D, Haidich B et al. Chest imaging and lung function impairment after long-term occupational exposure to low concentrations of chrysotile. *Arch Environ Occup Health* 2012;67(2):84–90.)

The most recent systematic review of the question as to whether pleural plaques alone, without diffuse pleural disease, pleural effusions, or asbestosis, can cause lung function impairment concluded that pleural plaques were not associated with changes in lung function over time in longitudinal studies. The weight of evidence indicates that pleural plaques do not impact lung function. Observed associations are most likely due to unidentified abnormalities or other factors. (Kerper LE, Lynch HN, Zu K, Tao G, Utell MJ, Goodman J. Systematic review of pleural plaques and lung function. *Inhal Toxicol* 2015;27(1):15–44.)

Asbestos-related benign pleural effusion is related to an intermediate or heavy level of exposure to asbestos and patients may be asymptomatic or symptomatic.

(Epler GR, McLoud TC, Gaensler EA. Prevalence and incidence of benign asbestos pleural effusion in a working population. *JAMA* 1982;247(5):617–22.) Epler et al. found that the prevalence was dose related with 7.0%, 3.7%, and 0.2% effusions with severe, indirect, and peripheral exposure, respectively. "The latency period was shorter than for other asbestos-related disorders. Benign effusion was the most common asbestos-related abnormality during the first 20 years after exposure. Incidence studies showed 9.2 effusions per 1000 person-years for level III exposure, 3.9 for level II, and 0.7 for level I. Most effusions were small; 28.6% recurred, and 66% were asymptomatic." More recent experience has noted that benign pleural effusions have a much longer latency than initially reported by Epler et al. It is not uncommon to see benign pleural effusions with a latency of 40–50 years after exposure. Benign asbestos-related pleural effusions was thought to suggest an intermediate level of exposure and a significant risk for mesothelioma. (Chapman SJ, Cookson WO, Musk AW, Lee YC. Benign asbestos pleural diseases. *Curr Opin Pulm Med* 2003;9(4):266–71; Jamrozik E, de Klerk N, Musk AW. Asbestos-related disease. *Intern Med J* 2011;41(5):372–80.)

The effusions are usually unilateral and small to moderate in size. The pleural fluid is an exudate with low concentrations of white cells and low concentrations of adenosine deaminase. The cytology is negative and biopsy shows only non-specific inflammation. An occult mesothelioma or lung cancer cannot be excluded until the condition has stabilized for 2–3 years. Long-term follow-up reveals a return of the effusion in about 20% and the development of a mesothelioma in approximately 5%. HB Eisenstadt, a practicing pulmonologist in Port Arthur, Texas, was one of the first to describe several cases of asbestos-related pleural effusions in asbestos-exposed refinery workers. (*Am Pract* 1962;13:573; *Dis Chest* 1964;46:78; *JAMA* 1965;192:419; *Ann NY Acad Sci* 1965;132:595; *N Engl J Med* 1974;290:1025.)

Rounded atelectasis, Blesovsky syndrome, pulmonary pseudotumour, or shrinking pleuritis with atelectasis is associated with chronic inflammatory pleural effusions from any cause, particularly following open-heart surgery, Dressler syndrome, pulmonary infarction, or parapneumonic or tuberculous effusions. Remember that rounded atelectasis is not specific for asbestos exposure. The inflammatory pleural reaction entraps the peripheral lung by infolding in a spiral fashion, often leaving a comet trail reaction in the adjacent lung. This appears as a swirling of vessels and bronchi converging at the hilum of the lung. The mass produced is commonly confused with various types of lung neoplasms. It usually presents as a single mass, but multiple lesions may occur. It was described in Germany in the 1920s but the association with asbestos exposure was not made until 1966 by Blesovsky. It is usually asymptomatic and must be differentiated from a lung cancer. Surgery may be indicated and helpful if there is significant physiological lung function impairment. (Loeschke H. *Storungen des Lufgehalis der lunge. In Henke-Lubarsch. Handbuck der Speceziellen Pathologischen Anataomie und Histologie III/I.* Berlin: Springer, 1928; Blesovsky A. The folded lung. *Br J Chest* 1966;60:19–22; Hillerdal G. Rounded atelectasis: Clinical experience with 74 patients. *Chest* 1989;95:836–41; Stahopoulos GT, Karamessini MT, Sotiriadi AE, Pastromas VG. Rounded atelectasis of the lung. *Respir Med* 2005;99:615–23;

Dernevik L, Gatzinsky P. Pathogenesis of shrinking pleuritis with atelectasis—"Rounded atelectasis." *Eur J Respir Dis* 1987;71:244–49; Menzies R, Fraser R. Rounded atelectasis: Pathologic and pathogenic features. *Am J Surg Pathol* 1987;11:674–81; Stathopoulos GT, Karamessini MT, Sotiriadi AE, Pastromas VG. Rounded atelectasis of the lung. *Respir Med* 2005;99(5):615–23; Batra P, Brown K, Hayashi K et al. Rounded atelectasis. *J Thorac Imaging* 1996;11:187–97; Mintzer RA, Cugell DW. The association of asbestos induced pleural disease and rounded atelectasis. *Chest* 1982;81:457–60; Chung-Park M, Tomashefski JF Jr, Cohen AM, el-Gazzar M, Cotes EE. Shrinking pleuritis with lobar atelectasis, a morphologic variant of "round atelectasis." *Hum Pathol* 1989;20(4):382–7; Sobocińska M, Sobociński B, Jarzemska A, Serafin Z. Rounded atelectasis of the lung: A pictorial review. *Pol J Radiol* 2014;79:203–9.)

Asbestos-related pleuritis may rarely involve the pericardium and cause asbestos-related *pericarditis, pericardial effusion, and constrictive pericarditis,* as can a malignant mesothelioma. In my clinical experience, mesothelioma involving the pericardium is the most common cause of pericardial disease in the asbestos-exposed population and must always be excluded prior to making a diagnosis of a benign asbestos-related pericardial effusion. (Davies D, Andrews MI, Jones JS. Asbestos induced pericardial effusion and constrictive pericarditis. *Thorax* 1991;46(6):429–32; Abejie BA, Chung EH, Nesto RW, Kales SN. Grand rounds: Asbestos-related pericarditis in a boiler operator. *Environ Health Perspect* 2008;116(1):86–9; Roggeri A, Tomasi C, Cavazza A, Serra L, Zucchi L. Haemorrhagic pericardial effusion in an asbestos worker. *Med Lav* 2003;94(4):391–4; Fernandes R, Nosib S, Thomson D, Baniak N. A rare cause of heart failure with preserved ejection fraction: Primary pericardial mesothelioma masquerading as pericardial constriction. *BMJ Case Rep* 2014; Belli E, Landolfo K. Primary pericardial mesothelioma: A rare cause of constrictive pericarditis. *Asian Cardiovasc Thorac Ann* 2015;23(5):599–600.)

Finally, there have been studies of the incidence of *retroperitoneal fibrosis* and asbestos exposure suggesting asbestos as a significant contributing factor. A history of asbestos exposure was associated with idiopathic retroperitoneal fibrosis (odds ratio: 4.22; 95% CI: 2.14–8.33). Exposure to asbestos and tobacco smoke resulted in strong risk factors for idiopathic retroperitoneal fibrosis. Coexposure to asbestos and smoke had a multiplicative effect on risk compared with single exposure. (Goldoni M, Bonini S, Urban ML et al. Asbestos and smoking as risk factors for idiopathic retroperitoneal fibrosis: A case–control study. *Ann Intern Med* 2014;161(3):181–8; Uibu T, Oksa P, Auvinen A et al. Asbestos exposure as a risk factor for retroperitoneal fibrosis. *Lancet* 2004;363(9419):1422–6.)

9

Disability and impairment in asbestosis and asbestos-related diffuse pleural disease

Why are lung function tests important? Lung function predicts not only disability but also mortality. Vehmas and coworkers studied a total of 590 workers, originally screened for occupational lung disease, including spirometry and pulmonary diffusing capacity measurements, and were followed-up for mortality data (International Classification of Diseases-10 classification). The mean follow-up time was 10.5 years. Associations of different lung function parameters with mortality from all causes and from cardiovascular and nonmalignant respiratory diseases were analyzed. Factor analysis was used to create obstructive and restrictive factors. A total of 191 deaths were found altogether. Most measured lung function variables were associated with increased mortality when studied separately. Both decreased forced expiratory flow in one second (hazard ratio/measurement unit: 0.977; 95% confidence interval [CI]: 0.969–0.988; $p < 0.001$) and impaired diffusing capacity (hazard ratio/measurement unit: 0.973; 95% CI: 0.965–0.981; $p < 0.001$) were independently associated with mortality from all causes, as well as from cardiovascular and nonmalignant respiratory diseases. Both, obstructive factor alone, and the sum of obstructive and restrictive factors, were associated with all studied mortality categories. The restrictive factor alone was associated with all-cause and respiratory mortality. Deteriorated lung function predicts deaths. (Vehmas T, Pallasaho P, Piirilä P. Lung function predicts mortality: 10-year follow-up after lung cancer screening among asbestos-exposed workers. *Int Arch Occup Environ Health* 2013;86(6):667–72; Moshammer H, Neuberger M. Lung function predicts survival in a cohort of asbestos cement workers. *Int Arch Occup Environ Health* 2009;82:199–207.)

Disability and impairment are confusing terms. Impairment means a reduction in a physiologic value below the lower limit of the normal predicted value, based on that person's age, sex, race, and height. An individual may have a significant impairment of lung function when compared with a normal person, but not have any evidence of any disability. Disability is a term used to describe an inability to perform normal activities. The amount of lung function impairment necessary to cause disability in a coal miner doing heavy work is going to be much more than a banker who may have very significant loss of function but not be disabled from his usual sedentary occupation. *Disability does not mean inability.* Motivation is critical if impaired individuals are likely to return to work. I have had patients continue to work with severe lung function impairment in a sedentary job on continuous oxygen therapy. This patient was physiologically disabled but not functionally disabled. Motivation, pain tolerance, and the importance of feeling needed in a job are parameters that affect employability but are difficult to quantitate. Disability is often multifactorial due to a constellation of medical problems that are also age related, such as peripheral vascular disease, pulmonary hypertension, cardiovascular disease, obesity, diabetic peripheral neuropathy, depression, cognitive problems, back problems, neuromuscular disease, previous strokes or other serious illnesses, and lack of general physical conditioning.

Impairment is a term that describes loss of organ function. The disability from the loss of lung function may be insignificant. Small reductions or impairments in lung function are often asymptomatic. The average person functions reasonably well if they have had a total removal of one lung, if the remaining lung is functionally normal. Once the lung function tests are below 50% of predicted, then small further reductions in lung function will produce disproportional increases in shortness of breath and disability. (Smith DD. Pulmonary impairment/disability evaluation: Controversies and criticisms. *Clin Pulm Med* 1995;2:334–43.)

Exercise intolerance is a condition in which the individual is unable to perform a physical exercise at the intensity or the duration that would be expected from someone of their age, sex, height, race, and general physical condition. The inability to perform exercise is generally related either to a cardiovascular, respiratory, neurological, or peripheral muscle disorder. When the inability to perform exercise is caused by impaired function of one or more of the major physiological systems, namely the respiratory, the cardiovascular, or the peripheral muscle metabolic system, the result is the amplification of the perceptions of respiratory discomfort, either alone or typically in conjunction with peripheral muscle discomfort/fatigue. In patients with chronic lung diseases, dyspnea sensations are exaggerated during exercise, secondary to the reduced breathing efficiency that results from the deteriorating ventilatory mechanics on the one hand and the increased ventilatory requirements on the other hand.

Exercise testing on a treadmill may produce a reduction in oxygen tension in early interstitial lung disease from a variety of causes. Unfortunately, this diagnostic test is not useful in detecting early asbestosis. Abnormalities in oxygen transport are more common in idiopathic pulmonary fibrosis (IPF). The differences in oxygen transport between asbestosis and IPF may reflect the lower level of inflammation in asbestosis as compared with IPF. (Smith D, Agostoni P, Butler J. The discriminatory value of gas transport abnormalities for asbestosis in asbestos workers. *Chest* 1987;9:305.) The test is abnormal late in the disease when other tests have already become abnormal. Breathlessness is very subjective and there is a poor correlation between a patient's complaint of breathlessness and their exercise performance on a treadmill. (Agostoni P, Smith D, Schoene R, Robertson T, Butler J. Evaluation of breathlessness in asbestos workers: Results of exercise testing. *Am Rev Respir Dis* 1987;135:812–6; Sue D, Oren A, Hansen JE, Wassserman K. Lung function and exercise performance in smoking and nonsmoking asbestos exposed workers. *Am Rev Respir Dis* 1985;132:612–8.)

In all chronic lung diseases, physical activity limitation is multifactorial, involving respiratory, hemodynamic, and peripheral muscle abnormalities. The mechanisms of limitation relate to (1) the imbalance between ventilatory capacity and demand; (2) the imbalance between energy demand and supply to working respiratory and peripheral muscles; and (3) the factors that induce peripheral muscle dysfunction. In practice, intolerable exertional symptoms (i.e., dyspnea) and/or leg discomfort are the main symptoms that limit physical performance in patients with chronic lung diseases. Furthermore, the reduced capacity for physical work and the adoption of a sedentary lifestyle in an attempt to avoid breathlessness upon physical exertion cause profound muscle deconditioning, which in turn leads to disability and loss of functional independence. Accordingly, physical inactivity is an important component of worsening the patient's quality of life and contributes importantly to poor prognosis. Identifying the factors that prevent a patient with lung disease from easily carrying out activities of daily living, provides a unique as well as important perspective for the choice of the appropriate therapeutic strategy. (Vogiatzis I, Zakynthinos G, Andrianopoulos V. Mechanisms of physical activity limitation in chronic lung diseases. *Pulm Med* 2012;2012:634761.)

The Cardiovascular Health Study, a longitudinal cohort of 5888 older adults, was performed in order to determine the confounding factors in pulmonary disability. Categories of lung function (normal, restricted, borderline, mild–moderate, and severe obstruction) were delineated by baseline spirometry (without bronchodilator). Disability-free years were calculated as total years alive and without self-report of difficulty performing at year 1. Instrumental activities of daily living were assessed over 6 years of follow-up. Using linear regression, the authors compared disability-free years by lung disease category, adjusting for demographic factors, body mass index, smoking, cognition, and other chronic comorbidities. Among participants with airflow obstruction, they examined the association of respiratory factors (forced expiratory volume in 1 second [FEV1] and dyspnea) and nonrespiratory factors (ischemic heart disease, congestive heart failure, diabetes, muscle weakness, osteoporosis, depression, and cognitive impairment) on disability-free years. The results showed that the average number of disability-free years were 4.0 out of a possible 6 years. Severe obstruction was associated with one fewer disability-free year compared to normal spirometry in the adjusted model. For the 1048 participants with airway obstruction, both respiratory factors (FEV1 and dyspnea) and nonrespiratory factors (heart disease, coronary artery disease, diabetes, depression, osteoporosis, cognitive function, and weakness) were associated with decreased disability-free years. The study concluded that severe obstruction is associated with greater disability compared to patients with normal spirometry. Both respiratory and nonrespiratory factors contribute to disability in older adults with abnormal spirometry. (Locke E, Thielke S, Diehr P et al. Effects of respiratory and nonrespiratory factors on disability among older adults with airway obstruction: The Cardiovascular Health Study. *COPD* 2013;10(5):588–96.)

Investigators from Thessaloniki, Greece, studied 266 out of a total of 317 employees who had worked in an asbestos cement factory during the period 1968–2004 with chest x-ray, high-resolution computed tomography (HRCT), and lung function tests. Abnormal HRCT findings were found in 75 subjects (67%) and were related to age, occupational exposure duration, and spirometric data. The presence of parenchymal or visceral pleural lesions (exclusively or as the predominant abnormality) was accompanied by lower total lung capacity and diffusion capacity. HRCT was much more sensitive than chest x-ray for occupational chrysotile exposure. Lung function impairment was related to parenchymal but not to pleural HRCT abnormalities. (Spyratos D, Chloros D, Haidich B et al. Chest imaging and lung function impairment after long-term occupational exposure to low concentrations of chrysotile. *Arch Environ Occup Health* 2012;67(2):84–90.)

Measurements of lung function are commonly used to determine physiologic impairment. These measurements have some limitations in that they require good patient cooperation and effort. Exercise testing is a better measurement of disability in a cooperative patient in that it incorporates the physiologic function of not only the lungs, but also the cardiovascular system, peripheral vascular system, and neuromuscular system. Lung function tests, such as spirometry with flow volume curves, bronchodilator tests, bronchial provocation tests, measurements of lung volumes, arterial blood gas studies at rest and during exercise, the determination of maximal inspiration and expiratory pressures, and measurements of diffusion are very useful as diagnostic tools in a variety of different lung conditions.

The single-breath carbon monoxide diffusing capacity is very useful in the diagnosis of interstitial lung disease. The test measures the capillary blood volume of the lungs. The test requires a good inspiration and a breath hold for 10 seconds since the measurement is proportional to the size of the breath of the participant and breath holding time. It is also affected by the amount of hemoglobin in the blood since it measures the uptake of carbon monoxide by hemoglobin in the red blood cells. The test should be corrected for anemia when present, and also corrected for carbon monoxide backpressure related to cigarette or cigar smoking. The prediction formula for diffusion should use values adjusted for cigarette smoking. Even when the predicted values are corrected for smoking, the actual values may be lower than predicted because smoking causes interstitial abnormalities related to respiratory bronchiolitis. (Caminati A, Cavazza A, Sverzellati N, Harari S. An integrated approach in the diagnosis of smoking-related interstitial lung diseases. *Eur Respir Rev* 2012;21(125):207–17; Caminati A, Graziano P, Sverzellati N, Harari S. Smoking-related interstitial lung diseases. *Pathologica* 2010;102(6):525–36.)

The value of the single-breath diffusion test, when properly corrected for anemia, inspiratory breath volume, and resting carboxyhemoglobin, is that it may indicate pulmonary vascular disorders, emphysema, or early interstitial disease when the spirometry and lung volumes are normal. When the test values are reduced in the presence of a restrictive type of lung disease, it is often suggestive of some type of interstitial lung disease. Severe restrictive disease, such as those related to diffuse pleural disease, may also be associated with a reduction of diffusion largely related to a low inspiratory capacity rather than interstitial lung disease. Increased lung volumes in the company of airflow obstruction and the presence of a reduced diffusing capacity suggest significant emphysema. An elevated diffusing capacity can occasionally be seen in asthma, obesity, and intrapulmonary hemorrhage. (Puente Maestú L, García de Pedro J. Lung function tests in clinical decision-making. *Arch Bronconeumol* 2012;48(5):161–9.)

James Pearle investigated the radiologic–physiologic correlations in 131 asbestos-exposed shipyard workers in 1982. He found that both, exposure to asbestos and smoking, contributed to the frequency of abnormalities in forced expiratory volume in one second (FEV1) and forced vital capacity (FVC). In contrast, airways obstruction (FEV1/FVC less than 70%) was unrelated to exposure, but correlated closely with smoking. Abnormalities in DLCO were minimally associated with asbestos exposure, but were strongly related to smoking history, suggesting that diffusion impairment in these workers is more likely to be related to smoking and emphysema than to interstitial disease. Significant roentgenographic pleural abnormalities were associated with both duration of exposure and smoking. Interstitial disease did not correlate with exposure and was only mildly associated with smoking. Smoking contributes to many of the functional and roentgenographic abnormalities in asbestos-exposed workers. Subsequent to this article, several other epidemiologic studies have confirmed that cigarette smoking without asbestos exposure caused increased interstitial markings and reduced diffusion. (Pearle JL. Smoking and duration of asbestos exposure in the production of functional and roentgenographic abnormalities in shipyard workers. *J Occup Med* 1982;24(1):37–40; Cullen MR, Barnett MJ, Balmes JR et al. Predictors of lung cancer among asbestos-exposed men in the Beta-Carotene and Retinol Efficacy Trial. *Am J Epidemiol* 2005;161(3):260–70.)

Algranti and coworkers studied the decline in lung function in asbestos cement workers and its relation to cigarette smoking. A group of 502 former asbestos cement workers with at least two spirometry tests 4 years apart was assessed. Repeated evaluations included respiratory symptoms questionnaire, spirometry, and chest imaging. Asbestos exposure was ascertained as years of exposure, an index of cumulative exposure and latency time. The mixed-effects model was used to evaluate the effect of exposure on the level and rate of change in FEV1 and FVC. The FEV1 level was significantly related to pack-years of smoking at entry and during the follow-up, the index of cumulative asbestos exposure at entry, and the presence of asbestosis at follow-up. The FVC level was also significantly related to pack-years of smoking during the follow-up, cumulative asbestos exposure at entry, asbestosis and pleural thickening at follow-up, and body mass index at entry. Asbestos exposure was not associated with increasing rates of FEV1 and FVC decline. However, FEV1 regression slopes with age, estimated by terciles of cumulative exposure, showed significant differences. The combined effects of smoking and exposure conferred further acceleration in lung function decline. Occupational exposure in the asbestos cement industry was a risk factor for increased lung function decline. The effect seemed to be mostly concentrated during the working period. Smoking and exposure had synergic effects. (Algranti E, Mendonça EM, Hnizdo E et al. Longitudinal decline in lung function in former asbestos exposed workers. *Occup Environ Med* 2013;70:15–21.) Based on a study of 3600 workers, Ameille and colleagues presented results that did not support a causal relationship between asbestos exposure alone and airway obstruction. (Ameille J, Letourneux M, Paris C et al. Does asbestos exposure cause airway obstruction, in the absence of confirmed asbestosis? *Am J Respir Crit Care Med* 2010;182(4):526–30.)

Restrictive lung function does increase mortality. A total of 590 workers originally screened for occupational lung disease, including spirometry and pulmonary diffusing capacity measurements, were followed-up for mortality data. Both obstructive factor alone and the sum of obstructive and restrictive factors were associated with all studied mortality categories. The restrictive factor alone was associated with all-cause and respiratory mortality. The authors' conclusions were that deteriorated lung function predicts deaths. (Vehmas T, Pallasaho P, Piirilä P. Lung function predicts mortality: 10-year follow-up after lung cancer screening among asbestos-exposed workers. *Int Arch Occup Environ Health* 2013;86(6):667–72.)

British authors evaluated thin-section computed tomography (CT) to determine the extent of asbestos-induced pleuropulmonary disease and emphysema. They found that these factors correlated significantly with physiologic impairment ($p < 0.001$). Combined CT variables predicted 58% and 57% of the variability in total lung capacity (TLC) and DLCO, respectively, despite considerable variation in the proportion of coexisting pathologic conditions. When predictive equations with CT variables derived from the initial study group were applied to the subsequent study group, predicted TLC (rho = 0.75; $p < 0.001$) and DLCO (rho = 0.64; $p < 0.001$) correlated strongly with measured values. This correlation between radiologic abnormalities and lung function was to be expected. Radiologic findings suggest the need for more accurate pulmonary function assessment. (Copley SJ, Lee YC, Hansell DM et al. Asbestos-induced and smoking-related disease: Apportioning pulmonary function deficit by using thin-section CT. *Radiology* 2007;242(1):258–66.)

The measurement of static lung compliance has been suggested as a more sensitive method for evaluating restrictive lung disease in asbestos-exposed workers. A comparative study was performed in patients having only parietal pleural plaques, and those having asbestosis and visceral pleural fibrosis showed significant decreases in static lung compliance, diffusing capacity, and vital capacity. Visceral pleural thickening was also associated with significantly reduced FEV1, mid expiatory flow at 50% of FVC [MEF(50)], and FEV1:FVC ratios. Multiple regression analyses indicated that the existence of visceral pleural fibrosis ($p = 0.017$) is the most important factor accounting for a decrease in static compliance. Reference values of static lung compliance differ notably. In comparison with mean reference values, the sensitivity of detecting reduced lung compliance was calculated to be between 9.7% and 45.5%. Other respiratory function variables failed to show any significant differences. The authors concluded that their data indicated that the measurement of static compliance is not sufficient or as senative as hoped for the early detection of pulmonary function impairment in patients with parietal pleural plaques. (Schneider J, Arhelger R, Raab W, Hering KG. The validity of static lung compliance in asbestos-induced diseases. *Lung* 2012;190(4):441–9.)

The determination of a diffusing capacity is also dependent on the use of appropriate prediction values. The diffusing capacity rises with elevation. The use of values obtained in Salt Lake City, Utah, which are elevated compared to values obtained near sea level, may produce a false appearance of abnormality. (Smith DD. Pulmonary impairment/disability evaluation: Controversies and criticisms. *Clin Pulm Med* 1995;2:334–43; Smith DD. What is asbestosis? *Chest* 1990;98:963–4; American Thoracic Society. ATS/ERS Task Force: Standardisation of lung function testing. *Eur Respir J* 2005;26:319–38; Hankinson JL, Odencrantz JR, Fedan KB. Spirometric reference values from a sample of the general US population. *Am J Respir Crit Care Med* 1999;159:179–87.)

Age is important when obtaining cooperation and reliable results. About 5% of adults screened for respiratory impairment are unable to perform pulmonary function testing. It is also important to define abnormality as below the lower limit of normal for every test. Decramer and colleagues found that if using the 80% of predicted threshold for abnormality, this misclassified 24% of patients. (Decramer M, Janssens W, Derom E et al. Contribution of four common pulmonary function tests to diagnosis of patients with respiratory symptoms: A prospective cohort study. *Lancet Respir Med* 2013;1:705–13.) Spirometry also has limitations and 10%–18% of patients, mainly the very young and the aged, cannot perform good-quality spirometry. (Pezzoli L, Giardini G, Consonni S et al. Quality of spirometric performance in older people. *Age Ageing* 2003;32:43–6; Enright P. Spirometer + body box = VW Beetle + Mercedes? *Respir Med* 2011;105:957–58; Miller MR, Hankinson J, Brusaco V et al. Standardisation of spirometry. *Eur Respir Dis* 2005;26:319–38.)

10

The evolution of workers' compensation and employer responsibility

We all tend to view history from our own prejudices and contemporary understanding of how things are now or should be now. It is difficult to grasp the ignorance and inertia of government agencies and medical science in failing to protect workers from industrial diseases. What deemed a reasonable industrial health standard relied on those experts who lived and worked at the time of the evolving medical and scientific information on asbestos.

At the turn of the twentieth century, the common understanding of work-related diseases was that the responsibility for prevention was largely that of the worker to protect themselves. It was assumed that if you were working in a dusty area, you should take whatever precautions you felt were necessary and if you felt the work exposure was dangerous, then you should work elsewhere. It was the worker who assumed the responsibility for their own health and not the employer, unless it could be proved that the employer was negligent. It was risk for wages. The first workers' compensation laws were enacted in 1911 in the United States and in 1915 in Canada. During the 1920s and 1930s, there was increasing awareness about the health effects of free silica in coal and hard-rock miners, and also the risk to workers in the asbestos textile industry. Studies were done that demonstrated health risks but it was not until the end of the 1930s that an occupational standard for asbestos exposure was recommended by the Public Health Service in 1938, and by the American Conference of Governmental Industrial Hygienists (ACGIH) in 1946.

Beginning in the late 1800s and early 1900s, industrial technology rapidly improved efficiency by providing machinery that produced huge amounts of dust. This new equipment in asbestos textile plants and modern pneumatic rock drills that greatly improved mining and tunnel drilling, produced large amounts of lethal silica dust.

The issue of worker versus employer responsibility came to a head in 1927 in Gauley Bridge, West Virginia, at what was called the Hawks Nest Tunnel.

The tunnel was bored under Gauley Mountain for 3 miles through high silica-containing granite rock to provide a channel for river water and power for a large industrial plant in West Virginia. The workers were often poor black or migrant workers who were not supplied with any respiratory protection or warning about the hazards of their work. Nearly all of the 3000 tunnel workers developed silicosis, and while the official death rate was 109 deaths, a Congressional investigation estimated there were more than 467 deaths while other resources suggested there were as many as 700–1000 deaths out of the 3000 workers. This was the largest industrial accident in West Virginian history and one of the largest in the history of industrial medicine in the United States. The results of this disaster were a call for government regulations, not only on silica exposure, but also a provision for safety regulations on all occupational diseases.

Shortly after this disaster, the Depression began in 1929, which resulted in a flurry of lawsuits against employers by a large pool of unemployed dependent and disabled workers who sought redress from former employers through the courts. This resulted in a variety of compromises, resulting in a workers' compensation system in which the employer agreed to pay damages based on a schedule for different work-related diseases, in exchange for not being sued by the employee. Initially, the compensation offered through workers' compensation was quite scanty and of a short duration. Over the years, and with increasing pressure from unions, the compensation system began to provide greater compensation and eventually lifelong benefits for injured workers. (Dust Disease and Workers Compensation. U.S. Department of Labor, Bureau of Labor Standards, August 1964. *Ann NY Acad Sci* 1965;132:722–44; Borron SW, Forman SA, Lockey JE et al. An early study of pulmonary asbestosis among manufacturing workers: Original data and reconstruction of the 1932 cohort. *Am J Ind Med* 1997;31:324–34.)

During the early years of workers' compensation, there were many hurdles for the worker with a dust-related disease to jump over. Many state government requirements included a timeline for minimal exposure before the worker was considered to have a sufficient exposure to receive compensation. This varied from state to state. In addition, the worker had to make a claim within a specified time limit, usually 2 years. This acted against workers because many of the dust-related diseases such as silicosis and asbestosis produce x-ray changes and physical symptoms many years after leaving the exposure. Therefore, the worker may have been excluded from compensation because they did not apply for compensation during the stated time limit. Many states provided disability compensation only if the disability was total. There often were no awards for partial disability in the case of dust diseases. Some states required workers to provide uncontestable proof of a work-related disease related to asbestos, which basically required an autopsy and pathological evidence that the interstitial fibrosis was related to asbestos exposure. It was very difficult for a living worker with asbestosis to get compensated under many state workers' compensation systems. For instance, Arizona, a large mining state, in the 1960s, did not authorize benefits for any occupational disease, and neither did Florida for any dust disease. Other states provided only a specific payment in the 1950s and 1960s. For instance, Maryland provided a payment of only $1000 if the worker had demonstrable evidence of a pulmonary dust disease, and their capacity for work had been impaired, but the impairment was less than total. In Vermont, another large mining state and producer of granite, during the 1960s had a maximum compensation for silicosis or asbestosis that was limited to $6000. The response of the state governments was largely related to the fact that the cost for dust diseases was quite burdensome compared to other occupational diseases. Many states were very reticent to give out large awards. In 1972, a National Commission on State Workmen's Compensation Laws concluded that State Workmen's Compensation Laws were "not living up to their potential" and the Commission made 84 recommendations for change. In 1976, another task force made further recommendations for reform, which were merged into the Division of State Workers' Compensation Standards in the Office of Workers' Compensation Programs of the U.S. Department of Labor. (Analysis of Workers' Compensation Laws 1984, Chamber of Commerce of the United States, Washington DC, Publication #6707.)

The next problem facing the workers' compensation system was defining what constituted a work-related disease. For workers with silicosis, one of their largest problems was tuberculosis. Those workers with mild silicosis who developed tuberculosis often developed severely disabling and fatal disease. There was much argument as to whether tuberculosis, a common infectious disease at that time, should be considered a nonwork-related disease in workers with dust-related disease, therefore exonerating the employer from responsibility. In addition, no one knew how to determine disability, and various political interests and unions tried unsuccessfully to establish competent impartial medical tribunals, free from political influences to answer these questions. (Markowitz G, Rosner D. The illusion of medical certainty: Silicosis and the politics of industrial disability 1930–1960. *Milbank Q* 1989;67:228–53.)

One of the first attempts at establishing some type of federal regulation for safety and health conditions was the Walsh Healey Act of 1938, which gave federal labor officials authority to impose safety regulations on work sites of industries doing business with the federal government. In addition, this provided a limit to workdays of 8 hours and time and one-half for overtime, as well as other benefits for workers in federal projects.

It was during the 1930s, 1940s, 1950s, and 1960s, with the passage of various workers' compensation programs that state and federal government officials had to decide what was safe and what was dangerous as it related to exposure to a various known occupational toxic agents. In 1938, at the time of the public health-recommended standard by Dreesen, a standard that reduced the risk of asbestosis or silicosis to 5% or potentially five deaths in 100, was a great step forward. In 1946, the Fleischer–Drinker study projected only three deaths out of nearly 1100 workers from asbestosis, which was very acceptable for the safety standard of that day. Also in 1946, the ACGIH published their first recommendation for various types of dust exposure.

In 1968, the British Industrial Hygiene Society recommended a standard in which only 1%, or 1 out of 100 asbestos workers, would be likely to develop asbestosis at an exposure limit of 5 fibers/cc of asbestos. This was accepted as a safe standard by the ACGIH in 1970 and the U.S. Department of Labor, Occupational Safety and Health Administration (OSHA)/National Institute for Occupational Safety and Health (NIOSH) in 1972. Later, in the 1970s, the exposure standard was gradually lowered, culminating in approximately 1 death in 10,000 in 1990–1994. Government agencies are currently trying to reduce the risk of significant illness from any occupational disease down to 1 death in 100,000 workers. The ability to reduce exposures to toxic substances to these low exposure levels has been related to large advances in medicine, industrial hygiene, and engineering practices that have greatly reduced exposures to a variety of potential toxins.

I remember a patient of mine who worked at the Puget Sound Naval Shipyard in Bremerton, Washington, as a ship builder from 1939 to 1968. When I saw him in 1977, he had advanced asbestosis. Government physicians refused to diagnose asbestosis until I intervened on his behalf. He sought help with his medical bills, but was rejected, like thousands of others, because of a 1974 amendment to the Federal Employees Compensation Act making anyone exposed prior to 1974 ineligible for an award. This was passed 4 years after the shipyards began to impose more rigorous safeguards to protect workers from asbestosis. This story is not atypical of problems with state and federal workers' compensation systems in the 1970s. The Department of Labor and Industry of the State of Washington required/recognized proof of asbestosis only by lung biopsy or autopsy during this same decade. Fortunately, largely by my effort, they accepted less rigorous diagnostic criteria by the end of the 1970s.

Since the advent of a new round of plaintiff lawsuits in the mid-to-late 1970s, state workers' compensation systems have been more amenable to accepting workers' compensation claims for injury. Workers pay a certain amount of money out of their paycheck that is matched by the employer to pay for insurance related to workers' compensation for future work-related claims. Currently, some state governments try to shift the cost of providing for these claims to industry by suggesting or requiring workers to contact plaintiff law firms. If the plaintiff lawsuit is successful, then the state workers' compensation system places a lien on the litigation award in order to get back the money awarded initially to the worker. In this way, the state pays nothing for the work-related injury by *cost shifting* indirectly to other parties. The money that was given to the state workers' compensation system for insurance premiums, through an assessment of the worker's salary, is never returned to the worker. This is indeed unfortunate and makes state government and nongovernmental workers' compensation systems enablers of plaintiff lawsuits.

The increasing cost of normal medical care, combined with decreasing insurance payment to medical providers, has prompted many providers to *cost shift* medical costs to workers' compensation programs, by claiming that the claimant has an occupational disease. This provides great financial savings, particularly to various group health programs, which results in inflated statistics on the incidence of all occupational disease.

Different countries responded differently to the recognition of asbestosis as a work-related disease. Germany accepted asbestos as a cause of lung cancer in 1943, but Spain did not list asbestosis and asbestos-related cancer of the lung and pleura in the list of occupational disease, as specified by Royal Decree, until 1978. (Isidro Montes I, Abu Shams K, Alday E et al. Guidelines on asbestos-related pleuropulmonary disease. *Arch Broncopneumol* 2005;41(3):153–68.)

Progress has been made, but attempts to develop a national workers' compensation program in the United States have been unsuccessful.

11

Does asbestos cause additional malignancies other than lung cancer and mesothelioma?

ASBESTOS AND RENAL CANCER

Some of the more practical aspects of the question of whether asbestos exposure causes an increased risk of renal cancer relate not only to respiratory exposure, but also asbestos fibers in drinking water. In the Northwest United States, most drinking water that comes from the Cascade Mountains is caught in mountain valleys, which are often dammed to form basins where the water sits before being transported to communities for domestic use. In Everett, Washington, the water comes from a watershed where a large amount of naturally occurring asbestos rock is constantly being eroded by snow, ice, and rain, becoming part of the snowmelt and rainwater that is captured in a catch basin for transport into the Everett water system. Large amounts of asbestos are found in Northwest rivers and water supplies. (Craig W. A flood of asbestos: How much should residents worry? *Seattle Times* September 4, 2010.) Various studies have been done of the incidence of colon cancer, renal cancer, and gastric cancer in Western Washington, particularly in Snohomish County, looking for an increased risk of colon cancer or renal cancer related to naturally occurring asbestos in the drinking water. No such increased risk has been demonstrated, even though it has been carefully searched for. The question about gastrointestinal (GI) penetration of the gut, from asbestos, was raised by many workers, and the studies on the penetration of the gut by asbestos fibers were reviewed by Philip Cook in *Environmental Health Perspectives* 1983;53:121–30.

There is no question that asbestos fibers can penetrate the GI tract. Asbestos bodies were found in the cancer of the colon of an insulation worker with asbestosis, the findings of which were published by Erlich, Rohl, and Holstein. (*JAMA* 1985;254:2932–3.) The cancer incidence following exposure to drinking water with asbestos leachate was reviewed by Holly L Howe, and others associated with the Division of Epidemiology of the New York State Department of Health, and for the state of Illinois. They looked at the town of Woodstock, where they found an average of 3.2 million fibers of asbestos per liter of drinking water, and looked at the cancer incidence using the New York State cancer registry. They found no evidence of elevated cancer incidence in sites that were associated with asbestos exposure. This was published in *Public Health Reports* 1989;104:251–6. MacRae reviewed the issue of asbestos in drinking water and cancer in the *Journal of the Royal College of Physicians in London* 1988;22:7–10. Again, the question was whether cement pipes were releasing asbestos, and the possibility of this causing an increased incidence of cancer, such as GI or renal cancer. Again the conclusion was that there were no data showing that the drinking water was carcinogenic.

Further studies on ingested mineral fibers and cancer were reviewed by Kanarec in the IARC publication, "Non-occupational exposure to mineral fibers" 1989;90:428–37. He thought there was some association between ingested asbestos fibers and cancer of the stomach and pancreas, but not colon or kidney, similar to the data published by Polissar et al. (*Am J Epidemiol* 1984;119:456–71) from an epidemiological study of Puget Sound. At the time of these studies in the Puget Sound area, the measured concentration of asbestos fibers ranged between 7.3 and 206.5 million fibers per liter of drinking water. In Connecticut, the level was below detectable levels at 0.7 million fibers per liter of drinking water.

Most people are unaware that the average individual, particularly in Western Washington, ingests large amounts of asbestos fibers regularly through drinking water. There is no good evidence that this is harmful. This issue has been carefully monitored by state and federal authorities. There is no evidence that further exposure in the workplace is associated with increased risk of colon cancer or renal cancer, based on my review of most of the world's literature. While there is no evidence that exposure to asbestos is associated with an increased risk of lymphoma, there is good evidence that asbestos exposure is associated with increased risk of lung cancer and peritoneal and pleural mesothelioma.

The most recent article on this issue was published by Varga, entitled "Asbestos fibers and drinking water: Are they carcinogenic or not?" This was published in *Medical Hypothesis* 2000;55:225–226. He points out that animal experiments have failed to demonstrate carcinogenicity of ingested asbestos, even though penetration of the fibers through the gut wall have been proven, and asbestos fibers are found in the kidney and urine. He raised the question of whether there still could be a carcinogenic effect of drinking water contaminated by asbestos, but pointed out that there was no epidemiologic proof of this association.

If ingestion of asbestos is carcinogenic for colon cancer and renal cancer, then animal studies should be able to confirm asbestos carcinogenicity as they have done for lung cancer and mesothelioma. This has been attempted by Donham et al. in "The effects of long-term ingestion of asbestos on the colon of F344 rats" (*Cancer* 1980;15(Suppl.):1073–84) and Ward JM et al. in "Ingested asbestos and intestinal carcinogenesis in F344 rats" (*J Environ Pathol Toxicol* 1980;3:301–12). The results have been negative. There are no data from Snohomish County,

Washington, or other areas with high asbestos water content, demonstrating a higher incidence of renal cancer compared with the national average.

The summary of this literature review indicates that while there have been some studies that have purported to show an increased risk of renal cell cancer, later studies have been unable to support this allegation. Two large studies by Selikoff and Enterline reported an increased risk of renal cell cancer in very heavily exposed insulators and employees of asbestos manufacturing plants. These studies have been faulted because the authors chose a national database to compare with the number of cancers observed in these different groups. Critics of the papers have pointed out that any local or regional database of deaths, related to different cancers in the general population, would have been much more suitable, since comparison with national database statistics tends to underestimate the risk of the variety of cancers locally. These two authors, Selikoff and Enterline, found elevated risk not only of kidney cancer, but also cancers of the larynx, stomach, esophagus, colon, and other organs. Their findings have not been replicated in a variety of very large studies that were done over the last 30 years. Many experts believe that the increased number of abdominal cancers found by death certificates, was based on misdiagnosis of peritoneal mesothelioma, and confused with a variety of other abdominal neoplasms, such as cancers of the esophagus, ovary, stomach, colon, and kidney. This is called a diagnostic bias and is responsible for the false diagnosis of a variety of abdominal cancers.

At least 70 epidemiologic studies of asbestos-exposed workers have been published. If asbestos was an important factor in the causation of renal cancer, one would expect many other epidemiologic studies to confirm this association. There is a glaring lack of support for the association between asbestos exposure and renal cancer in many other large epidemiologic studies. The strength of association, experimental evidence, consistency, and dose effect are lacking. A positive relationship has not been observed between the exposure to asbestos and cancer in studies in which chance, bias, and confounding, could be ruled out with reasonable confidence.

The available studies I have reviewed in the world's literature, have been of insufficient quality, consistency, or statistical power to permit a positive conclusion regarding the presence of a causal association between asbestos exposure and renal cancer.

There is limited evidence of carcinogenicity in animals: the data suggest a carcinogenic effect but are limited for making a definitive evaluation because, for example, (a) the evidence of carcinogenicity is restricted to a single experiment; (b) there are unresolved questions regarding the adequacy of the design, conduct, or interpretation of the study; or (c) the agent or mixture increases the incidence only of benign neoplasms or lesions of uncertain neoplastic potential, or of certain neoplasms which may occur spontaneously in high incidences in certain strains. The animal studies have been performed using rats ingesting asbestos rather than inhalation studies.

In order to prevent confounding in epidemiologic studies, other evidence judged to be relevant to an evaluation of carcinogenicity and of sufficient importance to affect the overall evaluation, must be recognized. This may include data on preneoplastic lesions, tumor pathology, genetic and related effects, structure–activity relationships, metabolism and pharmacokinetics, physicochemical parameters, and analogous biological agents. Various factors that need to be considered include smoking, obesity, hypertension, diuretic usage, arsenic exposure, and genetic diseases.

Various government agencies such as the International Agency for Research on Cancer (IARC), Lyon, France, have not found convincing evidence of an increased risk from asbestos exposure in causing renal cell cancer. Many others have reviewed the literature extensively. Lipworth and others, published a recent review in 2009 concluding that the weight of the evidence for asbestos contributing to the causation of renal cancer could not be supported by epidemiological studies. (Lipworth L, Tarone RE, Lund L, McLaughlin JK. Epidemiologic characteristics and risk factors for renal cancer. *Clin Epidemiol* 2009;1:33–43.)

A large multi-nation European epidemiological study evaluated the relationship between various dust exposures and renal cancer. Occupational exposures to dusts have generally been examined in relation to cancers of the respiratory system, and have rarely been examined in relation to other cancers, such as renal cell carcinoma (RCC). Although some previous epidemiological studies, though few, have shown certain dusts, such as asbestos, to increase renal cancer risk, the potential for other occupational dust exposures to cause kidney damage and/or cancer may exist. The authors investigated whether asbestos, as well as 20 other occupational dust exposures, were associated with RCC risk, in a large European, multi-center, hospital-based, renal case–control study. Among participants ever exposed to dusts, significant associations were observed for glass fibers (odds ratio [OR]: 2.1; 95% confidence interval [CI]: 1.1–3.9), mineral wool fibers (OR: 2.5; 95% CI: 1.2–5.1), and brick dust (OR: 1.5; 95% CI: 1.0–2.4). Significant trends were also observed with exposure duration and cumulative exposure. No association between renal cell cancer risk and asbestos exposure was observed. (Karami S, Boffetta P, Stewart PS et al. Occupational exposure to dusts and risk of renal cell carcinoma. *Br J Cancer* 2011;104(11):1797–803.)

ASBESTOS AND UPPER GI TRACT CANCER

An important issue in all cancer epidemiologic studies is confounding. It is difficult to control for confounders such as *Helicobacter pylori* infection in gastric cancer, or esophageal reflux in esophageal cancer. Some subtypes of cancer, such as lung cancer, may have different confounders such as the role of human papillomavirus (HPV) in the causation of squamous cell cancer of the lung, oropharynx, and rectum. Race, ethnicity, sex, age at the time of first exposure, genetic susceptibility, tobacco exposure, and socio-economic factors are important. Many important confounders have not been identified. Exposure information such as heavy, prolonged, or intermittent heavy exposure is often confusing. Information on fiber type, fiber length, and fiber diameter is usually not reported. Many authors report "asbestos exposure" as if any and all asbestos exposure has equal carcinogenicity! For instance, exposure to occasional brake or clutch dust is often included as a significant asbestos exposure in various epidemiologic studies, in spite of the fact that this is not supported in the scientific medical literature. Other authors assume that any asbestos exposure is a significant exposure. The difficulty in distinguishing between GI neoplasms and epithelial peritoneal mesotheliomas is usually not mentioned in many published papers.

Irving Selikoff and others published a landmark article in 1964 entitled "Asbestos exposure and neoplasia." (*JAMA* 1964;188:22–6.) This study that was done of New York and New Jersey insulators showed an increased risk of lung cancer mesothelioma, and it raised the possibility as to whether there was a relationship between asbestos exposure and an increased risk of GI cancer. They found 12 deaths from gastric cancer as compared to 4.3 expected. Seventeen deaths from colon cancer occurred where 5.2 were expected. There were no increased risks of lymphoma. In 1968, a further analysis of their data entitled "Asbestos exposure, smoking, and neoplasia" (*JAMA* 1968;204:106–12) suggested a relationship between cancers of the stomach, colon, and rectum in which 9.4 deaths were expected and 29 were observed. However, they stated that the numbers were so small that they could not make definite conclusions at that time.

Further studies by the same group on amosite workers from Paterson, New Jersey, were published in the *Archives of Environmental Health* 1972;25:184, where they again thought there was an increased risk of stomach, colon, and rectum cancer, but felt again that further observations would be required. There are a lot of problems with this cohort because many of the coworkers in this cohort had previous exposure from other industrial plants, and also probably were also exposed to crocidolite asbestos.

In 1974, Meurman and others studied 1092 Finnish anthophyllite workers, and they found no increase of GI cancers. (*Br J Ind Med* 1974;31:105–12.)

Lumley studied British dockyard workers (*Br J Ind Med* 1976;33:108–10) and noted no significantly increased risk of GI cancers, in that he found 416 cases, and expected 408, which is not a significant difference. They also looked at the incidence of lymphomas, and found 24 where they expected 28, again demonstrating no increased risk of lymphoma in this group.

Peto, Doll, and others evaluated 1106 men and women who worked in an English textile factory (*Br J Ind Med* 1977;34:169–73) and they found no excess of GI cancers, in that they found 16 cases where 15.7 were expected.

A study of 162 men who were working as insulators in 1940 was done by Elmes and Simpson as published in the *British Journal of Industrial Medicine* 1977;34:174–180. Their conclusion was that up until 1965, there had been an overall excess of deaths, and that they were due to asbestos, with or without tuberculosis, and to elementary cancer as well as to bronchial cancer and mesothelioma. From 1965 onwards, the overall death rate among survivors was not so excessive, but was only related to bronchial cancer and mesothelioma. This is an interesting article because one must recognize that it was not until the 1960s that pathologists recognized peritoneal and pleural mesotheliomas as distinct diseases, and therefore it is easy to understand how deaths that occurred in the 1940s and 1950s were diagnosed as colon cancer and GI cancer, rather than primary peritoneal mesothelioma.

Harrington and others studied the use of asbestos cement pipe for public water supply, and the incidence of GI cancer, in Connecticut between 1935 and 1973. They published this article in the *American Journal of Epidemiology* 1978;107:96–103, and found there was no association noted between asbestos exposure and the risk of GI cancer.

AB Miller, from the University of Toronto, studied the relationship between asbestos fiber dust and GI malignancy, and did a review of the literature in regard to the cause-and-effect relationship. Miller published his findings in the *Journal of Chronic Disease* 1978;31:22–33, concluding that the degree of risk of GI cancer in asbestos workers, 20 or more years following their first exposure, was increased by around 3:1, but then stated,

> There is no doubt that an association has been demonstrated between the exposure to asbestos and the subsequent develop-ment of cancers of the gastrointestinal tract, particularly that of the esophagus, stomach, colon, and rectum. The important question is the extent to which this association can be interpreted as being causal.

He then went to look at the criteria of Sir Bradford Hill on making the association between an occupational and environmental exposure and disease. He felt the strengths of the association between GI cancer and asbestos exposure were weak. There was a lack of consistency and no specificity. He felt that temporality had been demonstrated, but there was a lack of a clear biological gradient. He pointed out it was potentially plausible that asbestos could be absorbed through the intestinal tract and cause GI cancer, but there was really a lack of experimen-tal proof and coherence. Finally, there was a lack of good analogy. This paper was a landmark paper, because it set the stage for further studies and analysis of the relationship between asbestos fiber dust exposure and GI cancer, by carefully outlining the scientific questions that needed to be answered, to establish proof of an association between asbestos dust and GI cancer.

The research continued, and in 1979 the Advisory Committee of Asbestos in Great Britain published a report that gave perhaps cautious acceptance to the idea that alimentary tract cancers may sometimes be caused by asbestos in condi-tions of heavy industrial exposure. (*Lancet* 1979;2:887.)

Dr. Selikoff reviewed his own data and published a book called *Asbestos and Diseases* in 1978, and his comment at that time was "the evidence for carcino-genic or cocarcinogenic action of asbestos in tumors developing in the gastro-intestinal tract is highly suggestive but not conclusive, and for tumors and other sites, the evidence is so far equivocal" (p. 301).

The same group in 1979 studied 544 asbestos miners and published this in the *Annals of New York Academy of Sciences* 1979;330:11–21, and found no increased incidence of GI cancer and no mention of lymphoma.

These data were further supported by a study by Rubino, Piolatto, Newhouse, and others, in chrysotile workers from northern Italy, published in the *British Journal of Industrial Medicine* 1979;36:187–94.

Dr. Selikoff and his group again studied U.S. shipyards in 1979, and published their results in the *Annals of New York Academy of Sciences* 1979;330:295–311. They found three GI cancers where they expected 3.1, and there was no mention of any increased risk of lymphoma. Also in the same journal and the same year, he looked at deaths among 12,051 insulation workers in the United States and Canada with 20 or more years from onset of exposure. He found three GI cancers where he expected 2.8. In people who worked in shipyards and other insulators, he found 90 where he expected 50.4 cancers. This would not be a clinically significant difference. Based on different changes and the analysis of their data, the proportionate mortality ratio (PMR) ranged from 1.59 to 1.81, and again they concluded that "it would be folly to suppose that we have precisely determined the degree of association in this group of asbestos workers," as mentioned in their article in the *New York Academy of Sciences* 1979;330:91–116 (p. 94).

Hillerdal studied the relationship between GI cancer and the occurrence of pleural plaques on a chest x-ray, in a study published in the *Journal of Occupational Medicine* 1980;22:806–9. He felt that there was a slight, but significant, excess of pleural plaques in patients with GI cancer, particularly cancer of the stomach. When one looks at these numbers, the numbers are very small. He studied 108 patients with colon cancer, and the patients with colon cancer had three pleural plaques versus 1.8 expected. This indicates very small numbers and they are not statistically significant changes.

Following that study, Beaumont and Weiss (*Am J Epidemiol* 1980;112:775–86) reviewed the mortality in welders and ship fitters in two shipyards and various field construction sites, and found the standardized mortality ratio (SMR) for lymphoietic cancer to be 0.92, which means that there was no association found whatsoever, and the SMR for malignant neoplasms of the digestive organs was 0.84, again indicating no association.

Rossiter and Coals looked at a similar population of 6300 shipyard workers in England, published in *IARC* 1981;II:713–21, and they found a SMR for GI cancer of 76, and there is no mention of increased incidence of lymphoma.

McDonald, Liddell, Gibbs, and others, studied 11,379 asbestos miners and millers in Canada, and found there to be an SMR for carcinoma of the esophagus that was slightly elevated at 1.36, and for colon and rectal cancer, it was very low with an SMR of 0.56. There was no mention of increased risk of lymphoma. The risk did not really change significantly for colon and rectal cancer with increasing dose, as one would expect with other types of cancer. It did rise slightly with carcinoma of the esophagus and stomach, but did not rise significantly with colon cancer, in that at medium risk it was 0.43, at high risk it was 0.18, and at very high risk it was 1.39, which is not significant. Therefore, not only was the risk low, there was no dose–response. This article was published in the *British Journal of Industrial Medicine* 1980;37:11–24.

Thomas, Benjamin, and others published a similar study of 1592 Welsh asbestos cement factory workers in the *British Journal of Industrial Medicine* 1982;39:273–6, and they found no excess of GI cancer. The SMR for the total population was 92.

Dement, Harris, and others, studied the mortality among chrysotile asbestos textile workers in North Carolina, and they found no statistically significant increase in cancer of the digestive system, with an SMR of 131, as published in the *American Journal of Industrial Medicine* 1983;4:421–33.

Acheson, Gardner, and others, studied 5969 men involved in the manufacture of asbestos-containing products, and again found no increase in GI cancer. With an SMR for colon cancer of 137, they found six cases where 4.4 were expected, and the controlled group had an SMR of 142. This was published in the *International Journal of Epidemiology* 1984;13:3–10.

Berry and Newhouse studied 13,460 British friction product workers and found no excess of GI cancer in the whole cohort, with 103 GI cancers found and 107 were expected. This was published in the *British Journal of Industrial Medicine* 1983;40:3–4.

Kolonel and others looked at the cancer occurrence in shipyard workers exposed to asbestos in Hawaii, and published an article in *Cancer Research* 1985;45:3927, finding no significant increase of GI cancers in this group, in which they observed 45 cases and expected 47.

Lavine published a review article entitled "Does asbestos exposure cause gastrointestinal cancer?" in *Digestive Diseases and Sciences* 1985;30:1189–97, in which he concluded that there was no proof that asbestos exposure caused GI cancer.

In the same year, the British government commissioned a study on the health effects of asbestos, and this was done by Richard Doll and Dr. Peto, who published a study entitled "Asbestos, effects on health of exposure to asbestos," published by the Health and Safety Commission of Her Majesty's Stationery Office in 1985. This exhaustive review concluded that the laboratory evidence weighed against the possibility that asbestos caused cancer in sites other than lung pleura or peritoneum. They also pointed out that asbestos had failed to produce GI cancer in any type of animal when given by mouth. Furthermore, they felt that where there was an increased risk of GI cancer, this was most likely a misdiagnosis of cancer of the lung or mesothelioma of the pleura or peritoneum.

In 1985, Drs. Morgan, Foliart, and Wong reviewed 45 published articles relating to the incidence of cancer from asbestos exposure, and found that when all of these groups were combined the SMR for colon cancer was not increased. They published their article in the *Western Journal of Medicine* 1985;143:61–5.

Hodgson and Jones, from the Epidemiology and Statistics Unit in England, published a review of 31,150 male asbestos workers in England and Wales. They found an increased death rate from lung cancer and mesothelioma, but there was no evidence of any increased risk of cancer from the GI tract, and the risk of colon cancer actually showed a statistically significant deficit, with an SMR of 54. The total SMR for carcinoma of the colon before asbestos regulations came into place was 36, and of the rectum was 77. This article was published in the *British Journal of Industrial Medicine* 1986;43:158–64.

Botha, Irwig, and Strebel reviewed the incidence of all types of cancer, including GI cancer, from that area of South Africa where there was the highest incidence of mesothelioma due to the mining of crocidolite asbestos. This area was compared to other areas in South Africa to determine if there was an increased risk of colon cancer as well as other cancers. They then compared the various crocidolite-mining districts with these controlled districts, and found an elevated risk for asbestosis, mesothelioma, cancer of the lung, and cancer of the stomach, but not cancer of the colon. (*Am J Epidemiol* 1986;123:30–40.) A more recent study reviewed 32 studies and confirmed that being male with exposure to crocidolite, and working as a miner, was associated with a slight increase in the rate of stomach cancer, with a SMR of 1.19 (95% CI: 1.06–1.34). (Peng WJ, Jia XJ, Wei BG et al. Stomach cancer mortality among workers exposed to asbestos: A meta-analysis. *J Cancer Res Clin Oncol* 2015;141(7):1141–9.)

The World Health Organization reviewed the health effects of asbestos in its publication of 1986 "Asbestos and other natural mineral fibers" published in *Environmental Health Criteria 53*. The international panel of experts reviewed the animal ingestion studies, and concluded that there was no conclusive evidence in several studies performed by that time, that ingested asbestos in animals was carcinogenic (pp. 87–90). Human cohort studies on the risk of GI cancer were analyzed, and in 18 out of 30 studies of asbestos workers, the number of deaths from GI cancer exceeded the expected. The panel concluded, "These excesses are difficult to assess because of confounding factors such as social class and geographical variations, and possible misdiagnosis. Moreover, there is no evidence of dose-related effects. Thus, a causal relationship with asbestos has not been established" (p. 118).

Enterline, Hartley, and Henderson, did a review of 1074 white men who worked in an asbestos company between 1941 and 1967 here in the United States. The SMR for colon cancer was 98, and for the rectum was 159. This was published in the *British Journal of Industrial Medicine* 1987;44:397.

Sir Richard Doll and Julian Peto reviewed the question of asbestos exposure and other associated neoplasms in a chapter in the book, *Asbestos-Related Malignancy* by Antman, Aisner, Grune, and Stratton (1987; pp. 81–96). They looked at the results of 18 studies that evaluated lung, GI, and other cancers that had been published at that time. They then compared the SMRs for lung and GI cancers. They did find an excess risk of GI cancer associated with an excess risk of lung cancer, but they also found an excess risk of other cancers associated with an excess risk of lung cancer. They pointed out that when necropsy studies with histological exams were performed from 185 subjects that were personally reviewed, which they summarized in their Table 4.2, the numbers of deaths attributed to different types of cancer were reduced, by half for GI cancers from 14 to 7, increasing the number of mesotheliomas fourfold from 5 to 20.

These authors went on to quote Selikoff (Selikoff IJ, Hammond EC, Seidman H. Mortality experience of insulation workers in the United States and Canada 1943–1976. *Ann NY Acad Sci* 1979;330:91–116) and state,

> Selikoff in his review, concludes that the excess of cancer of the pancreas in his own series of insulation workers was an artifact due to miscertification, but that there were true excesses of cancers of the larynx, pharynx, and buccal cavity, esophagus, stomach, colon, rectum, and kidney that could be attributed to the men's

occupation. The simple explanation of the excess mortality of gastrointestinal cancer, however in our opinion the most likely, is it results largely or wholly from misdiagnosis of cancer of the lung and mesothelioma of the pleurae and peritoneum. We cannot, of course, rule out the possibility that asbestos may cause a small number of cancers in many different organs, even though there is no strong evidence that it does.

Sanden and Jarvholm looked at a group of Swedish shipyard workers 20 or more years after first exposure to asbestos, and found the incidence of colon and rectal cancer to be three cases when 7.8 were expected. Thus, again there was a negative SMR. There was no mention of increased risk for lymphoma. (*Int Arch Occup Environ Health* 1987;59:4–12.)

David Edelman from Chapel Hill, North Carolina, did a review entitled "Exposure to asbestos and the risk of gastrointestinal cancer: A reassessment" as published in the *British Journal of Industrial Medicine* 1988;45:75–82. He concluded that there was no dose–response relationship between exposure to asbestos and the risk of GI cancer, and that asbestos workers are not at an increased risk of GI cancer. His article was based on a review of 32 different cohorts of asbestos-exposed workers in which he analyzed the risk of GI cancer.

In another study of asbestos cement workers in Sweden, Albin, Attewell, Jakobsson, and others, reviewed a cohort of asbestos cement workers and published it in the *Arh Hig Rada Toksikol* 1988;39:461–7, and found a slight increase in the standard mortality ratio (SMR) for GI cancer of 140, but did not break it out as to the number with colon cancer.

Frumkin and Berlin published an article entitled "Asbestos exposure and gastrointestinal malignancy: Review and meta-analysis," published in the *American Journal of Industrial Medicine* 1988;14:79–95 with an erratum in *American Journal of Industrial Medicine* 1988;14:493 and a response concerning the article was published by RW Morgan in the *American Journal of Industrial Medicine* 1991;19:407–11, and then a response to Dr. Morgan's response was published in the *American Journal of Industrial Medicine* by Dr. Frumkin and Dr. Berlin in the *American Journal of Industrial Medicine* 1991;19:409–11. The basic argument in this series of patients is whether there is an association between increased lung cancer risk and increased risk of GI cancer as shown by Dr. Doll and Dr. Peto. However, they disagree with Dr. Doll and Dr. Peto, and conclude that this indicates that asbestos exposure does increase the risk of colon cancer. Dr. Frumkin does not believe that there is enough misclassification of the diagnosis of mesothelioma to cause a 1.6-fold increase in the incidence of colon cancer, whereas Dr. Doll and Dr. Peto in their own analysis of the data have shown that this indeed could be an explanation, since in their study the misclassification of the diagnosis of GI cancer reduced the incidence of GI by half or by twofold. Therefore, I disagree with Dr. Frumkin's and Dr. Berlin's assumption that this could not happen, since this has already been documented in an earlier study in the literature. I also forgot to mention in my analysis of Dr. Doll's and Dr. Peto's article that they also concluded that the association between asbestos exposure and lymphoma was not supported by the experience in Sweden or by Selikoff's own massive study of insulation workers in North America.

Mossman, Vignon, Corn, Seaton, and Gee, published a review on the health hazards of asbestos in the journal *Science* 1989;247:295–6. Their conclusions were that

> Tumors of the gastrointestinal tract, larynx, and other organs, including kidney, ovary, pancreas, pericardium, eye, and lymphatic system have been reported in some cohorts of asbestos workers. In general, the enhanced SMR's for these tumors are not statistically distinguishable from normal SMR's, and have not been confirmed in most cohorts.

The World Health Organization published a statement on the occupational exposure limit for asbestos in 1989. The World Health Organization brought together an international panel to review this subject. In annex 1, page 2 under "asbestos-related diseases," the question of whether cancer of the GI tract was related to asbestos exposure was discussed. The panel pointed out the difficulties of interpreting the data and highlighted that laboratory experiments had failed to produce GI tumors in animals exposed to asbestos. They summarized their data in a table on page 22 of annex 1 under "evidence relating asbestos to various diseases." They felt that the evidence was certain that asbestosis, mesothelioma, and lung cancer were related to asbestos exposure. They felt that the relationship between GI cancer and ovarian cancer was unclear, the relationship to laryngeal cancer was doubtful, and the relationship with other cancers, which would include lymphoma, was probably nonexistent.

William Weiss of Philadelphia reviewed the association between asbestos exposure and colorectal cancer specifically in an article published in *Gastroenterology* 1990;99:876–84. He reviewed the literature on 21 cohorts of workers exposed to asbestos up to 1988, and summarized the SMRs for all 21 cohorts, and this was 0.97. There was no dose–response relationship in the two studies in which such data were published. Therefore, he concluded that there was no evidence of an association between asbestos exposure and colorectal cancer. This article again used the same strategy of the earlier article of Miller in looking at the evidence as proposed by Sir Bradford Hill, and again he felt that the evidence was inadequate to show a causal relationship.

Dr. Selikoff reviewed the 17,800 insulation workers that were originally studied in 1967–1972, and hypothesized that such a relationship may exist between asbestos exposure and GI cancer, but with progressive follow-up of this cohort, the data suggesting a possible relationship weakened. His data were summarized in a study published in 1994 entitled "Asbestos disease—1990–2020: The risks of asbestos assessment" published in *Advances in Modern Environmental Toxicology* Volume XXII edited by Melman and Upton, 1994. Table 3 on page 140 examines the observed versus the expected rate of GI cancer over three periods of time. The SMR for GI cancer was 189 for 1967–1972 and dropped to 131 between 1973 and 1979 and dropped further to 117 between 1980 and 1986. The progressive drop in the SMR suggests that the earlier death certificates were confounded by confusion regarding the clinical/pathologic diagnosis of GI malignancy with peritoneal mesothelioma, since the actual number of peritoneal mesotheliomas increased while the diagnosis of GI neoplasm decreased. His data in very heavily exposed workers do not support any causal relationship between asbestos exposure and GI cancer.

The argument went on, in that Neugut and others claimed an association between asbestos exposure with colorectal adenomatous polyps and cancer in a study published in the *Journal of National Cancer Institute* 1991;83:827–8. They felt that there was an elevated risk for adenomatous polyps in subjects exposed to asbestos.

Later on, Garabrant, Peters, and Homa published a review on asbestos and colon cancer in the *American Journal of Epidemiology* 1992;135:843–53. Based on a study of 746 histologically confirmed cases of colon cancer with matched controls from Los Angeles County, California, they concluded that there was a lack of association with asbestos exposure. Their study concluded that occupational exposure to asbestos is not a risk factor for colon cancer.

In 1994, Jakobsson, Albin, and Hagmar, published an article entitled "Asbestos, cement, and cancer in the right part of the colon" in *Occupational and Environmental Medicine* 1994;51:95–101. It was their conclusion that there was an increased incidence of cancer in the right part of the colon in these asbestos cement workers. This study is of interest in that it looked at the incidence of the cancer in the right colon versus the left colon and rectum, and found that the incidence of cancer in the right colon was elevated with a total of 24 cases when about 9.63 were expected. In the left colon they found five cases of colon cancer with 9.3 expected, and in the rectum they found 24 cases with 15 expected. The overall morbidity from colorectal cancer among asbestos cement workers was increased to 1.4, and the combined standardized incident rate (SIR) was increased in the whole group to 1.49. The overall mortality for the asbestos cement workers was slightly higher than the general population, with a SMR of 1.14, and the overall incidence of cancer among the workers revealed a SIR of 1.38. When they compared it with other industrial workers, the SIR for cancer for the right side of the colon was low at 0.44. Thus, the so-called increased rate for cancer of the right side of the colon in asbestos workers is largely related to a comparison population, which had a much lower rate than expected. There is no mention of an increased risk of lung cancer in this population. The data certainly suggest that the increased risk found in this population was related to methodological error.

Another study published in the *Journal of Occupational Medicine* 1994;36: 1027–31 entitled "Construction occupations, asbestos exposure and cancer of the colon and rectum" by Demers, and others, looked at the association between employment, asbestos exposure, and colon cancer risk, in the state of Michigan. A total of 261 cases of colorectal cancer and 183 controlled cases were identified within the state of Michigan, and then correlation was made to occupations historically known to involve heavy exposure to asbestos. The cancers of the colon actually showed a reduced OR, again in conflict with some other studies that had claimed that there was an association between occupational exposure to asbestos and colon cancer. The ORs for exposure in colon cancer ranged from 0.4 to 0.6 based on duration of exposure; again, an OR of less than 1 means a negative association between the exposure and risk.

John Gamble published a review entitled "Asbestos and colon cancer: A weight of evidence review," published in *Environmental Health Perspectives* 1994;102:1038–50. Dr. Gamble weighed all the current epidemiologic studies and pointed out that the major evidence for a causal association at high exposure was a combined colorectal SMR of 1.5 for asbestos cohorts where the lung cancer SMR was greater than twofold. He went on to highlight that misdiagnosis may spuriously elevate the SMR. He pointed out

> The strongest evidence against the causal association between colon cancer and asbestos exposure is the lack of exposure–response gradient in asbestos cohorts where trends for lung cancer are observed. Population-based case–control studies of colon cancer do not show any consistent risk associated with asbestos exposure. Long-term ingestion studies show no evidence of increased incidence of colon cancer in animals by this route of exposure, and do not provide biological plausibility for a causal association between asbestos exposure and colon cancer.

Dr. Gamble reviewed the recent evidence again in 2008, and concluded that none of the various methods for estimating asbestos exposure yielded consistent exposure–response trends, and the strengths of the associations were consistently weak or nonexistent for the four types of GI cancers and asbestos exposure. (Gamble J. Risk of gastrointestinal cancers from inhalation and ingestion of asbestos. *Regul Toxicol Pharmacol* 2008;52(1 Suppl.):S124–53.)

A meta-analysis of the risk of colon cancer and its relationship with asbestos exposure, was performed by Homa, Garabrant, and Gillespie, as published in the *American Journal of Epidemiology* 1994;139:1210–22. They studied 20 asbestos-exposed cohorts and summarized the data, stating that

> After stratifying the cohorts based on mortality due to all cancers excluding those known or specified to be associated with asbestos exposure, lung cancer mortality was not clearly associated with colorectal cancer mortality, suggesting that the crude association between these factors may be due to misdiagnosis of lung cancer.

William Weiss of Philadelphia published a second article entitled "The lack of causality between asbestos and colorectal cancer" in the *Journal of Occupational Environmental Medicine* 1995;37:1364–73. He reviewed 30 cohort studies, and again the overall relative risk summarized in all 30 cohorts for colorectal cancer was 0.99, which indicates no association.

A more recent review was performed in 1997 by Seong-Kyu Kang and others from the Division of Surveillance of the National Institutes of Occupational Safety and Health in Cincinnati. They looked at GI cancer mortality of workers in occupations with high asbestos exposures, and published their study in the *American Journal of Industrial Medicine* 1997;31:713–8. They looked at 15,524 cases of GI cancer, in 12 occupations with elevated proximal mortality ratios (PMRs) for mesothelioma. The PMR for colorectal cancer was felt to be significantly elevated at 108, which is a very small change. Their conclusions were that rectal cancer incidence was elevated in mechanical and electronic engineers. However, high-exposure occupations, such as insulation, construction painter supervision, plumbing, furnace operation, and construction electric installation, showed no elevation of GI cancers. In conclusion, while this death certificate study supports an association between asbestos exposure and some GI cancer, the magnitude of this effect was thought to be very small. They went on to point out that the death certificates that were used in the study did not provide information on confounding factors, such as diet, exercise, drinking, smoking, social and economic status, and other possible confounding factors for GI cancer. Since they were unable to control for these confounding factors, it is very difficult to be sure that the very small increase in PMR of 108 was truly due to occupational exposure to asbestos.

The World Health Organization again reviewed the health effects of chrysotile asbestos in 1998 in a monograph entitled *Environmental Health Criteria 203 Chrysotile Asbestos*. On page 126, it states, "In predominately 'chrysotile'-exposed cohorts, there is no consistent evidence of excess mortality from stomach or colorectal cancer."

A more recent meta-analysis of asbestos-exposed cohorts was done by Goddman, Morgan, Ray, and others, and published in *Cancer Causes and Control* 1999;10:453–65. They looked at 69 asbestos-exposed occupational cohort studies that reported on cancer morbidity and mortality. They not only looked at GI cancer, they also looked at urinary and lymphohematopoietic cancers. Increased risk, of course, for lung cancer and mesothelioma was established, and there was a slight increase for laryngeal cancer. *The data for GI cancer showed no evidence of a significant association or dose–response effect.* No association between asbestos exposure and lymphoma was found. This article is particularly important since it is the most comprehensive of any to be published, and it included the largest number of asbestos-exposed cohorts in its data analysis.

Small studies continue to be published. There was a study from Poland published in the *International Journal of Occupational Medicine and Environmental Health* 2000;13:121–30. This study was on the mortality of workers at two asbestos cement plants in Poland, by Szeszenia-Dabrowska and others, who found an SMR for GI cancer of 264. However, but that was only seven cases, which means that the numbers are so small that the study lacks statistical power. This is similar to the studies of the mortality of all cancers from an asbestos factory in east London between 1933 and 1980 that was published by Berry, Newhouse, and Wagner, and republished in the *Journal of Occupational Environmental Medicine* 2000;57:782–5, in which they found an increased incidence of cancer of the lung and pleural and peritoneal mesothelioma, and also observed an excess of cancer of the colon, in that they found 27 cases when 15 were expected. This gave them an SMR of 1.83, which again is not statistically significant.

A Norwegian study focused on the incidence of asbestos-related cancers among 28,300 officers and enlisted servicemen in the Royal Norwegian Navy. Until 1987, asbestos aboard the vessels potentially caused exposure to 11,500 crew members. Increased risk of mesothelioma was seen among engine room crews, with SIRs of 6.23 (95% CI: 2.51–12.8) and 6.49 (95% CI: 2.11–15.1) for personnel who served less than 2 years and those with longer service, respectively. Lung cancer was nearly 20% higher than expected among both engine crews and non-engine crews. An excess of colorectal cancer bordering on statistical significance was seen among nonengine crews (SIR: 1.14; 95% CI: 0.98–1.32). Land-based personnel and personnel who served aboard after 1987 had a lower lung cancer incidence than expected (SIR: 0.77; 95% CI: 0.64–0.92). No elevated risk of laryngeal, pharyngeal, or stomach cancers was seen. The overall increase (65%) of mesotheliomas among military Navy servicemen was confined to marine engine crews only. The mesothelioma incidence can be taken as an indicator of the presence or absence of asbestos exposure, but the study offered no consistent explanation of the variation in incidence of other asbestos-related cancers. (Strand LA, Martinsen JI, Koefoed VF et al. Asbestos-related cancers among 28,300 military servicemen in the Royal Norwegian Navy. *Am J Ind Med* 2010;53(1):64–71.)

A Spanish study of pathologically diagnosed stomach cancer, exploring the relationship between stomach cancer, by histological type, occupation and occupational exposure, was performed on 399 incident histologically-confirmed stomach cancer cases (241 intestinal and 109 diffuse adenocarcinomas) and 455 controls, with frequency matched by sex, age, and province of residence. Occupation was coded according to the Spanish National Classification of Occupations, 1994. Occupational exposures were assessed by the FINJEM Job Exposure Matrix. ORs were estimated by unconditional logistic regression, adjusting for matching variables and education, smoking, alcohol, and diet. In men, a statistically significant increased risk of the diffuse subtype was found for "cooks" (odds ratio [OR]: 8.02), "wood-processing-plant operators" (OR: 8.13) and "food and related products machine operators" (OR: 5.40); for the intestinal subtype, a borderline association was found for "miners and quarry workers" (OR men: 4.22; 95% CI: 0.80–22.14). Significantly increased risk was observed between the diffuse subtype of stomach cancer and the highest level of exposure to "pesticides" (OR both sexes: 10.39; 95% CI: 2.51–43.02; p(trend) = 0.02) and between the intestinal subtype and asbestos (OR men: 3.71; 95% CI: 1.40–9.83; p(trend) = 0.07). Restricted analyses of exposures of 15 years and longer showed significant associations between the diffuse subtype and the exposure to "wood dust" (OR men: 3.05). This study supports the relationship previously suggested between stomach cancer and occupational exposure to dusty and high-temperature environments. Several occupations may also increase the risk of diffuse stomach cancer, but not the intestinal subtype. The CI for asbestos exposure was too wide to be statistically significant. (Santibañez M, Alguacil J, de la Hera MG et al. Occupational exposures and risk of stomach cancer by histological type. *Occup Environ Med* 2012;69(4):268–75.)

Another multicenter hospital-based Spanish case–control study was conducted in two Mediterranean provinces of Spain. Occupational, sociodemographic, and lifestyle information, was collected from 185 newly diagnosed male esophageal cancer patients (147 squamous cell carcinoma and 38 adenocarcinoma), and 285 frequency-matched controls. Occupation was coded according to the Spanish National Classification of Occupations, 1994. Occupational exposure to a selection of carcinogenic substances was assessed by the FINJEM job exposure matrix. ORs were calculated by unconditional logistic regression adjusted for age, education, alcohol intake, and cigarette smoking. For the squamous cell variety, statistically significant associations were found for waiters and bartenders (OR: 8.18; 95% CI: 1.98–33.75) and miners, shot-firers, stone cutters, and carvers (OR: 10.78; 95% CI: 1.24–93.7) in relation to other occupations. For the adenocarcinoma variety, statistically significant associations were observed for carpenters and joiners (OR: 9.69), animal producers and related workers (OR: 5.61), and building and related electricians (OR: 8.26), although these observations were based on a low number of cases. Regarding specific exposures, the study found a statistically significantly increased risk of squamous cell carcinoma for ionizing radiation, and of adenocarcinoma for high exposure to volatile sulfur compounds (OR: 3.12) and lead (OR: 5.30). For all histological types of occupational cancers (OC) combined, a threefold increase in risk was found with a significant trend for asbestos exposure (OR: 3.46; 95% confidence interval [CI]: 0.99–12.10). The data suggest that some occupational exposures may specifically increase the risk of esophageal squamous cell carcinoma or adenocarcinoma, while other exposures such as asbestos may increase the overall risk of esophageal cancer. This increased risk may be due to coincidental exposure related to asbestos exposure. (Santibañez M, Vioque J, Alguacil J et al. Occupational exposures and risk of oesophageal cancer by histological type: A case–control study in eastern Spain. *Occup Environ Med* 2008;65(11):774–81.)

The assessment of causation in GI cancer is complicated by many other factors and exposures that have not been controlled for in large historical epidemiologic studies. Shipyard and construction workers are exposed to a variety of chemicals, gases, fumes, and dusts, other than asbestos, which are also carcinogenic. It is because these same groups of workers that are exposed to asbestos are also exposed to many strong carcinogens that epidemiologic data results have been confusing and inconsistent. (Oddone E, Modonesi C, Gatta G. Occupational exposures and colorectal cancers: A quantitative overview of epidemiological evidence. *World J Gastroenterol* 2014;20(35):12431–44.)

Greenberg and Roggli summarized the literature as of 1992 in the textbook *Pathology of Asbestos Related Diseases*, page 213, as follows: "…for the reasons just noted, the relationship between asbestos exposure and colorectal cancer remains unconvincing."

Andrew Churg and Francis Green speak to the same issue in Chapter 10, page 381, of the second edition of their book *Pathology of Occupational Lung Disease* in 1998:

At various times claims that laryngeal, esophageal, gastric, and colorectal carcinomas are associated with occupational asbestos exposure have been advanced. These are purely epidemiologic issues, since even if an association was demonstrated, no specific pathologic findings would allow attribution of causation in a specific case. All of these tumors are common in the general population and have various well documented causes, including smoking (larynx, esophagus), alcohol (larynx, esophagus), diet (stomach, colorectal), and social class. Recent summaries have concluded that there is no consistent evidence for an elevated risk of any of these tumors, in asbestos-exposed cohorts, nor is there evidence for a dose response. Claims regarding a possible association between asbestos exposure and lymphoproliferative malignancies have similarly not been borne out on further study.

Colon cancer and asbestos exposure

Finally, I would like to comment on some of the more practical aspects of this question of whether asbestos exposure causes an increased risk of colon cancer. As you know, the water that comes from the Cascade Mountains is caught in mountain valleys, which are often dammed to form basins where the water sits before being transported to communities for domestic use. In Everett, the water comes from a watershed where a large amount of naturally occurring asbestos rock is constantly being eroded by snow, ice, and rain, becoming part of the snowmelt and rainwater that is captured in the catch basin for transport into the Everett water system. Various studies have been done of the incidence of colon cancer and gastric cancer in western Washington, particularly in Snohomish County, looking for an increased risk of colon cancer related to naturally occurring asbestos in the drinking water. No such increased risk has been demonstrated, even though it has been carefully searched for. The question about GI penetration of the gut from asbestos was raised by many workers, and the studies on the penetration of the gut by asbestos fibers were reviewed by Philip Cook in *Environmental Health Perspectives* 1983;53:121–30.

There is no question that asbestos fibers can penetrate the GI tract. Asbestos bodies have been found in cancer of the colon in an insulation worker with asbestosis, and was published by Erlich, Rohl, and Holstein in *JAMA* 1985;254:2932–3. The cancer incidence, following exposure to drinking water with asbestos leachate, was reviewed by Holly L Howe and others associated with the Division of Epidemiology of the New York State Department of Health, and for the state of Illinois. They looked at the town of Woodstock, where they found an average of 3.2 million fibers of asbestos per liter of drinking water, and looked at the cancer incidence using the New York State cancer registry. They found no evidence of elevated cancer incidence in sites that were associated with asbestos exposure. This was published in *Public Health Reports* 1989;104:251–6. MacRae reviewed the issue of asbestos in drinking water and cancer in the *Journal of the Royal College of Physicians in London* 1988;22:7–10. Again, the question was whether asbestos was being released by cement pipes, and if so, whether this causes an increased incidence of cancer. Again the conclusion was that there were no data suggesting or confirming that drinking water was carcinogenic.

Further studies on ingested mineral fibers and cancer were reviewed by Kanarec in the IARC publication, "Non-occupational exposure to mineral fibers" 1989;90:428–37. He thought that there was some association between ingested asbestos fibers, and cancer of the stomach and pancreas, but not the colon, similarly to the data published by Polissar et al. (*Am J Epidemiol* 1984;119:456–71) from an epidemiological study of Puget Sound. At the time of these studies in the Puget Sound area, the measured concentration of asbestos fibers ranged from 7.3 to 206.5 million fibers per liter of drinking water. In Connecticut, the level was below detectable levels at 0.7 million fibers per liter of drinking water.

Most people are unaware that the average individual, particularly in Western Washington, ingests large amounts of asbestos fibers regularly through drinking water. There is no good evidence that this is harmful. This issue has been carefully monitored by state and federal authorities. There is no evidence that further exposure in the workplace is associated with increased risk of colon cancer based on my review of most of the world's literature. There is no evidence that exposure to asbestos is associated with an increased risk of lymphoma. There is good evidence that asbestos exposure is associated with increased risk of lung cancer and peritoneal and pleural mesothelioma.

The most recent article on this issue was published by Varga entitled "Asbestos fibers and drinking water: Are they carcinogenic or not?" which was published in *Medical Hypothesis* 2000;55:225–6. He points out that animal experiments have failed to demonstrate carcinogenicity of ingested asbestos, but that penetration of the fibers through the gut wall have been proven. He raised the question of whether there still could be a carcinogenic effect of drinking water contaminated by asbestos, but pointed out that there was no epidemiologic proof of this association.

If asbestos is carcinogenic for colon cancer, then animal studies should be able to confirm asbestos carcinogenicity, as they have done for lung cancer and mesothelioma. This has been attempted by Donham et al. (Donham KJ, Berg JW, Will LA, Leininger JR. The effects of long term ingestion of asbestos on the colon of F344 rats. *Cancer* 1980;15(Suppl.):1073–84) and Ward et al. (Ward JM, Frank AL, Wenk M, Devor D, Tarone RE. Ingested asbestos and intestinal carcinogenesis in F344 rats. *J Environ Pathol Toxicol* 1980;3:301–12). The results have been negative.

Berry, Newhouse, and Wagner published a review of 557 deaths from exposure to crocidolite asbestos. (Berry G, Newhouse ML, Wagner JC. Mortality from all cancers of asbestos factory workers in east London 1933–80. *Occup Environ Med* 2000;57(11):782–5.) Most of the deaths were from lung cancer and mesothelioma. There was an excessive risk of colon cancer, finding 27 cases with only 12 expected. The authors concluded that some of these deaths were labeled as colon cancer but were actually peritoneal mesotheliomas. Therefore, what appeared to be an excessive risk of colon cancer could not be proven to a reasonable degree of scientific certainty.

One of the more recent reviews on colon cancer was published in the second edition of *Clinical Oncology* in 2000, edited by Abeloff, Armitage, Lichter, and Niederhuber, and does not mention any association between asbestos exposure and colon cancer in the written text. Table 13.1 from the IARC mentions the association between asbestos and GI cancer, but this is from old, nonupdated material. The most recent review was published in *Cancer Principles and Practice of Oncology*, sixth edition, edited by Devita et al. and published by Lippincott William & Wilkins in 2001. The section by Skibber, Minsky, and Hoff does not mention any association between asbestos and colon cancer.

A consensus report was prepared by a group of experts convened at the IARC meeting held on 9–11 January 1996. The first part of the report addresses the strengths, weaknesses, and gaps in the present knowledge on fiber character-ization, genotoxicity, cell proliferation, and activation, in animal studies. The second part of the report provides answers to specific questions concerning the relevance of mechanistic data from *in vitro* and *in vivo* assays, in the assessment of the carcinogenic risk of fibers to humans. Finally, the relevance of mechanis-tic data in the evaluation of fiber carcinogenicity is discussed (see Appendix for criteria).

> Cancers other than of the lung or mesothelioma have been con-sidered in many studies. Some indicated an approximately two-fold risk with regard to gastrointestinal cancer in connection with shipyard work and some increased risk was also seen in associa-tion with exposure to both chrysotile and crocidolite, to crocidolite or to chrysotile. Cancer of the colon and rectum was associated with asbestos exposure during chrysotile production, with an approximately two-fold risk; a similar excess was found for unspec-ified asbestos exposure. Some excess of ovary cancer has been reported in two studies but not in another; exposure to crocido-lite was probably more predominant in the studies that showed excesses. Bile duct cancer appeared in excess in one study based on record-linking, and large-cell lymphomas of the gastrointestinal tract and oral cavity appeared to be strongly related to asbestos exposure in one small study covering 28 cases and 28 controls, giving a risk ratio of 8; however, ten cases and one control also had a history of malaria [ref. 106 of the report]. An excess of lym-phopoietic and haematopoietic malignancies has been reported in plumbers, pipe fitters, sheet metal workers and others with asbestos exposure [refs. 17, 54, 107, and 108 of the report].

Since this consensus report, more recent studies have been performed. Perhaps one of the more interesting studies that was performed was by the group at McGill University in Montreal, who performed a case–control study on the relationship between occupational exposure and colon cancer. (Goldberg MS, Parent ME, Siemiatycki J et al. A case–control study of the relationship between the risk of colon cancer in men and exposure to occupational agents. *Am J Ind* 2001;39:531–46.) The authors discovered an increased risk of colon cancer with a variety of occupational exposures to 21 agents, including asbestos, mineral wool, polystyrene, polyurethanes, polyacrylates, cellulose, glass fibers, inorganic insu-lation dust, iron oxide, xylene, diesel engine emissions, etc. This means that when assessing risk from asbestos fibers, consideration must be given to the many other substances that may increase the risk for colon cancer that act as confounders in epidemiologic data.

The largest epidemiologic study to date has been performed in Finland on occupational exposures and GI cancers in women. (Weiderpass E, Vainio H, Kauppien T et al. Occupational exposures and gastrointestinal cancers among Finnish women. *J Occup Environ Med* 2003;45:305–15.) The authors evaluated 413,877 women born between 1906 and 1945. They found 2009 cases of colon cancer. There was an increased risk of colon cancer for sedentary work, but not for asbestos exposure.

A more recent study on the association between GI cancers and asbestos exposure, has been published from Australia, in a group of heavily exposed crocidolite workers. (Reid A, Ambroini, de Klerk N et al. Aerodigestive tract cancers and exposure to crocidolite (blue asbestos): Incidence and mortality among former crocidolite workers. *Int J Cancer* 2004;111:757–61.) The study did not show an association between cumulative asbestos exposure and GI cancers, or a dose–response effect. Smoking status was strongly associated with the incidence of upper GI cancers.

Perhaps, the best recent review on the subject of GI cancer and asbestos exposure has been done by Gamble:

This paper summarizes the weight of epidemiological evidence to evaluate the hypothesis that asbestos exposure is causally associated with increased risk of gastrointestinal (GI) cancers as suggested by Selikoff in an early study of insulation workers. This review looks at populations that develop GI cancers, namely stomach, colorectal, colon and rectal. Guidelines for assessing causality are strength of association, biological gradient and consistency of the associations. Exposure-response (E-R) was evaluated using three methods to estimate exposure. Rate ratios (RRs) for lung cancer and percent of mesothelioma are used as surrogate measures of asbestos exposure for all the cohorts of exposed workers. Quantitative or semi-quantitative estimates of cumulative exposure to asbestos were also used to assess E-R trends and were compared to E-R trends for lung cancer and mesothelioma in individual studies. Surrogate measures are important since there are few individual studies that have assessed E-R. None of the various methods to estimate asbestos exposure yielded consistent E-R trends and the strength of the associations were consistently weak or non-existent for the four types of GI cancers. The epidemiological evidence detracts from the hypothesis that occupational asbestos exposure increases the risk of stomach, colorectal, colon, and rectal cancer. (Gamble J. Risk of gastrointestinal cancers from inhalation and ingestion of asbestos. *Regul Toxicol Pharmacol* 2008;52(1 Suppl.):S124–53.)

There is ample data in the literature to suggest that there may be a familial predisposition to a variety of malignancies related to genetic changes that predispose people to a variety of tumors. There are three major categories of genes that have been implicated in the causation of cancer. These are oncogenes, tumor-suppressor genes, and mismatch repair genes.

One path for causing colon cancer is the inactivation of a tumor-suppressor *APC* gene, and a second cause is replication errors associated with alterations in DNA mismatch genes. The association with the genetic condition called "multiple polyposis coli" was recognized as early as 1934, and is an autosomal dominant condition. Patients who have a family history of colon cancer should be evaluated to see if they have the *FAP* and *APC* genes present, since this is going to be very important in evaluating their children and grandchildren for a very high risk of colon cancer.

A recent large epidemiological study from The Netherlands has suggested that high prolonged exposure to asbestos produces a small increased risk of all types of GI and colorectal cancer. The limitation of this study is the lack of information on confounders that have been mentioned earlier in this chapter. When an increase in epithelial abdominal neoplasms is found only in those workers with heavy exposure, this suggests that there may be pathological confusion with epithelial peritoneal mesotheliomas. (Offermans N, Varmeulan R, Burdorf A et al. Occupational asbestos exposure and risk of esophageal, gastric, and colorectal cancer in the prospective Netherlands Cohort Study. *Int J Cancer* 2014;135(8):1970–7.)

In conclusion, there have been many epidemiologic studies that have studied asbestos exposure and the risk of colon cancer. Most of these studies found no increased risk. Those studies that have claimed a positive association have not been corrected for many important confounding variables such as a positive family history, diet, socioeconomic factors, and exposure to other GI carcinogens. Many of the older studies that have relied on data from death certificates have overestimated the risk of GI malignancy, because of misdiagnosis related to the confusion between GI cancers pathologically and abdominal peritoneal epithelioid mesotheliomas in asbestos exposed individuals. This issue has been studied for nearly 40 years. The lack of animal data, a dose–response effect, and convincing consistent epidemiologic data, act as strong evidence against causation. An overview and analysis of the world's literature has been performed and the evidence is very strong that asbestos exposure is not associated with a significantly increased risk of colon cancer.

CARCINOMA OF THE LARYNX: THE ROLE OF ASBESTOS

Cancer of the larynx was rarely noted in the medical literature prior to the invention of the laryngoscope by Garcia in 1860. Environmental factors in causation were not established until the 1950s, when Wynder (1956) and his associates identified cigarette smoking as the major factor in the causation of laryngeal cancer. The identification of cigarette smoking as a single cause of laryngeal cancer has been now proven to be simplistic.

The causation of carcinoma of the larynx is very complex. The early studies were unaware of the complexity of the imbibing of alcohol and its synergistic effect with cigarette smoking, and the causation of carcinoma of the larynx. Many of the controlled studies that have been done over the years have tried to control for smoking, but have not generally controlled well for alcohol. An alcohol history is much more difficult to obtain because of the social stigmata associated with being an alcoholic. In addition, we now recognize that other factors may play a role, such as chronic gastroesophageal reflux, and infection with HPV. Factors such as race and sex also play a significant role in the risk of developing cancer of the larynx. I will discuss these and other factors later, but I would like to begin this discussion with a review of some of the important papers that have been published over the years, particularly concerning a possible association between asbestos exposure and carcinoma of the larynx. Interest in the United States in the association between cigarette smoking and lung cancer, and its association with asbestos exposure, was stimulated by the seminal work by Hammond and Selikoff in 1965, and later papers in 1968. A study was done in three urban counties in South Carolina by Caston and others. It was noted that certain counties had a significantly higher incidence of laryngeal cancers. (Caston JC, Finklea JF, Sandifer SH. Cancer of the larynx and lung in three urban counties in South Carolina. *South Med J* 1972;65(6):753–6.)

The concern about asbestos exposure and its contribution to laryngeal cancer was first brought up by Stell and McGill in 1973. Since then, there has been a considerable interest in this issue. The most recent review of the subject was the review by Browne and Gee in the *Annals of Occupational Hygiene*, published in 2000. They concluded that there is not sufficient evidence to indicate that asbestos exposure increases the risk for laryngeal cancer. My review of the literature on the subject, including all of the references in their article, which includes the major epidemiologic studies on asbestos exposure and cancer, is that the Browne and Gee are correct in their analysis of the data published by the year 2000. (Stell PM, McGill T. Exposure to asbestos and laryngeal carcinoma. *Lancet* 1975;89(5):513–7; Browne K, Gee JBL. Asbestos exposure and laryngeal cancer. *Am Occup Hyg* 2000;44(4):239–50.)

Stell and McGill, from Liverpool, England, wrote three papers in the early 1970s regarding studies of patients with laryngeal cancer, and possible exposure to asbestos. They noted that while the smoking habits of these patients were similar, the patients with cancer of the larynx had an increased frequency of possible exposure to asbestos. Similar associations were made by Newhouse and Berry in the *Lancet* in 1973. (Newhouse ML, Berry G. Asbestos and laryngeal carcinoma. *Lancet* 1973;2(7829):615.) This was commented on further by Libshitz and others from Philadelphia, when they reported three patients with carcinoma of the larynx, and a history of asbestos exposure, with intrathoracic changes characteristic of asbestosis.

Shettigara and Morgan did a retrospective study of 43 pairs of patients with laryngeal cancer, and managing to control for smoking, age, and sex, seemed to find an association between asbestos exposure and laryngeal cancer, as well as cigarette smoking. They did not find a relationship with alcohol exposure. (Shettigara PT, Morgan RW. Asbestos, smoking, and laryngeal carcinoma. *Arch Environ Health* 1975;30:517–9.)

An animal study was done by Wehner and colleagues at the Batelle Laboratories in Richland, Washington, and published in *Environmental Research* in 1975. In the study, they looked at 102 male Syrian golden hamsters, who received chronic exposure to Canadian chrysotile asbestos and cigarette smoke. They found that the incidence of laryngeal lesions and malignant tumors was significantly lower in the asbestos plus smoke-exposed group, than a controlled group that received smoke alone. They could not find any evidence of a carcinogenic effect of asbestos in this animal model. (Wehner AP, Busch RH, Olson RJ et al. Chronic inhalation of asbestos and cigarette smoke by hamsters. *Environ Res* 1975;10:368–83.)

Freifeld, from the New Jersey College of Medicine, published an article in *JAMA* in September 1977, because of the possibility that there was an association between epidermoid cancer of the larynx, and exposure to asbestos. No in-depth literature review was done and it was simply a report of one case. (Freifeld S. Asbestos exposure and laryngeal carcinoma. *JAMA* 1977;238(12):1280.)

Ward Hinds, in cooperation with David Thomas and HP O'Reilly, did a study of three counties in Washington State, and found smoking and alcohol consumption to increase the risk of laryngeal cancer independently, with a clear dose–response relationship. Neither asbestos exposure nor exposure to other substances was found to significantly increase the risk of laryngeal cancer. This important paper was published in *Cancer* in 1979. Later, in December 1979, Bignon, Hirsch, and others from France, reported significant concentrations of asbestos fibers in samples of laryngeal tissue from two patients with past exposure to asbestos and associated asbestosis. One patient had a polyp on the vocal cord, and the other had laryngeal cancer. They again speculated whether asbestos as an irritant might be responsible for the causation of laryngeal cancers. (Hinds MW, Thomas DB, O'Reilly HP. Asbestos, dental X-rays, tobacco, and alcohol in the epidemiology of laryngeal cancer. *Cancer* 1979;44:1114–20; Bignon J, Monchaux G, Sebastien P et al. Human and experimental data on translocation of asbestos fibers through the respiratory system. *Ann NY Acad Sci* 1979;330:745–50.)

A study published in September 1980, by Blot and colleagues, was a case–control study involving interviews with relatives of males who died of lung and laryngeal cancer in Tidewater, Virginia. No increase in lung cancer was found among the smaller number of men who began work in the shipbuilding industry after 1949, and no overall excess of laryngeal cancer was associated with shipbuilding. He noted an increased risk of laryngeal and lung cancer in blacks. He felt that his studies demonstrated that exposure to asbestos, in association with smoking, gave rise to a higher incidence of laryngeal cancer. He felt that patients who had been exposed to asbestos, and developed laryngeal cancer, could be said to be suffering from an occupational disease. (Blot WJ, Morris LE, Stroube R et al. Lung and laryngeal cancers in relation to shipyard employment in coastal Virginia. *J Natl Cancer Inst* 1980;65(3):571–5.)

Hillerdal and Lindholm reviewed the issue of laryngeal cancer and asbestos in 1980, and stated at that time that tobacco smoking and the use of alcoholic beverages were the main known carcinogens causing laryngeal cancer, but their data suggested that laryngeal cancer was an occupational disease. (Hillerdal G, Lindholm CE. Laryngeal cancer and asbestos. *ORL J Otorhinolaryngol Relat Spec* 1980;42(4):233–41.)

Also in 1980, Victor Roggli and others, performed an autopsy study on five patients with occupational asbestos exposure and proven asbestos-associated pulmonary disease, in which sections of larynx were examined. They found asbestos bodies in two of the five larynges, but none in ten larynges obtained in autopsy controls. This suggested that asbestos exposure might result in retention of asbestos fibers in laryngeal tissue. (Roggli VL, Greenberg SD, McLarty JL et al. Asbestos body content of the larynx in asbestos workers: A study of five cases. *Arch Otolaryngol* 1980;106(9):533–5.)

A review of the epidemiology of laryngeal cancer was published by Rothman and others from the Harvard School of Public Health in *Epidemiologic Reviews* in 1980. They again reviewed the data indicating that cigarette smoke and alcohol were the major factors associated with carcinoma of the larynx. They felt that the evidence supporting the association between asbestos and laryngeal cancer was more substantial than that for other risk factors. Unfortunately, the few studies provided for the effects of occupational exposure were nonconfounded by smoking and alcohol consumption. In other words, the studies were not adequately controlled for the major known causes of laryngeal cancer. They also mention that other studies had suggested that nickel and wood dust had been associated with laryngeal cancer, including a Japanese study showing that mustard gas might also cause laryngeal cancer, and that other exposures to a lesser degree may have an impact on the pathogenesis of carcinoma of the larynx. (Rothman KJ, Cann CI, Flanders D et al. Epidemiology of laryngeal cancer. *Epidemiol Rev* 1980;2:195–209.)

A paper was published in December 1981 from the National Cancer Institute in Toronto, Canada, by Burch and others, evaluating the effects of tobacco, alcohol, asbestos, and nickel on the etiology of carcinoma of the larynx. This was a case–control study, and the attributable risk potential for males using tobacco products and alcohol together, was estimated to be 94%. The relative risk for the effects of exposure to asbestos after the effects of cigarette smoking was controlled, was 2.3, and the effects were only seen in cigarette smokers. The findings on asbestos were based on very small numbers and controls, and therefore it was felt that these numbers were very subject to large sampling errors. However, they felt there was a possible causal role between asbestos exposure and cancer of the larynx. (Burch JD, Howe GR, Miller AB et al. Tobacco, alcohol, asbestos, and nickel in the etiology of cancer of the larynx: A case–control study. *J Natl Cancer Inst* 1981;67(6):1219–24.)

A follow-up study of workers from an asbestos cement factory was published in the *British Journal of Industrial Medicine*, by Thomas and others, in 1982, in which they followed workers who had been exposed to both crocidolite and chrysotile asbestos. They found an excess of lung cancers, and two pleural mesotheliomas, but no cancers of the larynx were found. (Thomas HF, Benjamin IT, Elwood PC et al. Further follow-up study of workers from an asbestos cement factory. *Br J Ind Med* 1982;39:273–76.)

A later paper by Elwood and others from Great Britain, published in the *International Journal of Cancer* in 1984, looked at the effects of alcohol, smoking, and social and occupational factors on the etiology of cancer of the oral cavity, pharynx, and larynx. Increased risks were seen with alcohol consumption, and less strongly with smoking, but together, there was either a multiplicative or additive model for the relationship between alcohol combined with tobacco. Increased risks were found with low socioeconomic status, unmarried state, and poor dental hygiene, but there was no significant association with specific occupational exposures, such as asbestos. (Elwood JM, Pearson JCG, Skippen DH et al. Alcohol, smoking, social and occupational factors in the aetiology of cancer of the oral cavity, pharynx and larynx. *Int J Cancer* 1984;34:603–12.)

Another contribution published in 1984 was by Flanders, Cann, Rothman, and Fried, in the *American Journal of Epidemiology*. They conducted a case–control study to identify employment-related risk factors for laryngeal cancer in Richmond County, Georgia, trying to match their control subjects based on sex, age, area of residence, smoking, and alcohol drinking history. From lifetime employment histories, laryngeal cancer rate ratios were estimated, comparing the incidence among subjects who had ever worked in an occupation, with an incidence rate among subjects who had never worked in that occupation. The highest risk was in farmers, particularly grain farmers, and there was increased risk in textile processors as well. There was a lower risk for drivers of electric engines, while laborers and maintenance personnel had a very significantly increased risk. It is possible that some of these textile workers had exposure to asbestos, but one would not have thought that there would have been exposure to asbestos in some of these other groups, such as farmers. (Flanders WD, Cann CI, Rothman KJ, Fried MP. Work-related risk factors for laryngeal cancer. *Am J Epidemiol* 1984;119:23–32.)

In 1984, Olsen and Sabroe published an article on the occupational causes of laryngeal cancer, based on a case–control study of all new cases of laryngeal cancer in Denmark, from 1980 until 1982. Questionnaires were used to obtain information on education, occupation, and number of occupational exposures, as well as smoking and drinking habits. High risk ratios for laryngeal cancer were found for semi-skilled and unskilled workers, as well as workers exposed to dust, out-of-doors workers, drivers, and people working in the cement industries and port services. The study hypothesis was that exposure to chromium or nickel increases the incidence rate of laryngeal cancer. While there was no support for an increased risk from chromium, exposure to nickel had a statistically significant risk ratio of 1.7. The relative risks for cancer of the larynx were 1.8 for asbestos and 1.6 for any occupational dust. A risk ratio of 1.8 was of borderline statistical significance, according to the authors. (Olsen J, Sabroe S. Occupational causes of laryngeal cancer. *J Epidemiol Community Health* 1984;38:117–21.)

Ohlson and Hogstedt did a study of 1176 Swedish chrysotile asbestos cement workers in 1985. They were unable to demonstrate any increased risk of lung cancer, or other cancers of the respiratory tract, which would include laryngeal cancers, in this cohort with a median exposure of somewhere between 10 and

20 fiber-years. (Ohlson CG, Hogstedt C. Lung cancer among asbestos-cement workers: A Swedish cohort study. *Br J Ind Med* 1985;42:397–402.)

A later study of asbestos cement workers was published in 1994 by Giaroli and coworkers from Italy. This was a cohort that included workers from ten factories that used both chrysotile and crocidolite asbestos. There was a definite increased risk of lung cancer in this series, in which there was exposure to amphibole asbestos. Mortality for laryngeal cancer was not increased in this cohort, even though there was an increased incidence of lung cancer. There was also no increase in GI neoplasms. (Giaroli D, Belli S, Bruno C et al. Mortality study of asbestos cement workers. *Int Arch Occup Health* 1994;66:7–11.)

A review of the mortality of factory workers in East London that was reported by Newhouse, Berry, and Wagner in the *British Journal of Industrial Medicine* in 1985, looked at the mortality of 3000 male factory workers, 1400 laggers, and 700 women factory workers in East London, employed between 1933 and 1964. The women studied were employed between 1936 and 1942. They found, of course, an increased number of mesothelial tumors and carcinomas of the lung. They felt there was an excess of GI tumors, but no dose–response relationship could be shown. Among the severely exposed male factory workers, there was an excess of death from cancer of the larynx and among the severely exposed women, there was an excess of death from carcinoma of the breast and ovary. 2% of the deaths were due to asbestosis. Again, in this type of study, there could not be adequate control for both alcohol and cigarette smoking; therefore, it is unclear from this study whether the proposed increased risk of laryngeal cancers was indeed a true increase of risk, because of the lack of the adequate controls. (Newhouse ML, Berry G, Wagner JC. Mortality of factory workers in East London 1933–80. *Br J Ind Med* 1985;42:4–11.)

Doll and Peto, in 1985, agreeing with Newhouse, felt that the information available at that time suggested a relationship between asbestos exposure and laryngeal cancer. (Doll R, Peto J. *Effects on Health Exposure to Asbestos.* London: HMSO, 1985.)

The following year, in the *American Journal of Epidemiology*, Botha and others from the Institute of Biostatistics of the South African Medical Research Council, tried to evaluate the excess mortality from stomach cancer, lung cancer, and asbestosis or mesothelioma, in crocidolite mining districts in South Africa. They found increased numbers of all these cancers, but did not mention any increased risk of cancer of the larynx. (Botha JL, Irwig LM, Strebel PM. Excess mortality from stomach cancer, lung cancer, and asbestosis and/or mesothelioma in crocidolite mining districts in South Africa. *Am J Epidemiol* 1986;123:30–40.)

Rebecca Zagraniski and others, evaluated the occupational risk factors for laryngeal cancer in Connecticut between 1975 and 1980, publishing their findings in 1986, in the *American Journal of Epidemiology*. They felt that there was an increased risk for those who worked in rubber product manufacturing and transportation manufacturing other than shipbuilding, and for men who had ever been machinists, bartenders, farmers, masons, and metal grinders. Only one occupation—machinists—had a significantly increased OR. Asbestos and nickel were not found to be risk factors for laryngeal cancer in this study in which there was adequate control for the effects of tobacco and alcohol. (Zagraniski RT, Kelsey JL, Walter SD. Occupational risk factors for laryngeal carcinoma: Connecticut, 1975–1980. *Am J Epidemiol* 1986;124:67–76.)

Ross Brownson evaluated various risk factors for laryngeal cancer, using a case–control design from the Missouri Cancer Registry between 1984 and 1985. He felt that the risk for laryngeal cancer was increased synergistically by both alcohol and tobacco. He noted that after controlling for alcohol and tobacco, the only occupational category with an elevated risk was nonconstruction laborers. (Brownson RC, Chang JC. Exposure to alcohol and tobacco and the risk of laryngeal cancer. *Arch Environ Health* 1987;42(4):192–6.)

Viallat and coworkers from Marseille, France, did a study on 200 subjects to determine possible links to asbestos, including 50 patients with cancer of the larynx, 50 patients with cancer of the lung, and 100 controls. They then rated the exposures to asbestos in the cancer patient cases, compared to the controls, and found that the cancer patients had an increased risk due to asbestos exposure. Their study found that time between first exposure to asbestos and the development of cancer of the larynx was 28.5 years on average, as compared to 46 years for cancer of the lung. They stated that this study confirmed an etiologic role of asbestos in the pathogenesis of cancer of the larynx. This study, published in 1986, is fraught with methodological problems, and obviously there was no effort to control many factors, including alcohol and tobacco use in the cancer population, as compared to the control population. We would now recognize in retrospect also that this somewhat simplistic study is methodologically not a valid method for trying to determine the role of asbestos in the causation of cancer of the larynx, because of the inadequacy of control for many of the factors that are also associated with increased risk of cancer of the larynx besides asbestos, such as diet, socioeconomic status, tobacco consumption, alcohol consumption, HPV infection, etc. (Viallat J, Farisse P, Rey F et al. Amiante et cancer du larynx. *Annales d'oto-laryngologie* (Paris) 1986;103:63–6.)

Eduardo De Stefani and others from the Departments of Pathology and Otolaryngology in Uruguay, and the Department of Pathology at Louisiana State University in New Orleans, published a study of 107 patients afflicted with laryngeal cancer compared to 290 controls with diseases considered not related to tobacco and alcohol exposure, who were interviewed at the University Hospital in Montevideo, Uruguay. Tobacco smoking was the greatest risk factor, and while alcohol exposure displayed lesser effects, its interaction with tobacco resulted in very high risks, perhaps 100 times higher. Also, the habit of drinking a local tea called "mate," was associated with a threefold increased risk after controlling for the effects of age, tobacco, and alcohol consumption. Infrequent consumption of vegetables and fruit increased the risk by 2.7-fold, suggesting the role of diet in the causation of laryngeal cancer. (De Stefani E, Correa P, Oreggia F et al. Risk factors for laryngeal cancer. *Cancer* 1987;60:3087–91.)

Linda Brown and others from the Division of Cancer Etiology at the National Cancer Institute in Bethesda, Maryland, did a study which was published in *Cancer Research* in 1988, on the occupational risk factors for laryngeal cancer on the Texas gulf coast. Occupational exposures were examined, and controlled for possible confounding by cigarette smoking and alcohol consumption. And slightly elevated risks were seen for men employed in public services industries, such as transportation, communication, utilities, and sanitary services, with a relative risk was 1.6. Metal fabricating had a relative risk of 2.1, construction 1.7, and maintenance had a relative risk of 2.7. Occupations in which there was exposure to paint had a relative risk of 1.8, while exposure to diesel and gasoline fumes had a relative risk of 1.5. Elevated risks of borderline significance, were seen for men employed as wood workers and furniture makers—the numbers were small but the risk was 8.1—and those with occupational exposure to asbestos, had a risk of only 1.5. If they categorized the asbestos exposure by intensity of the exposure, they felt that there was a positive association between asbestos exposure and increased risk. (Brown LM, Mason TJ, Pickle LW et al. Occupational risk factors for laryngeal cancer on the Texas Gulf Coast. *Cancer Res* 1988;48:1960–4.)

Charles Chan and J Bernard Gee, from Yale did, a critical analysis of the available epidemiologic investigations on the causal relationship between asbestos exposure and laryngeal cancer. They reviewed the nine case–control studies that indicated that the estimated risk attributable to asbestos exposure alone was negligible, when smoking and ethanol intake were properly controlled. They felt that the six longitudinal studies that showed an increased risk of laryngeal cancer due to asbestos exposure had had not made a proper adjustment for the confounding effects of smoking and ethanol consumption. (Chan CK, Gee JBL. Asbestos exposure and laryngeal cancer: An analysis of the epidemiologic evidence. *J Occup Med* 1988;30(1):23–7.)

Steenland and others from the University of California at Davis, published an article in 1988 on the incidence of laryngeal cancer and exposure to acid mists. Sulfuric acid mist was the primary exposure for most men in this cohort, and these people had worked in a pickling operation for a minimum of 6 months before 1965, with an average exposure duration of 9.5 years. They felt that, when using data corrected for their smoking, the incidence of laryngeal cancer was definitely increased related to chronic acid mist exposure. This study was followed by a paper by Tola and others from the Institute of Occupational Health in Helsinki, Finland, and published in the *British Journal of Industrial Medicine* in 1988, on the incidence of cancer among welders, platers, machinists, pipe fitters, shipyard workers, and machine shop workers. The smoking habits of the cohorts appeared to be similar. While the incidence of laryngeal cancer was slightly raised among the shipyard workers, it was not among the machine shop workers. No excessive risk of mesothelioma was observed among the welders. There was a small excess risk of lung cancer, but this was thought to be possibly due to chance alone. (Steenland K, Schnorr T, Beaumont J et al. Incidence of laryngeal cancer and exposure to acid mists. *Br J Ind Med* 1988;45:766–76; Tola S, Kalliomaki PL, Pukkala E et al. Incidence of cancer among welders, platers, machinists, and pipe fitters in shipyards and machine shops. *Br J Ind Med* 1988;45:209–18.)

Finally, another case–control study of carcinoma of the larynx and hypopharynx was carried out in six populations in Italy, Switzerland, and France, and published by the IARC. The effect of tobacco was similar at all sites, and the risk associated with never smoking was one tenth of the risk of smokers. The risk from alcohol and smoking depended on the site, but they were similar for the epilarynx and hypopharynx, and lower for the endolarynx. For all sites, the risk decreased after quitting. Exclusive use of filtered cigarettes was thought to be somewhat protective. The authors felt that the relative risk of exposure to alcohol and tobacco were consistent with a multiplicative model. This study was particularly important because it is the largest one reported, looking at the risk associated with 1147 male cases and 3057 male controls.

David Edelman published a review article on laryngeal cancer and occupational exposure to asbestos in 1989. Based on his review, in only two of the 13 cohort studies, were the SMRs significantly increased. He mentions that smoking as a risk factor for laryngeal cancer may have been more prevalent among asbestos workers than comparison populations. Murray Finkelstein evaluated the mortality rates among employees potentially exposed to chrysotile asbestos in two automotive parts factories in Canada, and published his findings in the *Canadian Medical Association Journal* in 1989. He looked at the mortality rates among 1657 employees of these plants, and found a significantly increased rate of death from laryngeal cancer and lung cancer, and only one or two deaths from mesothelioma. A case–control analysis of this population, however, showed no association between the risk of laryngeal cancer and the total duration of employment, which was a surrogate for asbestos exposure. (Edelman DA. Laryngeal cancer and occupational exposure to asbestos. *Int Arch Occup Environ Health* 1989;61:223–7; (Finkelstein MM. Mortality rates among employees potentially exposed to chrysotile asbestos at two automotive parts factories. *CMAJ* 1989;141:125–30.)

Because of the increasing interest in the association between asbestos exposure and carcinoma of the larynx, the Department of Social Security in Great Britain, evaluated the world's literature in an effort to determine whether workers who had been exposed to asbestos and developed carcinoma of the larynx should be compensated for having an occupational disease. The review, done by the "Industrial Injuries Advisory Council," concluded that the evidence received did not enable them to believe that the statutory requirements were met in the case of laryngeal cancer. They decided to continue monitoring the situation. They pointed out in the text of their report that in most of the case–control studies, asbestos exposure was associated with a small increase in risk that was not statistically significant, at the 5% level, to demonstrate an association that would be considered significant enough to be a probable cause. They went on to mention that one of the problems with the cohort studies was that they used mortality rather than cancer incidence as an endpoint. Deaths from laryngeal cancer are relatively uncommon, and in five of the eight studies, the risk estimates were based on fewer than five cases. Therefore, there was considerable statistical uncertainty. Furthermore, they mention that there were other causes, such as the exposure to mustard gas and acid mists, but they did not feel the evidence concerning sulfuric acid mist was sufficiently strong to justify calling it an occupational carcinogen. (Harrington JM. *Cancer or the larynx. Report by the Industrial Advisory Council; Social Security Act 1975*, 1989.)

The World Health Organization evaluated the occupational exposure limit for asbestos in a report published in 1989. They listed the evidence relating asbestos to various diseases, and under laryngeal cancer, they felt that the evidence was doubtful, but felt certainty for lung cancer. They went on to say

A recent review by Chan and Gee (1988) has concluded that the epidemiologic evidence does not support a causal relationship between asbestos exposure and laryngeal cancer, whereas Doll and Peto (1985) concluded that asbestos should be regarded as one of the causes of laryngeal cancer. [Chan CK, Gee JBL. Asbestos exposure and larnyngeal cancer. *J Occ Med* 1988;30:23–7; Doll R, Peto J. *Effects on Health Exposure to Asbestos.* London: HMSO, 1985.] One difficulty here is that a number of studies have reported raised levels of cancer of the larynx—although in most case–control studies the excess disappeared when smoking and alcohol were taken into account, and in the cohort studies such adjustment has not been made—there are even more cohort studies where the relevant figures have not been published. So the available evidence is selective at present—and it may be that the unavailable evidence is similar to that published or was possibly not published because it did not show excess. The Industrial Injuries Advisory Council in the United Kingdom has recently concluded that the evidence does not support a causal association. (WHO. *Occupational Exposure Limit for Asbestos.* Geneva: Office of Occupational Health World Health Organization, 1989; Annex p. 3,22; Regular p. 8,9.)

A group from Yugoslavia evaluated the laryngeal mucosa of 195 workers in an asbestos cement factory in Yugoslavia. The cement contained 13% asbestos, which was a mixture of amosite, crocidolite, and chrysotile. They looked at patients with chronic laryngitis, and biopsied ten out of 195 workers. While no cases of laryngeal cancer were seen, they noted irritation of the larynx, and felt that the term laryngeal asbestosis was justified for this nonspecific picture. (Kambic V, Radsel Z, Gale N. Alterations in the laryngeal mucosa after exposure to asbestos. *Br J Ind Med* 1989;46:717–23.)

The UK Industrial Injuries Advisory Council declined to classify laryngeal cancer in patients exposed to asbestos as a prescribed disease, or acceptable for a compensation award in 1989.

A study in Madrid, Spain, by Bravo and associates, looked at occupational risk factors for cancer of the larynx in Spain, since Spain is one of the countries with the highest incidence of laryngeal cancer. They did a case–control study and found that 56.5% of the laryngeal cancer patients had a sedentary occupation working in a service sector. Exposure to insecticides or silica were the strongest risk factors for laryngeal cancer. Associations between laryngeal cancer and exposure to fumes, chemical products, mineral dust, or wood dust were not found. (Bravo MP, Espinosa J, Calero JR. Occupational risk factors for cancer of the larynx in Spain. *Neoplasma* 1990;37:477–81.)

Later, a study by Cauvin and others from Paris, France, was published in *Clinical Otolaryngology* in 1990, in which they did an epidemiologic case–control study of occupational risk factors and cancers of the upper respiratory and digestive tract, finding that cancer of the supraglottis was associated with exposure to oil and grease, with an OR of 2.4, and with exposure to cement, with an OR of 4.2. Cancer of the glottis was associated with exposure to dye with an OR of 6.4. Also, exposure to flour occurred more frequently among controls and among patients with pharyngeal or oral cancer. At the same time, a national longitudinal study was done in Denmark, and published by Guenel and others in the *British Journal of Industrial Medicine* in 1990. They did a multivariate analysis of the risk factors for laryngeal cancer and felt that the risk was strongly related to sociodemographic factors. They noted that the risk for workers living in Copenhagen was almost five times higher than for the risk for men who were self-employed in agriculture, and living in rural areas. They felt that tobacco and cigarette smoking alone could not explain all of the cases. They noted that marital state was a risk factor for laryngeal cancer, with an excess risk for widowed or divorced and married persons, compared with unmarried persons. The highest risks were found in bricklayers, slaughterhouse workers, drivers, various retail salespeople, and a variety of other occupations, while shipyard workers had a risk that was lower, but increased depending on the trade. (Cauvin JM, Guenel P, Luce D et al. Occupational exposure and head and neck carcinoma. *Clin Otolaryngol* 1990;15:439–45; Guenel P, Engholm G, Lyng E. Laryngeal cancer in Denmark: A nationwide longitudinal study based on register linkage data. *Br J Ind Med* 1990;47:473–79.)

Another study from Italy was reported by Piolatto, Negri, and others in the *British Journal of Industrial Medicine* in 1990, on the mortality of a cohort of chrysotile miners employed since 1946 in Balangero, Italy. There were a total of 427 deaths out of 27,010 man-years at risk. There was a substantial excess mortality from all causes, which was related mainly to the high rates of the use of alcohol, including deaths from hepatic cirrhosis and accidents. The mortality from cancer was increased, and the SMR for carcinoma of the larynx was 267 based on eight deaths. This barely reached statistical significance. No consistent associations between the duration or cumulative exposure to asbestos dust and oral cancer were seen, but the laryngeal and pleural cancer cases were in the highest category of duration and degree of exposures. They agreed that part of laryngeal cancer cases were probably attributable to the high alcohol consumption in this group of workers, but they still felt that there was some, perhaps moderate, risk of asbestos exposure for causing laryngeal cancer. There was no way in this death certificate study to control for actual amount of smoking or actual alcohol consumption, other than to point out that because of the excessive deaths from alcohol-related causes, it was clear that this population consisted of heavy drinkers. Since the actual consumption of alcohol and tobacco and other factors could not be controlled, this type of study is really of little value, in that it is in conflict with other studies of a similar type, which failed to demonstrate any increased risk of laryngeal cancer. Here again, another study is published without adequate control for tobacco and alcohol, trying to estimate the actual risk of laryngeal cancer, which, of course, is impossible without adequate controls. (Piolatto G, Negri E, La Vecchia C et al. An update of cancer mortality among chrysotile asbestos miners in Balangero. *Brit J Ind Med* 1990;47:810–4.)

FD Liddell reviewed the literature on laryngeal cancer and asbestos in an editorial published in the *British Journal of Industrial Medicine* in 1990. His conclusions were that the data did not support a significantly increased risk of laryngeal cancer related to asbestos exposure. (Liddell FD. Laryngeal cancer and asbestos. *Br J Ind Med* 1990;47:289–91.)

A contrary opinion on the epidemiologic evidence was published by Smith, Handley, and Wood in the *Journal of Occupational Medicine* in 1990, in which they felt that the epidemiologic evidence did indicate that asbestos causes laryngeal cancer. They felt that the case–control studies gave mixed results but generally supported the hypothesis. (Smith AH, Handley MA, Wood R. Epidemiological evidence indicates asbestos causes laryngeal cancer. *J Occup Med* 1990;32(6):499–507.)

Steven Parnes also evaluated the relationship between asbestos exposure and carcinoma of the larynx in an article in *Laryngoscope*, published in March 1990. He evaluated 322 people in a plant manufacturing brake linings, in which asbestos was a major component. He noted an increased incidence of laryngitis in those with asbestos exposure, compared to a low-risk group. He noted that there were three cases of laryngeal cancer observed when only 0.77 cases were expected. These cases involve smokers with limited asbestos exposure; therefore, neither the longitudinal nor cross-sectional data could support asbestos as an etiologic factor for laryngeal cancer, but Parnes felt it might be an irritant. (Parnes SM. Effects of Asbestos on the larynx. *Laryngoscope* 1990;100:254–61.)

A group from Germany published a review of a hospital-based case–control study of laryngeal cancer conducted in Bremen, Germany, between 1986 and 1987. The OR was increased for heavy smoking and consumers of alcohol, but no increased risk could be shown for exposure to asbestos, coal tar, or welding fumes. On the other hand, excess risks were observed for exposures to diesel oil, gasoline, and mineral oil, when controlling for smoking and alcohol. (Sturm W, Menze B, Krause J et al. Use of asbestos, health risks and induce occupational diseases in the former East Germany. *Toxicol Lett* 1994;72:317–24.)

Another epidemiologic study was done in Seoul, Korea, at the Korea Cancer Center Hospital, by Choi and Kahyo. They noted that the risk for cancers of the oral cavity, pharynx, and larynx rose for current smokers and declined for ex-smokers. The relationship was strongest for laryngeal cancer. Heavy drinkers who drank 90 g of ethanol daily, had a 15-fold increased risk of cancer of the oral cavity, and an 11-fold risk of pharyngeal cancer compared to nondrinkers. However, alcohol was a weaker risk factor for laryngeal cancer than cigarette smoking. The relative risk from smoking two packs of cigarettes a day over several decades is 20 or more. The synergy index, or the effect of the combination of cigarette smoking and alcohol consumption of 200 mL/day, is as high as 3.3, and the combination of smoking and alcohol consumption may lead to between a 20- and 50-fold increased risk of developing laryngeal cancer, compared to non-smokers and nondrinkers, according to Muscat and Wynder. (Muscat JE, Wynder

EL. Tobacco alcohol, asbestos, and occupational risk factors for laryngeal cancer. *Cancer* 1992;69:2244–51; Choi SY, Kahyo H. Effect of cigarette smoking and alcohol consumption in the aetiology of cancer of the oral cavity, pharynx and larynx. *Int J Epidemiol* 1991;20:878–85.)

Fischbein and others from Mount Sinai in New York City reported one patient with asbestosis, laryngeal cancer, and malignant peritoneal mesothelioma. This patient was an insulation worker, and they felt that all three conditions were related to asbestos exposure. They quoted a review by Doll and Peto on other asbestos-related neoplasms, published in 1986, in a book by Antman, entitled *Asbestos-Related Malignancy* at which time Doll and Peto felt that asbestos should be regarded as perhaps one of the causes of laryngeal cancer. (Fischbein A, Luo JCJ, Pinkston GR. Asbestosis, laryngeal carcinoma, and malignant peritoneal mesothelioma in an insulation worker. *Br J Ind Med* 1991;48:338–41.)

A study by Tom Vaughan and Scott Davis from the Fred Hutchison Cancer Research Center in Seattle, Washington, evaluated the contribution of wood dust exposure to squamous cell cancers of the upper respiratory tract. They did not find a significantly increased risk for cancer of the oropharynx and larynx, but their numbers were small, and did suggest increased risk for sinonasal and nasopharyngeal squamous cell cancers. (Vaughn TL, Davis S. Wood dust exposure and squamous cell cancers of the upper respiratory tract. *Am J Epidemiol* 1991;133:560–4.)

Joshua Muscat and Ernst Wynder, from the Division of Epidemiology of the American Health Foundation in New York, looked at the data from a hospital-based case–control study between 1985 and 1990, to examine the effects of tobacco, alcohol, asbestos, and other occupational exposures on laryngeal cancer risks in 194 white males with primary cancer of the larynx. A dose-dependent effect of cigarette smoking was observed, which was not unexpected, but they found that the effects of cigarette smoke were greater for supraglottic cancer than cancer of the glottis. The effects of alcohol showed a dose-dependent effect, with the highest risk for supraglottic cancer as opposed to glottic cancer. A slightly elevated but nonsignificant association was seen from asbestos exposure and glottic cancer. The relative risks did not increase linearly with the number of years employed in an asbestos-related occupation. No relationship was observed between asbestos and cancer of the supraglottis. When examining the data for the synergistic effect of cigarette smoking and asbestos exposure, no excessive risk was found. However, a significantly elevated risk was found for a man exposed to diesel fumes, with a relative risk of 5.2. An elevated but not statistically significant risk was seen for men chronically exposed to rubber and wood dust. (Muscat JE, Wynder EL. Tobacco, alcohol, asbestos, and occupational risk factors for laryngeal cancer. *Cancer* 1992;69(9):2241–51.)

Another study was performed on occupational exposure and the incidence of laryngeal cancer in Edmonton, Alberta, by Soskolne and others and was published in 1992. They demonstrated that when exposed to tobacco and alcohol, there was a strongly positive association with sulfuric acid mists. Asbestos as a confounder was found to be nonsignificant. (Soskolne CL, Jhangri GS, Siemiatycki J et al.

Occupational exposure to sulfuric acid in southern Ontario, Canada, in association with laryngeal cancer. *Scand J Work Environ Health* 1992;18:225–32.)

Heinz Maier and coworkers from Heidelberg, Germany, published an article in 1992 on the risk factors of cancer of the larynx. This was a case–control study, and they pointed out that squamous cell cancer of the larynx is a multifactorial disease, firmly linked to several environmental risk factors. They noted that 90% of the patients were blue-collar workers, most of them working in dirty and dusty jobs, and this finding was consistent with some other published studies. Occupational exposure to cement dust was associated with increased risk. Exposure to coal and tar products was associated with a considerable risk of supraglottic cancer, with a relative risk of 6.11 adjusted for tobacco and alcohol. In addition, an increased risk was associated with chronic exposure to pinewood dust, and the authors mention that an increased incidence of laryngeal cancer in wood workers had been observed in other studies. Social class and educational factors played a role, in that the educational level in the patients with laryngeal cancer was lower than the general level, and poor housing conditions were observed in some patients, suggesting that lower socioeconomic status was associated with various cancers, particularly laryngeal cancers. Dietary factors were studied, and the patients with cancer had a low intake of fruit, salads, dairy products, and vitamin pills. The authors concluded that in this case–control study of 164 male patients compared to 656 male control patients, that tobacco and alcohol are the major risk factors. In addition, there were aspects of poor diet, occupational factors, and social status, as well as increasing evidence that viral infections and genetic predisposition are causes of laryngeal cancer. There is no mention of asbestos being found as a cause of cancer in this case–control study from Germany. (Maier H, Gewelke U, Dietz A et al. Risk factors of cancer of the larynx: Results of the Heidelberg case–control study. *Otolaryngol Head Neck Surg* 1992;107:577–82.)

Another study from the University of Washington in Seattle, Washington, was published in the *British Journal of Industrial Medicine* in 1992 by Wortley and others, looking at specific jobs and occupational exposures that were associated with increased risks of laryngeal cancer in Western Washington. They looked at 235 cases diagnosed between September 1983 and February 1987 and 547 controls. They tried to control for alcohol use, cigarette smoking, age, and education, and found increased risks for painters, construction supervisors, miscellaneous mechanics, construction workers, and metal-working and plastic-working machine operators, as well as handlers, equipment cleaners, and laborers. Potential exposures to asbestos, chromium, nickel, formaldehyde, diesel fumes, and cutting oils, were assessed by using a job–exposure matrix developed for this study. No significantly raised risks were seen, although there might have been an increased risk suggesting that those exposed to long-term formaldehyde at the highest exposures were at increased risk. (Wortley P, Vaughan TL, Davis S et al. A case–control study of occupational risk factors for laryngeal cancer. *Br J Ind Med* 1992;49:837–44.)

William Blot of the Epidemiology and Biostatistics Program at the National Cancer Institute in Bethesda, did a study in cooperation with the Department of Epidemiology in Shanghai, China, on diet and other risk factors for laryngeal cancer in Shanghai, China, published in the *American Journal of Epidemiology* in 1992. Here, cigarette smoking was a major risk factor accounting for 86% of the male and 54% of the female cases. After adjusting for smoking, there was a small increase in risk associated with drinking alcoholic beverages, and among men, cases more often reported occupational exposures to asbestos and coal dust. A protective effect was associated with the intake of fruits, particularly oranges and tangerines, certain dark green and yellow vegetables, and garlic, but there was an increased risk with the intake of salt-preserved meat and fish. They felt that these data showed that dietary factors play an important etiologic role. (Zheng W, Blot WJ, Shu XO et al. Diet and other risk factors for laryngeal cancer in Shanghai, China. *Am J Epidemiol* 1992;136:178–91.)

Franco Berrino, from the National Tumor Institute in Milan, Italy, did a very large study for the IARC evaluating cancer of the larynx and occupation. They published the preliminary results at the 9th International Symposium on Epidemiology and Occupational Health in a National Institute of Occupational Safety and Health (NIOSH) publication in 1992. Dr. Berrino published a book chapter in 1993 on occupational factors in upper respiratory tract cancers. This very extensive review was largely based on his own data. Berrino points out that misclassification of laryngeal cancer is really quite common. In the Lombardy Cancer Registry in Italy, up to one-third of the deaths coded as laryngeal cancer were not due to laryngeal cancers but to cancers of other sites. This is quite important since most experts believe that cancer of the oropharynx demonstrates different strengths of etiological factors at different anatomical subsites. This means that the effects of tobacco and alcoholic beverages, etc., are greater or lesser based on the location of the tumor in the oropharynx. Therefore, it is very important to properly classify the location of the tumor. (Berrino F. Occupational factors of upper respiratory tract cancers. In: A Hirsch (Ed.), *Prevention of Respiratory Diseases*. New York: M. Dekker, 1993, pp. 81–96.)

The IARC international case–control study that began in the early 1980s of a large population base, was an incidence case–control study that was carried out in six areas of Southern Europe, in which cancers of the larynx and hypopharynx were known to be especially prevalent. The main purpose of this study was to clarify the role of tobacco smoking, intake of alcoholic beverages, and their interaction. Information on alcoholic beverages, diet, and smoking was analyzed in a total of 1010 incident cases in which the actual anatomic site was accurately described. The occupational history was recorded from 1945 for each job lasting at least 6 months. A job matrix for 13 agents, including asbestos, polycyclic aromatic hydrocarbons (PAH), chromium, nickel, and other substances was carefully evaluated. In this study, when there was adequate control for tobacco and alcohol, the relative risk for asbestos in the endolarynx was 1.7 and 2.1 in the hypopharynx. It was 1.2 for PAH in the endolarynx and 2.2 in the hypopharynx. Gas fumes and vapors gave a risk of 1.3 in the endolarynx and 2.5 in the hypopharynx. Solvents gave a risk of 1.9 in the endolarynx and 1.5 in the hypopharynx. Formaldehyde increased the risk to 1.7 in the endolarynx and 1.4 in the hypopharynx. All dust except asbestos gave a risk of 1.5 in the endolarynx and 1.9 in the hypopharynx.

Dr. Berrino and colleagues, in their review of the effects of asbestos exposure, pointed out that the relationship between asbestos and laryngeal cancer remained a highly controversial issue. They highlighted that most studies did not reach statistical significance, and the observed relative risk values were mutually inconsistent from one study to another, and of course, the other major problem was that tobacco and alcohol use had not always been taken into account in many of the studies that had reported an increased risk of laryngeal cancer from asbestos exposure. He felt that the relationship between asbestos exposure and laryngeal cancer was one of the "soundest results that can be achieved when occupational epidemiology is based on retrospective assessment of exposure." He further pointed out that there was a high risk of laryngeal cancer for carpenters and painters, and especially for jobs involving heavy dust exposure, such as masonry, tile laying, and plastering. It seemed that the construction industry entailed a high risk of pharyngeal cancer. (Berrino F, Richiardi L, Boffett P et al. Occupation and larynx and hypopharynx cancer: A job–exposure matrix approach in an international case–control study in France, Italy, Spain and Switzerland. *Cancer Causes Control* 2003;14:213–23.)

This study did not demonstrate a dose–response relationship between the alleged environmental factors because of its experimental design. When any exposure over 6 months is considered a significant exposure, then what normally would be considered an insignificant exposure now becomes a significant exposure for the purposes of the study. This means that the authors' evaluation of the relative risks of certain exposures are meaningless because they did not account for the intensity and duration of these exposures in a meaningful way.

William Blot and others published another paper in the *Journal of the National Cancer Institute* in March 1993 looking at racial differences in the risk of oral and pharyngeal cancer. In the United States, blacks have the highest rates for oral and pharyngeal cancer. What determines this racial disparity is not clear in the large population-based case–control studies consisting of 1065 oral cancer patients and 871 whites and 194 blacks, and it was felt that differences with respect to alcohol consumption, especially among current smokers, emerged as the most important explanatory variable. However, after adjusting for smoking and heavy drinking, there was a 17-fold increased risk among blacks and a ninefold increase among whites. Blacks tended to drink more than whites, but there did not appear to be any significant race-related variables in smoking. Whites tend to have a higher intake of protective dietary factors, such as fruits and vitamin C than blacks. It was felt that the data showed evidence that various environmental and lifestyle determinants may affect the risk of oral cancer, including laryngeal cancer in blacks and whites. The primary factor for the difference between races was alcohol consumption, and it was felt that if alcohol consumption could be reduced, the risk would be substantially reduced for laryngeal and oral cancer. (Day GL, Blot WJ, Austin DF et al. Racial differences in risk of oral and pharyngeal cancer: Alcohol, tobacco, and other determinants. *J Natl Cancer Inst* 1993;85(6):465–73.)

Hedberg and others from the Fred Hutchison Cancer Institute and the University of Washington published another paper in *Cancer Causes and Control* entitled "Alcoholism and cancer of the larynx—A case–control study in Western

Washington (United States)." Some of the problems in epidemiologic studies are mentioned, including that alcoholics may give less valid reports of cigarette consumption than nonalcoholics, making this a confounder. Also, nutritional factors are known to be related to alcohol consumption, such as decreased consumption of fruits and vegetables. Genetic factors were also thought to play a role. Perhaps the risk of alcoholism may measure the risk of susceptibility to the carcinogenic effects of alcohol and cigarettes. (Hedberg K, Vaughan TL, White E, Davis S, Thomas DB. Alcoholism and cancer of the larynx: A case–control study in Western Washington (United States). *Cancer Causes Control* 1994;5:3–8.)

Douglas Liddell reviewed the cancer mortality statistics in chrysotile mining and milling in Quebec, as published in the *Annals of Occupational Hygiene* in 1994. In the Quebec, cohort, there were 18 cases of laryngeal cancer, when only 13.8 were expected in the follow-up of 10,925 men born between 1891 and 1920, who had worked for at least 1 month or more in the mines and mills of the Eastern townships of the Providence of Quebec. The excess laryngeal cancer was concentrated in smokers, and any association between dust measurements was negative. No information was available on alcohol consumption. A similar type of chrysotile mine and mill exposure had been reported from the Balangero chrysotile mine in Northern Italy by Rubino and others in 1979, and by Piolatto and others in 1990. In the latter group, there were five more laryngeal cancers than the three laryngeal cancers that were expected, and there was also an excess of lung cancer, but in this population there was also an increased incidence of alcoholism. Therefore, we cannot conclude that there was a true increased risk of laryngeal cancer in this group when controlling for both alcohol and cigarette smoking. The data from this group are basically uninterpretable. The incidence of cancer of the lung, pleura, larynx, and pharynx was evaluated in an asbestos cement plant in Croatia, and published in 1995 by Curin and Saric, who included data on smoking and alcohol consumption of residents in the area, as well as educational levels, among other factors, and this showed that the mortality rates were actually lower for carcinoma of the lung and larynx than expected, while rates for mesothelioma were increased. (Liddell D. Cancer mortality in chrysotile mining and milling: Exposure–response. *Ann Occup Hyg* 1994;38(4):519–23; Rubino GF, Newhouse M, Murray R et al. Radiologic changes after cessation of exposure among chrysotile asbestos miners in Italy. *Ann NY Acad Sci* 1979;330:157–61; Piolatto G, Negri E, La Vecchia C et al. An update of cancer mortality among chrysotile asbestos miners in Balangero. *Br J Ind Med* 1990;47:810–4; Curin K, Saric M. Cancer of the lung, pleura, larynx and pharynx in an area with an asbestos-cement plant. *Arh Hig Rada Toksikol* 1995;46:289–300.)

Ellen Eisen and coworkers from the Massachusetts Institute of Technology, did a mortality study of machining fluid exposure in the automotive industry, and did a case–control study of laryngeal cancer. They studied automobile workers exposed to metalworking fluids, and found 108 cases of laryngeal cancer. They felt that mineral oils were associated with a twofold excess of laryngeal cancer risk. There was also some evidence of an association with elemental sulfur, which was commonly added to straight machining fluids to improve the integrity of the materials under extreme pressure and heat. They pointed out that high-stress operations requiring machining fluids, enriched with sulfur, are more likely to produce polycyclic aromatic hydrocarbons during the process. This study, published in 1994, is just another one of many other studies highlighting the role of machining fluids as possible causative agents in laryngeal cancer. (Eisen EA, Tolbert PE, Hallock MF et al. Mortality studies of machining fluid exposure in the automobile industry III: A case–control study of larynx cancer. *Am J Ind Med* 1994;26:185–202.)

Saric and Vujovic did a study on the incidence of malignant tumors in the area of an asbestos-processing plant in Croatia and published this in 1994. They presented some unusual findings, in which they demonstrated that the actual incidence of cancer of the lung and bronchus was lower in the area of the asbestos factory, than the general area of Croatia. The actual incidence of cancer of the lung was about half that found in the rest of Croatia. Fewer malignant tumors of the pharynx and peritoneum were found in that area, but there was increased incidence of mesothelioma, and laryngeal tumors were about twice as prevalent as in other areas of Croatia. In the area of the asbestos factory, an incidence of four of the five laryngeal cancers was found in farmers, indicating that they were not actually workers in the factory, but were people who lived in the area of the factory, so they did not work primarily with the asbestos. The authors concluded that since the farmers worked in an area where there was a higher amount of asbestos in the air, asbestos was responsible. Obviously, if the asbestos was responsible, one would expect the incidence of tumors to be highest in people directly working in the factory, where they would have gotten the highest dose, and not in people who worked in the area of the factory, and were not directly exposed to asbestos. Therefore, the data from the paper fail to support the authors' conclusion that asbestos might play a role in the causation of laryngeal cancer. (Saric M, Vujovic M. Malignant tumors in an area with as asbestos processing plant. *Public Health Rev* 1994;22:293–303.)

A very large study was reported of an analysis of a case–control study of a cohort of workers in the electricity and gas industry in France, by Imbernon and colleagues in 1995, which included 1,400,000 person-years in a study of 117,000 men. They found 116 cases of laryngeal cancer, but the association between laryngeal cancer and asbestos exposure showed a tendency towards a nonsignificant increase in OR in the highest cumulative exposure categories, and that this tendency to a slight increase disappeared when adjusting for other occupational confounders. In this extremely large study, there was no evidence that asbestos exposure, which is quite significant in this type of industry, was associated with increased risks of laryngeal cancer. There was a slight increase of laryngeal cancer with exposure to cadmium, coal tar, and crystalline silica noted. The Germans reviewed, again, the association between occupational asbestos, dust exposure, and laryngeal cancer in an article published in 1995, based on a review of 31 cohort studies, and 24 case–control studies, and the conclusions of 11 more recent reviews, and found that these reviews were somewhat contradictory. In most studies, there was no statistically significant indication of a causal relationship. They observed that it was very noteworthy that an increased risk of laryngeal cancer among persons exposed to asbestos dust was reported mostly in older studies in which smoking habits and/or alcohol consumption as the most important nonoccupational risk factors were usually not taken into account. In addition, since most of the calculated positive associations were very weak, no reliable conclusion could be reached. Their conclusion was that "while there may be a causal relationship between occupational exposure to asbestos dust and the occurrence of laryngeal cancer, this cannot be regarded as certain on the basis of the evidence reviewed." (Imbernon E, Goldberg M, Bonenfant S et al. Occuptional respiratory cancer and exposure to asbestos: A case–control study in a cohort of workers in the electricity and gas industry. *Am J Ind Med* 1995;28:339–52.)

A Spanish group evaluated occupational risks for laryngeal cancer in Spain and published their study in 1995. Spain has one of the highest incidence rates of laryngeal cancer in the world, and during recent decades, the mortality rate among males has risen slightly and then leveled off. The authors looked at occupational history and lifetime consumption patterns for cigarettes and alcohol, and made risk estimates adjusted for tobacco and alcohol consumption. The highest risk was for wood workers. The OR for wood workers exposed for over 20 years was 5.63, being even greater in furniture workers, in whom the OR was 6.67. Other occupational categories with high ORs were transport drivers, with an OR of 3.31, and bricklayers and masons with an OR of 2.3. Wood dust or chemical compounds used in the treatment of wood could underlie the strongest association discovered between a work exposure and carcinoma of the larynx. (Pollan M, Lopez-Abente G. Wood-related occupations and laryngeal cancer. *Cancer Detect Prev* 1995;19(3):250–7.)

Steven Parnes from the Division of Otolaryngology at Albany Medical College, reviewed the effects of asbestos on the larynx in a paper published in 1996, in which he reviewed 33 cohort studies and pointed out that the majority did not demonstrate any increase in SMRs, and those that did, often failed to take into account the compounding effects of cigarette smoking and alcohol consumption. Twenty-six case–control studies were also examined, and again very few demonstrated that those patients who presented with laryngeal cancer had an increased exposure to asbestos. He pointed out that there had also been three cross-sectional studies performed, with on-site head and neck examinations, in which no specific laryngeal cancer had been seen in high-risk patients. The on-site studies, however, did demonstrate a higher incidence of harmful effects of the larynx, noting edema, inflammation, or specific lesions. Thus, there would be some support that asbestos may be an irritant, although a causal relationship between asbestos exposure and laryngeal cancer could not be definitely established. (Parnes SM. Effects of asbestos on the larynx. *Curr Opin Otol Head Neck Surg* 1996;4:54–8.)

Dario Agudelo and others from Spain (1997) evaluated a group of patients with laryngeal cancer without a history of tobacco and alcohol use, and noted the patients who had no exposure to tobacco and alcohol developed laryngeal cancer about 10 years later than smokers and drinkers. They showed no male predominance, and their lesions were mostly located in the glottis, which permitted early diagnosis and a higher survival rate. (Agudelo D, Quer M, Leon X et al.

Laryngeal carcinoma in patients without a history of tobacco and alcohol use. *Head Neck* 1997;19(3):200–4.)

James Koufman and Alan Burke, from Wake Forest University, published an article on the etiology and pathogenesis of laryngeal cancer, in *Otolaryngologic Clinics of North America*, in February 1997. This is a very nice review of the subject in which the authors point out the male-to-female ratio for this disease as being approximately 5:1, and that there was an increasing incidence of laryngeal squamous cell cancer in black male patients. They reviewed the various studies looking at the relative risks of developing laryngeal cancer associated with tobacco use, including cigarettes, chewing tobacco, cigars, and pipes. In various studies, the relative risks for cigarettes ranged from 5.6 for less than 50 pack-years to 34.4 when smoking more than two packs a day. The risk is 40-fold if you smoke and chew tobacco, and the risk for cigars and pipes was 3.9 for cigars or pipe alone, and 10 for cigars, pipes, and cigarettes in a study by Wynder, and 22 for the study by Rothman. They also reviewed the studies of the effects of alcohol, which increases risk by 5.6-fold based on Wynder's series. He examined the occupational risk factors showing that risk was greater in blue-collar workers. Besides occupational factors, he discusses the effects of the consumption of fruits, vegetables, dairy products, and supplemental vitamins, and the protective effect that fruits and vegetables have. Some authors have reported a 4.75-fold increased risk of laryngeal cancer when fruits and vegetables were consumed less than 40 times a month compared to those who consumed these fruits and vegetables more than 80 times a month. He also discusses the role of HPV and the role of gastroesophageal reflux in laryngeal carcinogenesis. (Koufman JA, Burke AJ. The etiology and pathogenesis of laryngeal carcinoma. *Otolaryngol Clin North Am* 1997;30(1):1–19.)

In 1976, Glanz and Kleinsasser were the first to suggest that inflammatory disease related to esophageal reflux could have a causal relationship with laryngeal carcinoma, by causing chronic inflammation. They briefly reviewed this literature. They concluded with a discussion of a multifactorial theory of aero-digestive carcinogenesis, which takes into account the fact that many of these carcinogens coexist in the same patient, and all contribute to the causation of laryngeal cancer. These different factors have a synergistic effect and thus, for instance, people who smoke have an increased incidence of esophageal reflux. Alcoholics may also reflux more often, and therefore the effects of alcohol and tobacco may in part be mediated by the effects of esophageal reflux on causing chronic irritation, which in combination with alcohol and tobacco, may be an important factor in the induction of laryngeal carcinogenesis. Factors such as HPV and its role is unclear, but we know that between 80% and 90% of cervical cancers are related to this same virus, so we know that it has great potential for the induction for carcinogenesis. Women who smoke are more likely to get cervical cancer, suggesting that this particular virus, in combination with the effects of cigarette smoking, is more likely to induce tumors. This particular paper does a very nice job of bringing together many different factors that have been considered potential carcinogens, and pointing out that it is unlikely that any one factor is the major cause of laryngeal cancer, in that probably several different factors are working together in the causation of the average laryngeal tumor. (Glanz H, Kleinsasser O. Chronic laryngitis and carcinoma. *Arch Otorhinolaryngol* 1976;212(1):57–75; Agudelo D, Quer M, Leon X et al. Laryngeal carcinoma in patients without a history of tobacco and alcohol use. *Head Neck* 1997;19:200–4.)

Obviously, this raises serious questions about the simplistic view of many epidemiologists that if a population could be adequately controlled for tobacco and alcohol consumption, then any increased incidence in cancer of the larynx is going to be due to some sort of environmental or occupational factor. Controlling for alcohol and tobacco does not control for dietary factors, esophageal reflux, HPV, and many other exposures, which may also be contributory.

Another German study was published in 1997 on the epidemiology of laryngeal cancer. This was the result of a Heidelberg case–control study in which the authors state that squamous cell carcinoma of the larynx is a multifactorial disease, predominately found in males between the ages of 50 and 70 years. Chronic consumption of alcohol and tobacco independently increases the relative risk of this type of cancer in a dose-dependent manner, but they also found that low educational standards and occupational training were associated with high risk. The majority of the cancer patients were blue-collar workers who were exposed to a variety of hazardous working materials, such as polycyclic aromatic hydrocarbons, cement dust, metal dust, asbestos, varnish, lacquers, fossil fuels, and a whole variety of things, which may also be contributing to the risk of laryngeal cancer. They also concluded that the consumption of fruits, salads, and dairy products may decrease the incidence of laryngeal cancer. Therefore, they felt the laryngeal cancer was a multifactorial disease, firmly linked to lifestyle and environmental factors, as well as alcohol, tobacco, and a variety of possible occupational factors. (Koufman JA, Burke AJ. The etiology and pathogenesis of laryngeal carcinoma. *Otolaryngol Clin North Am* 1997;30(1):1–19.)

A hospital-based case–control study was carried out in 15 hospitals in France, by Goldberg and others, and published in 1997. This is a nice review of many of the other factors that have been reported to be associated with increased risk of laryngeal cancer, including agricultural workers, such as animal husbandry workers and metal processing and manufacturing workers. They found that the risk for blacksmiths was very high, at 4.6 times the risk for controls, and the risk for toolmakers and metal pattern makers was 4.1. Plumbers and pipe fitters previously had not been found to be at risk of laryngeal cancer, and their risk was thought to be around 1.8. It was mentioned by the authors that "although the role of asbestos in laryngeal cancer is still controversial, the excess risk found here for brick layers and stone masons (OR 3.1) for the hypopharynx might be due to exposure to asbestos. Asbestos might also be a potential risk factor for plumbers and other workers in the construction industry where asbestos is much used. In several studies, the occupations related to this industry showed associations with laryngeal cancer and pharyngeal cancer. They mention the potential risk from silica as a cause of laryngeal cancer and increased risk in mining operations, glass formers, and potters." (Goldberg P, Leclerc A, Luce D et al. Laryngeal and hypopharyngeal cancer and occupation: Results of a case–control study. *Occup Environ Med* 1997;54:477–82.)

Obviously, you cannot have your cake and eat it too. You cannot blame asbestos for increased risk in bricklayers and stonemasons, where there is minimal exposure, and then in the next paragraph say that there is an increased risk of laryngeal cancer from exposure to silica, which is the main mineral that is found in rocks and bricks. Actually, the only bricklayers that have exposure to asbestos are those that lay high-silica-containing bricks inside furnaces or other high heat-type facilities where they used asbestos-containing mortar in between the bricks. As a general trade, a very small percentage of bricklayers have any exposure to asbestos. I think the point of the paper is that there are many different trades that have been associated with an increased risk of laryngeal and hypopharyngeal cancer, including service workers, agricultural workers, animal husbandry workers, miners, and quarry men, as well as plumbers and pipe fitters. Glass formers and potters, transport equipment workers, and a variety of other occupations, including the manufacturing of metal products and being a blacksmith, all have increased risks of laryngeal cancer. How much of this risk is accounted for by differences in smoking habits, socioeconomic class, and diet is obviously very difficult to determine. One can see as we study the issue of occupation and laryngeal and hypopharyngeal cancer, that it is very difficult to say that one occupational exposure (i.e., asbestos) is a significant cause of laryngeal cancer, when all of these other factors have never been controlled for in most retrospective cohort or case–control studies.

More recently (1998), there has been some epidemiologic evidence that exposure to machining fluids imparts an increased risk of laryngeal cancer. In a recent study of 45,000 automobile production workers, workers exposed to machining fluids in one of three plants had an increased SMR for laryngeal cancer of 1.85. Because of this information, a death certificate case–control study was done on the Connecticut Tumor Registry, in the Connecticut Division of Vital Statistics, by Mark Russi and others and published in 1997. They felt that when cases were compared to population controls, no association between machining fluid exposure and laryngeal cancer was observed. This study was followed by another study from the National Institutes of Occupational Safety and Health, by Calvert and others, in the *American Journal of Industrial Medicine* in 1998. They did a systemic review on the data of the cancer risk among workers exposed to metal working fluids, and they felt that there was substantial evidence for increased risks of cancer at several sites, including the larynx, rectum, pancreas, skin, scrotum, and bladder, at least associated with metal working fluids used prior to the mid-1970s. It seemed that the role of metal working fluids was still unclear, and was a potential cause that had not been adequately controlled for epidemiologic studies. (Calvert GM, Ward E, Schnorr TM et al. Cancer risks among workers exposed to metalworking fluids: A systematic review. *Am J Ind Med* 1998;33:282–92.)

Another study reported in 1998 was of a correlation between laryngeal and pharyngeal carcinomas, and 24-hour pH monitoring of the esophagus and pharynx as a measure of chronic esophageal reflux. Over an 8-year period, the authors correlated the results of pH monitoring in 798 patients, with a variety of upper aerodigestive tract symptoms, and in this group were 63 patients who had laryngeal and pharyngeal cancer. They found a very high incidence of esophageal reflux of about 50%, but they found no significant difference between those with or without laryngeal or pharyngeal cancers, raising a question about the role of esophageal reflux in the causation of laryngeal cancer. (Chen MYM, Ott D, Casolo BJ, Moghazy KM, Koufman JA. Correlation of laryngeal and pharyngeal carcinomas and 24-hour pH monitoring of the esophagus and pharynx. *Otolaryngol Head Neck Surg* 1998;119:460–2.)

Two important papers were published in 2001 regarding gastroesophageal reflux disease (GERD) as a risk factor for laryngeal and pharyngeal cancer. One was by El-Serag and colleagues, from Houston, who did a case–control study of a total of 8228 hospital patients with laryngeal cancers, and 1912 with pharyngeal cancers, which were compared with controls. In this very large series of hospitalized patients, the prevalence of GERD was higher amongst patients with laryngeal cancer at 8.9% versus 4% and pharyngeal cancer at 6.2% versus 3.8%, with a p-value of 0.0001. When this population was controlled for age, gender, ethnicity, smoking, and alcohol, GERD was associated with an OR of 2.4 for laryngeal cancer in hospitalized patients, and for outpatients it was associated with an increased risk of 2.31. This study is particularly important since it is the largest study that has ever been done on this topic, particularly in lieu of a previous earlier study that I mentioned, in which no increased incidence of GERD was found in laryngeal cancer patients versus controls. (El-Serag HB, Hepworth EJ, Lee P et al. Gastroesophageal reflux disease is a risk factor for laryngeal and pharyngeal cancer. *Am J Gastroenterol* 2001;96(7):2013–8.)

A study was done in Sweden by Gustavasson and colleagues looking at the effects of occupational exposures and squamous cell cancer of the oral cavity, pharynx, larynx, and esophagus. In this study, exposure to asbestos was associated with an increased risk of laryngeal cancer, and a dose–response relationship was present with a relative risk of 1.8 in the highest-exposure group. They also found an increased risk from welding fumes and eye exposure to polycyclic aromatic hydrocarbons on esophageal cancer. They found that exposure to wood dust was associated with a decreased risk of cancer at the studied sites. These authors attempted to control for alcohol and tobacco use. There are some methodological problems; I note in this particular paper that they evaluated 157 patients with carcinoma of the larynx, and looked at the risk of those who were currently smoking and who had asbestos exposure, versus those who were currently smoking or who had stopped smoking and, who did not have asbestos exposure. The important issue of estimating pack-years of exposure, and age of initiation of tobacco smoking, were major factors that were not evaluated. The discussion and the methods sections in this paper were very superficial, and I found the data uninterpretable. (Gustavsson P, Jakobsson R, Johansson H et al. Occupational exposures and squamous cell carcinoma of the oral cavity, pharynx, larynx, and oesophagus: A case–control study in Sweden. *Occup Environ Med* 1998;55:393–400.)

Another Scandinavian study was published in *Cancer Causes and Control* in 1998 from Norway, in which Kjaerheim and others evaluated the role of alcohol, tobacco, and dietary factors in the causation of upper aero-gastric tract cancers in a study of 10,900 Norwegian men. They found that *dietary factors* were associated with a reduced cancer risk, particularly the high consumption of oranges and bread. (Kjaerheim K, Gaard M, Andersen A. The role of alcohol, tobacco, and dietary factors in upper aerogastric tract cancers: A prospective study of 10,900 Norwegian men. *Cancer Causes Control* 1998;9:99–108.)

A study by De Stefani and others, from Uruguay, assessed 107 patients with laryngeal cancer, and 290 control patients considered not to be related to tobacco and alcohol exposure in Uruguay. Epidemiologic analysis performed at Louisiana State University in New Orleans, demonstrated that dark tobacco smoking was the strongest risk factor at a 2.5 times higher risk than that of light tobacco smoking, and a 35 times risk than that of nonsmoking. The alcohol exposure displayed a lesser effect, but interaction with tobacco resulted in very high risk at more than 100 times higher than the controls. In this study, red wine showed relative risks similar to hard liquor consumption. In addition, the drinking of a local tea called "mate" was associated with a threefold increased risk of laryngeal cancer. This study is of particular interest in that it demonstrates that certain types of tobacco such as cigarettes, cigars, and chewing tobacco, are much more carcinogenic than others, and demonstrates a very high risk in patients who smoke and have heavy alcohol consumption. Occupations and the risk of laryngeal cancer published in the *American Journal of Industrial Medicine* in 1998, found that butchers, vintners, bakers, and car assemblers presented with increased risks of laryngeal cancer. Similarly, asbestos, the mist of strong inorganic acids, and pesticide exposures, were associated with an increased risk of laryngeal cancer, and the OR for strong acids was 1.8. (De Stefani E, Correa P, Oreggia F et al. Risk factors for laryngeal cancer. *Cancer* 1987;60:3087–91.)

A study by Prescott and coworkers from Denmark (1999), evaluated the influence of different types of alcoholic beverages on the risk of lung cancer, and they found that the high consumption of beer and liquor was associated with an increased risk of lung cancer, whereas wine might protect against the development of lung cancer. Whereas this study was not of laryngeal cancer, the application to laryngeal cancer is obvious, and further studies need to be done on the types of alcoholic beverages, and their associated risks in carcinoma of the larynx. (Prescott E, Gronbaek M, Becker U et al. Alcohol intake and the risk of lung cancer: Influence of type of alcoholic beverage. *Am J Epidemiol* 1999;149:463–70.)

Schlecht and others from Brazil evaluated the interaction between tobacco and alcohol consumption and the risk of cancers of the upper aerodigestive tract. The joint effects of tobacco and alcohol together exceeded the levels expected under a multiplicative model for moderate smokers. Among never-smokers, heavy drinkers had a 9.2 times greater risk of cancer of the mouth, pharynx, and supraglottis than never-drinkers, with a dose–response relationship with cumulative consumption. It was felt that alcohol might act as a promoter for tobacco and as an independent risk factor. The authors felt that alcohol might increase the permeability of mucosal cells to tobacco smoke carcinogens, due to solubilization by alcohol. Secondly, they felt that the presence of low levels of carcinogenic substances and alcoholic beverages, or the cellular injury produced by ethanol metabolites, might explain the increased risk of cancer. Predominately, it was felt that alcohol and tobacco work together in a synergistic fashion. (Schlecht N, Franco EL, Pintos J et al. Interaction between tobacco and alcohol consumption and the risk of cancers of the upper Aero-digestive tract in Brazil. *Am J Epidemiol* 1999;150(11):1129–37.)

A study from Switzerland and France (2000) looked at the role of alcohol dehydrogenase-3, and cytochrome P-450, on E-1 genotypes in the susceptibility to cancers of the upper aerodigestive tracts. The authors felt that genetic poly-morphisms of certain types of enzymes might influence susceptibility to alcohol-related cancers. It was felt that there was suggestive evidence that certain genetic polymorphisms were more susceptible to laryngeal cancers than others, but that the numbers in this study were too small to come to firm conclusions. (Hanna E, MacLeod S, Vural E, Lang N. Genetic deletions of glutathione-S-transferase as a risk factor in squamous cell carcinoma of the larynx: A preliminary report. *Am J Otolaryngol* 2001;22(2):121–3.)

A seminal review on the subject of asbestos exposure and laryngeal cancer was written by Kevin Browne and J Bernard Gee, and published in the *Annals of Occupational Hygiene* in 2000. They reviewed all of the identified studies of asbestos workers providing data on laryngeal disease that have been commonly used to evaluate the risk for laryngeal cancer in asbestos-exposed workers. They reported, as had others, that confounding of the data due to smoking and alcohol intake, and to a lesser extent diet and other socioeconomic factors, cre-ated a major difficulty in evaluating these studies. Among 24 prospective stud-ies for which a SMR was available, nine had an SMR at or below unity. Eleven studies were evaluated in which there was no SMR for comparison, and in only one of these was there a clear excess in risk. In 17 retrospective studies, only two showed a significantly increased relative risk. There was also evidence from animal experiments and studies in which associations with pleural plaques and autopsy findings appeared negative or inconclusive. (Browne K, Gee JBL. Asbestos exposure and laryngeal cancer. *Am Occup Hyg* 2000;44(4):239–50.)

Furthermore, Browne and Gee commented on the paper by AH Smith and others in 1990. (Smith AH, Handley MA, Wood R. Epidemiological evidence indicates asbestos causes laryngeal cancer. *J Occup Med* 1990;32(6):499–507.) The authors pointed out that on the first page of their paper, one important principal of meta-analysis is that all eligible studies should be considered. Their criticism of Smith's paper was that the authors drew up rules for eligibility for their study that effectively excluded most of the relevant studies, selecting only cohort studies showing a relative lung cancer risk greater than 2, before adjust-ing for smoking, despite the fact that this procedure is likely to create a bias that results in favor of groups with smoking habits higher than the control popula-tion. Among other criticisms that might be mentioned, principal is the disregard of the qualifications or results by the authors of other individual papers, and also their use of the number 4 as a relative risk for ethanol abuse. While this figure might be approximately correct when it is an independent risk factor, our previ-ous discussion shows that there is an interactive effect of smoking, and that the relative risk compared with nondrinking nonsmokers may reach as high as 40. Overall, Browne and Gee did a careful analysis of the world's literature including

24 prospective studies, and concluded there was not sufficient evidence to conclude that asbestos exposure was a risk factor for laryngeal cancer.

A South African study was published by Kielkowski, Nelson, and Rees, in *Occupational and Environmental Medicine* in 2000, providing an analysis of a group of white individuals who were studied in the Northern Cape Providence of South Africa. This is the area that was originally studied by JC Wagner, and it was a location of a large amount of crocidolite asbestos mining and milling. A survey of the death certificates was done and the authors found a very high incidence of mesothelioma in both men and women. They also found two cases of laryngeal cancer with a proportional cancer mortality rate of 1.8. However, in this study there was no adjustment for tobacco smoking, alcohol consumption, diet, or any other factors, and therefore the value of the study is rather limited. (Kielkowski D, Nelson G, Rees D. Risk of mesothelioma from exposure to crocidolite asbestos: A 1995 update of a South African mortality study. *Occup Environ Med* 2000;57:563–7.)

A later study from France, by Laforest (2000) and others, evaluated the occupational exposure information in a group of 201 workers with hypopharyngeal cancers, 296 with laryngeal cancers, as well as 296 controls. They then controlled for alcohol and cigarette smoking and looked at other occupational exposures, and found that hypopharyngeal cancer was associated with exposure to coal dust with an OR of 2.31, which was statistically significant at the p-value level of 0.005. When patients were exposed to formaldehyde, there was a fourfold increased risk at the highest exposure level. The authors mentioned in their article that "although the association between exposure to asbestos and laryngeal cancer has been repeatedly found, the existence of a causal relationship is still debated." (Laforest L, Luce D, Goldberg P et al. Laryngeal and hypopharyngeal cancers and occupational exposure to formaldehyde and various dusts: A case–control study in France. *Occup Environ Med* 2000;57:767–73.)

A case–control study from France by Marchand and Luce (2000), looked at the role of occupational exposures to asbestos and man-made vitreous fibers. This case–control study carefully controlled for tobacco and alcohol and the level of exposure to asbestos. Exposure to asbestos was associated with a slight, nonsignificant increase in risk of laryngeal cancer with an OR of 1.24 and a significantly increased risk of hypopharyngeal cancer with an OR of 1.8. The risk increased with increasing cumulative exposure for laryngeal cancer, but the OR did not differ significantly from unity. For hypopharyngeal cancer, a significant risk was associated with the highest cumulative exposure level, and the OR was 2.4. The OR by which laryngeal cancer was associated with asbestos exposure increased with a maximum probability of exposure, the total duration of exposure, the time since first exposure, and with a young age at first exposure, but no result was statistically significant. Their conclusion was that there was not enough evidence to demonstrate that asbestos was associated with laryngeal cancer, but that asbestos may have a carcinogenic effect on the epilarynx and the hypopharynx. Mineral wools also had a carcinogenic effect on the epilarynx and hypopharynx, but there was confounding because patients exposed to asbestos are often exposed to mineral wools, so it is very difficult to know how much of this is due to one type of mineral fiber versus another. (Marchand JL, Luce D. Laryngeal and hypopharyngeal cancer and occupational exposure to asbestos and man-made vitreous fibers: Results of a case–control study. *Am J Ind Med* 2000;37:581–9.)

An autopsy case series was reported from Japan, by Murai and Kitagawa from the Department of Pathology at Toyama, Japan, in 2000, based on a pathological evaluation of 525 autopsy cases of asbestosis. In the 525 cases with asbestosis, there were 174 lung cancers, 73 malignant mesotheliomas and six laryngeal cancers, or 2.4% of all the cancers and 1.1% of asbestosis cases. The control populations without asbestosis had a risk of 0.3% for laryngeal cancer, so that the number of cases was higher than expected at a p-value of 0.001. This indicates that this was a significant increase in the number of laryngeal cancers above that which was expected. The authors went on in their last paragraph to point out that they did not evaluate smoking habits and alcohol consumption or any other risk factors associated with laryngeal cancer, but they found more laryngeal cancers in this group of patients with asbestosis. They pointed out that they needed more data before they could arrive at a firm conclusion of any association between asbestosis and laryngeal cancer, and of course, the kind of data they needed is data that would have allowed them to control for other risk factors. (Murai Y, Kitagawa M. Autopsy cases of asbestosis in Japan: A statistical analysis on registered cases. *Arch Environ Health* 2000;55(6):447–52.)

A review of the history, etiology, and epidemiology of laryngeal cancer was published in *Clinical Otolaryngology and Allied Sciences* in 2001 by Rafferty, Fenton, and Jones, and they discussed the various causes of laryngeal cancer, and mentioned the data on asbestos. (Rafferty MA, Fenton JE, Jones AS. The history, aetiology and epidemiology of laryngeal carcinoma. *Clin Otolaryngol Allied Sci* 2001;26(6):442–6.) They quoted an article by Boyle and MacFarlane and others published in *Current Opinion Oncology*, at which time the authors had stated that the available evidence supported an association between occupational exposure and increased risk of laryngeal cancer. (Boyle P, Macfarlane GJ, Zheng T et al. Recent advances in epidemiology of head and neck cancer. *Curr Opin Oncol* 1992;4(3):471–7.) They mention a case–control study conducted in Shanghai by Zheng and colleagues that revealed an OR of 2.0 with asbestos exposure, but no dose–response relation with frequency or duration of exposure was observed. (Zheng W, Blot WJ, Shu XO et al. Diet and other risk factors for laryngeal cancer in Shanghai, China. *Am J Epidemiol* 1992;136:178–91.) Rafferty and colleagues also mentioned a study in New York, which revealed an elevated, but not statistically increased, association between glottic cancer and asbestos exposure with an OR of 1.3, and they pointed out that this study demonstrated neither a relationship between asbestos and supraglottic cancer, nor a synergistic effect between cigarette smoking and asbestos exposure, when quoting from the 1992 paper by Muscat and Wynder that I previously discussed. Basically, these comments indicate great ambivalence on the part of the authors from Liverpool, and not a deep understanding of the subject. (Rafferty MA, Fenton FE, Jones AS. The history, aetiology and epidemiology of laryngeal carcinoma. *Clin Otolaryngol Allied Sci* 2001;26:442–6.)

A paper was published in 2001 from the Departments of Otolaryngology and Head and Neck Surgery at the University of Arkansas. Hanna and others looked for genetic deletions of glutathione-S-transferase as a risk factor for squamous cell carcinoma of the larynx. They found that the glutathione-S-transferase *M-1* gene was deleted in 80% of patients with laryngeal squamous cell cancer and in 50% of control subjects, and they felt that this was significant, suggesting that this detoxifying enzyme that normally protects against cellular DNA damage from exogenous substances, had been affected by some type of oncologic process, and that this was another contributing factor in the pathogenesis of laryngeal cancer. (Hanna E, MacLeod S, Vural E, Lang N. Genetic deletions of glutathione-S-transferase as a risk factor in squamous cell carcinoma of the larynx: A preliminary report. *Am J Otolaryngol* 2001;22(2):121–3.)

A meta-analysis of alcohol drinking and cancer risk was published in the *British Journal of Cancer* in 2001 by Bagnardi and others from Italy, in which they did a meta-analysis of the association between alcohol consumption and the risk of 18 different neoplasms, reviewing the epidemiologic literature between 1966 and 2000. They found 235 studies covering 117,000 cases, and strong trends and risks were observed for cancers of the oral cavity, pharynx, esophagus, and larynx. This meta-analysis showed no evidence of a threshold effect for most alcohol-related neoplasms, which indicates that perhaps even low or modest levels of alcohol consumption, particularly in the presence of cigarette smoking, are significant contributing factors. (Bagnardi V, Blangiardo M, La Vecchia C. A meta-analysis of alcohol drinking and cancer risk. *Br J Cancer* 2001;85(11):1700–5.)

Also in 2001, a paper was published by Zang and Wynder evaluating the confounding effects of cigarette smoking on the relationship between alcohol use and lung cancer risk, with laryngeal cancer used as a positive control. The alcohol, it turns out, had very little effect on the rates of lung cancer, but by contrast, the effect of alcohol on laryngeal cancer remained high, even after an adjustment for smoking with an OR of 5.6. Parts of this paper that look at the effects of alcohol and cigarette smoking and laryngeal cancer are particularly interesting since they involve 521 male and 159 female laryngeal cancer cases, and 8169 male and 4154 female controls. Thus, the risk analysis and the study are of very good quality with very good controls. (Zang EA, Wynder EL. Reevaluation of the confounding effect of cigarette smoking on the relationship between alcohol use and lung cancer risk, with larynx cancer used as a positive control. *Prev Med* 2001;32:359–70.)

The Institute of Medicine published a document entitled *Asbestos: Selected Cancers* in 2006 and the authors concluded,

Considering all lines of evidence, the committee place greater weight on the consistency of the epidemiologic studies in the biologic plausibility of the hypothesis than on the lack of confirmatory evidence from animal studies or documentation of fiber deposition in the larynx. The committee concluded that the evidence is sufficient to infer a causal relationship between asbestos exposure and laryngeal cancer.

Basically, the committee ignored most of the nine steps of Bradford Hill's requirements for evidence of a cause-and-effect relationship. The association between asbestos exposure and laryngeal cancer is not *strong* or *consistent*, nor is there a *dose–response* relationship or *experimental evidence* of a cause-and-effect relationship. Other experts, as quoted below, came to the same conclusion about the Institute of Medicine Report. (Institute of Medicine Committee on Asbestos. *Asbestos: Selected Cancers*. Washington, DC: National Academic Press, 2006.)

Robert Sataloff commented as Editor-in-Chief of *Ear, Nose, & Throat Journal* with Sidrah Ahmed that

> Medicine is replete with assumptions and myths based on faulty reasoning. It is important for all of us to be aware of this problem and diligent about assessing evidence to draw the best possible conclusions. One of the most frequent errors results from *post hoc ergo propter hoc* reasoning. This classic error in logic assumes that because Event B happens after Event A, Event B is caused by Event A. Proof of causation requires considerably more rigorous evidence. The suggestion that asbestos exposure can cause laryngeal cancer appears to be an example of this flaw in logic... Otolaryngologists should recognize that patients who have been exposed to asbestos (or who have asbestosis) may develop laryngeal carcinoma; but in the absence of evidence, we cannot conclude that their asbestos exposure caused their cancers. As always, we must remain vigilant in distinguishing between the coexistence of two events and a causal link between them. The evidence must be studied carefully whenever a causal link is suggested. (Ahmed SM, Sataloff RT. Asbestos exposure and laryngeal cancer: Is there an association? *Ear Nose Throat J* 2009;88:1140–2.)

Edwin Sturgis, a noted ear, nose and throat physician and epidemiologist, replied in agreement with Dr. Sataloff:

> I read with interest your editorial in the October issue, 'Asbestos exposure and laryngeal cancer: Is there an association?' I completely agree with the central point that the simple association of two events does not prove that the first event causes the second. This point is important to understanding epidemiologic studies suggesting disease associations and highlights the timelessness of considering all of Koch's postulates and Hill's criteria of disease causality.

As to the specific question the authors raised regarding whether asbestos is a cause of laryngeal cancer, I share a concern that associations at a population/group level may be interpreted as proof that an individual's cancer has a specific cause. However, a critical monograph on the subject from the National Academies of Sciences was not referenced or reviewed. This monograph represents the review and conclusions of an Institute of Medicine multidisciplinary committee of 12 distinguished members, backed by research staff, as well as a separate and independent 12-person review committee. Dr. Sturgis commented that "neither I nor a member of my institution was a member of these committees. The conclusion of the committee regarding laryngeal cancer was that despite "...the lack of confirmatory evidence from animal studies or documentation of fiber deposition in the larynx... evidence is sufficient to infer a causal relationship between asbestos exposure and laryngeal cancer." In making this conclusion, the committee considered 35 cohort populations and 18 case–control studies. This work is a comprehensive review of this literature and a summary of the principal epidemiologic criteria supporting asbestos as a cause of laryngeal cancer, namely: (1) consistency of the epidemiologic studies; (2) biologic plausibility; (3) strength of association; (4) dose–response effect; and (5) effect modification." (Committee on Asbestos: Selected Health Effects. Laryngeal cancer and asbestos. In: *Asbestos: Selected Cancers*. Washington, DC: National Academies Press, 2006, pp. 173–92; Sturgis EM. Asbestos exposure and laryngeal cancer. *Ear Nose Throat J* 2010;89:104.)

In March 2009, 27 scientists from eight countries met at the IARC agency to review certain human carcinogens. They concluded that asbestos exposure was responsible as a causative agent in sufficient quantity to cause lung cancer, mesothelioma, carcinoma of the ovary, and carcinoma of the larynx. (Straif K, Benbrahim-Tallaa L, Baan R et al.; WHO International Agency for Research on Cancer Monograph Working Group. A review of human carcinogens—Part B: Biological agents. *Lancet Oncol* 2009;10(5):453–4.) Evidently, this group did not consult Drs. Sataloff or Sturgis.

Epidemiological studies continue to be published that simply evaluate the prevalence of various cancers in asbestos-exposed individuals as opposed to unexposed individuals. These types of studies prove nothing because they are not adequately controlled for the many other causes of laryngeal cancer and contributing factors. Again, these studies are examples of *"post hoc ergo propter hoc* faulty reasoning." (Offermans NS, Vermeulen R, Burdorf A et al. Occupational asbestos exposure and risk of pleural mesothelioma, lung cancer, and laryngeal cancer in the prospective Netherlands Cohort study. *J Occup Environ Med* 2014;56(1):6–19; Offermans NS, Vermeulen R, Burdorf A et al. Occupational asbestos exposure and risk of oral cavity and pharyngeal cancer in the prospective Netherlands Cohort Study. *Scand J Work Environ Health* 2014;40(4):420–7.)

Paget-Bailly, Cyr, and Luce from France, reviewed epidemiologic data on occupational exposures and laryngeal cancer. The authors performed a systematic literature search and a series of meta-analyses for agents with at least ten available studies with homogenous exposure. They analyzed 99 publications and found that significantly increased meta-relative risks (meta-RRs) were obtained considering exposure to polycyclic aromatic hydrocarbons (meta-RR: 1.29; 95% CI: 1.10–1.52), engine exhaust (meta-RR: 1.17; 95% CI: 1.05–1.30), textile dust (meta-RR: 1.41; 95% CI: 1.09–1.83), and working in the rubber industry (meta-RR: 1.39; 95% CI: 1.13–1.71). Exposures to wood dust, formaldehyde, and cement dust were not significantly associated with laryngeal cancer. In regards to the available epidemiologic data, they could not draw firm conclusions on the role of solvents. (Paget-Bailly S, Cyr D, Luce D. Occupational exposures and cancer of the larynx—Systematic review and meta-analysis. *J Occup Environ Med* 2012;54(1):71–84.)

Other authors mentioned earlier have found evidence of a variety of occupational exposures that are confounders to epidemiologic studies, including race, social class, diet, polycyclic aromatic hydrocarbon exposure, rubber industry workers, textile dust, engine exhaust, gastroesophageal reflux, cigarette smoking, chewing tobacco, alcohol ingestion, HPV, coal dust, mineral wool exposure, formaldehyde, welding fumes, pesticide exposure, inorganic acids, "mate" tea, metal machining fluids, silica dust, blacksmithing, plumbers and pipefitters, and genetic factors, to name a few of the purported causes of laryngeal cancer. The many different causes of laryngeal cancer make it very difficult to find a control population without confounding exposures to other laryngeal cancer-causing exposures or conditions to compare with an asbestos-exposed population.

A large prospective population-based study from The Netherlands and Finland of 58,279 men showed no convincing evidence of an association between asbestos and risk of oral cavity cancer, pharyngeal cancer and combined oral and pharyngeal cancer, as an exposure–response relation was lacking, and the results were not robust against the use of different job–exposure matrices. However, the potentially increased health risks of pharyngeal cancer and oral and pharyngeal cancer observed in this and previous studies were felt to warrant further research. (Offermans NS, Vermeulen R, Burdorf A et al. Occupational asbestos exposure and risk of oral cavity and pharyngeal cancer in the prospective Netherlands Cohort Study. *Scand J Work Environ Health* 2014;40(4):420–7.)

THE ROLE OF HPV: THE ELEPHANT IN THE ROOM

HPV is a very common virus and is also known as the wart virus since it causes warts. There are approximately 150 genotypes, and about a dozen of these genotypes are considered carcinogenic—specifically genotypes 16, 18, 31, 33, 39, 45, 51, 52, 56, 58, 59, and 68. Following the discovery that HPV causes squamous carcinoma of the cervix in women, HPV has been associated with the development of squamous cancer of the lung, head and neck, and larynx. (Bouvard V, Baan R, Striaf K et al. A review of human carcinogens—Part B: Biological agents. *Lancet Oncol* 2009;10:321–22; Tommasino M. The human papillomavirus family and its role in carcinogenesis. *Semin Cancer Biol* 2014;26:13–21; Gheit T, Abedi-Ardekani B, Carreira C et al. Comprehensive analysis of HPV expression in laryngeal squamous cell carcinoma. *J Med Virol* 2014;86(4):642–6.)

The new potential cause of carcinoma of the larynx began to be appreciated in the mid-1990s based on the paper by Anna Maria Pou and others on adult respiratory papillomatosis, which is related to the HPV. HPV papillomas are the most common benign neoplasms of the larynx, and HPV is a common cause of venereal warts in men and women. This sexually transmitted disease can also be transmitted into the oropharynx, and the glottis is the preferred site for the development of papillomas. The same subtypes of HPV that are thought to be major causes of squamous cell carcinoma of the cervix—types 16 and 18—are the same genotypes of papillomavirus that are now implicated as causes of laryngeal cancer. The data on the role of HPV and the risk of laryngeal cancer were further confirmed by Charles Moore and coworkers from the Department of Otolaryngology at the Emery Health System, and a group at the University of Alabama, and the University of Michigan as published in *Otolaryngology—Head and Neck Surgery* in 1999. (Pou AM, Rimell FL, Jordan JA et al. Adult respiratory papillomatosis: Human papillomavirus type and viral coinfections as predictors of prognosis. *Ann Otol Rhinol Laryngol* 1995;104:758–62; Moore CE, Wiatrak BJ, McClatchey KD et al. High-risk human papillomavirus types and squamous cell carcinoma in patients with respiratory papillomas. *Otolaryngol Head Neck Surg* 1999;120:698–705.)

These studies on HPV were confirmed by Badaracco and others from Rome, Italy, in an article published in *Anti-Cancer Research* in 2000. It certainly is clear that HPV infection may be related to a proportion of head and neck cancers, but its association was not as clear as it has been with cervical cancer. Certainly, most authors would agree that HPV infection would certainly be a very significant risk factor for cancer of the larynx. Kaya and others from Turkey, found a statistically significant correlation between HPV infection and tumor recurrence in laryngeal cancers, but not between HPV presence and tumor stage or grade. The implication of the HPV data is that there is a very significant risk factor for carcinoma of the larynx, which in the presence of or absence of cigarettes and alcohol may be a very significant contributor to carcinogenesis that has not been taken into account in any of the major epidemiologic studies. Epidemiologists have tried to control for other social, environmental, and occupational risk factors in the determination of whether asbestos is a cause of laryngeal cancer, but not HPV infection. (Badaracco G, Venuti A, Morello R et al. Human papillomavirus in head and neck carcinomas: Prevalence, physical status and relationship with clinical/pathological parameters. *Anticancer Res* 2000;20:1301–6; Kaya H, Kotiloglu E, Inanli S et al. Prevalence of human papillomavirus (HPV) DNA in larynx and lung carcinomas. *Pathologica* 2001;93:531–34.)

A series of articles came out between 2000 and 2002 regarding HPV and esophageal reflux as causes of laryngeal cancer. Smith, Summersgill, and others from Iowa published an article in the *Annals of Otology, Rhinology, and Laryngology* in November 2000, reviewing their studies on detecting HPV infection. They pointed out that HPV infection and laryngeal and pharyngeal squamous cell carcinomas have been reported in a wide frequency ranging from 22% to 83%, exhibiting a spectrum of oncogenic and nononcogenic HPV types. In their studies, patients with laryngeal cancer were not more likely to be identified with oncogenic versus nononcogenic HPV types. The limitation of this study was that it relied predominately on brush material rather than biopsy material. A previous study showed a positivity rate of 66% from biopsy material compared to 16.7% from brushing from tumors as published by Vowles and others in the *Journal of Laryngology and Otology* 1997;111:215–7. (Smith EM, Summersgill KF, Allen J et al. Human papillomavirus and risk of laryngeal cancer. *Ann Otol Rhinol Laryngol* 2000;109:1069–76.)

Another study was done in Rome, by Almadori and others, as published in *Clinical Cancer Research* in 2001. This was a study trying to detect epidermal growth factor receptor expression in primary laryngeal squamous cell carcinomas. They found HPV DNA in 35.7% of tumors, and it was almost exclusively that of the oncogenic varieties of HPV 16, 18, and 33 genotypes. They found evidence of enhanced epidermal growth factor receptor over-expression, and it was felt that this might be one of the steps that would be part of the multi-step process leading towards laryngeal cancer.

A Turkish study, published in *Pathologica* in 2001 by Kaya and others, found HPV virus DNA signals in 47.6% of the cases of laryngeal squamous cell carcinomas, and in 11.5% of the cases of lung cancer. The authors also found a significant correlation between HPV infection and tumor recurrence, but not between HPV presence and tumor stage or grade. (Kaya H, Kotiloglu E, Inanli S et al. Prevalence of human papillomavirus (HPV) DNA in larynx and lung carcinomas. *Pathologica* 2001;93:531–4.) In 2013, a large multinational study of the prevalence of HPV 16 virus antibodies was published, and the authors found evidence of HPV 16 virus infection in 34.8% of head and neck cancers. (Kreimer AR, Johansson M, Waterboer T et al. Evaluation of human papillomavirus antibodies and risk of subsequent head and neck cancer. *J Clin Oncol* 2013;31(21):2708–15.)

The major problem with analysis of these data, is that laryngeal cancer is not related to a single cause. This means that if one controls for tobacco and alcohol, and then evaluates the incidence of laryngeal cancer, it does not necessarily follow that any increased number of cases is by definition related to asbestos exposure. There are so many other factors that may contribute to the causation of laryngeal cancer that also are not controlled for, such as exposure to acid mists, various dusts, diet, race, sex, social class, oral hygiene, chewable tobacco products, Guta eaters or other chewable irritating plants, possibly formaldehyde, possibly heavy metals, possibly esophageal reflux, and certainly HPV infection. HPV infection appears to be a very significant contributing factor in a large percentage of carcinomas of the larynx, and therefore this particular cause of laryngeal cancer would have to be controlled for in the analysis of any data for the evaluation of the effects of asbestos exposure, and the subsequent development of laryngeal cancer. Obviously, the basic principle of epidemiology is that analysis of epidemiologic data is only of value if other variables of causation can be adequately controlled in the data analysis. I think it is very clear based on my review of the data that there has never been a paper published in which there has been adequate control for all of the variables of potential causation in the data analysis. Some authors have tried to control for alcohol, tobacco, diet, race, and sex, which are all important variables, but this is the extent of the level of the science at this point.

It is important to recognize that for the reasons stated above, the occasional finding of a slightly increased incidence of laryngeal cancer *per se* in a cohort of workers exposed to asbestos, does not necessarily mean that asbestos exposure *per se* is the cause of the increased incidence of these laryngeal cancers. Furthermore, there is a problem with biologic plausibility, in that there is no animal model indicating that cigarette smoking combined with asbestos exposure in animals, results in laryngeal cancer.

In summary, I do not believe that there is adequate information in the world's literature to suggest that asbestos exposure is a cause of laryngeal cancer. Finally, it is now recognized that 35% or more of laryngeal cancers are due to HPV. Molecular and epidemiologic evidence suggest a strong etiologic association of HPV with oropharyngeal cancers. The incidence of oropharyngeal cancers in the United States has increased between 1973 and 2007, whereas incidence of cancers at other head and neck sites have decreased steadily. Compared with HPV-negative cancers, HPV-positive oropharyngeal cancers are associated with certain sexual behaviors, occur more often among white men and people who do not use tobacco or alcohol, and may occur in a population younger by about 4 years (median ages: 52–56 years). Despite often having a later stage of diagnosis, people with HPV-positive oropharyngeal cancers have a lower risk of dying or recurrence than do those with HPV-negative cancers. The effectiveness of the HPV vaccine in preventing oropharyngeal cancers is unknown. (Cleveland JL, Junger ML, Saraiya M et al. The connection between human papillomavirus and oropharyngeal squamous cell carcinomas in the United States: Implications for dentistry. *J Am Dent Assoc* 2011;142(8):915–24.)

Previous epidemiologic studies corrected for cigarette smoking and alcohol ingestion in asbestos-exposed populations, but did not control for HPV. The failure to account for the most important cause of laryngeal cancer invalidates earlier studies that have claimed any association between asbestos exposure and laryngeal cancer. However, the major role of HPV has not stopped some unethical scientists from performing misleading epidemiologic studies controlling only for smoking and alcohol and not HPV or other know causes of laryngeal cancer. (Ramroth H, Ahrens W, Dietz A et al. Occupational asbestos exposure as a risk factor for laryngeal carcinoma in a population-based case–control study from Germany. *Am J Ind Med* 2011;54(7):510–4.) More recent data from the National Health and Nutrition Examination reveals an increased prevalence of HPV in older adults who smoke and consume alcohol—the very population that has the highest risk for laryngeal cancer! The possible synergistic effect of HPV, alcohol, and smoking has not been investigated, but remains an intriguing possibility. (Chaturvedi AK, Graubard BI, Pickard RK et al. High-risk oral human papillomavirus load in the US population, National Health and Nutrition Examination Survey 2009–2010. *J Infect Dis* 2014;210(3):441–7.)

Li and coworkers reviewed the medical literature, and performed a meta-analysis of a number of molecular epidemiological studies that had been conducted to explore the association of HPV infection with laryngeal cancer. In total, 55 eligible studies were included. The overall HPV prevalence in laryngeal cancer tissues was 28.0% (95% CI: 23.5–32.9%). (Li X, Gao L, Li H et al. Human papillomavirus infection and laryngeal cancer risk: A systematic review and meta-analysis. *J Infect Dis* 2013;207(3):479–88.)

Other scientists from Boston have tried to control for age, race, education, income, smoking, alcohol consumption and one HPV serotype, HPV 16, in performing a nested case–control study of men with pharyngeal cancer. Serum antibody tests correlated with tissue viral DNA, but not all patients with tissue infection had a positive serological test, limiting the usefulness of serological tests in epidemiological studies. (Mbulawa ZZ, Williamson AL, Stewart D et al. Association of serum and mucosal neutralizing antibodies to human papillomavirus type 16 (HPV-16) with HPV-16 infection and cervical disease. *Gen Virol* 2008;89(Pt 4):910–4; Mirghani H, Amen F, Moreau F et al. Human papilloma virus testing in oropharyngeal squamous cell carcinoma: What the clinician should know. *Oral Oncol* 2014;50(1):1–9.) Furthermore, some otherwise normal men and women may have positive oral IgA antibodies without disease. (Marais DJ, Sampson C, Jeftha A et al. More men than women make mucosal IgA antibodies to human papillomavirus type 16 (HPV-16) and HPV-18: A study of oral HPV and oral HPV antibodies in a normal healthy population. *BMC Infect Dis* 2006;6:95.)

Many of the previously reviewed studies were controlled for cigarette and cigar smoking, but did not mention chewing tobacco use and its strong association with HPV. In Pakistan, the incidence of oral cancer ranks second of all cancers in Karachi in both genders, according to World Health Organization statistics. This is attributed to the popularity of chewable tobacco products among the general population. Studies on Gutka eaters in a set population of Karachi, showed a high frequency of HPV (17%) and a high prevalence of HPV in squamous cell carcinoma in Pakistani patients (68%). The exposure of oral mucosa to chewable tobacco causes abrasions, making it susceptible to HPV. This authors' review strives to summarize the role of HPV in chewable tobacco-related precancerous and cancerous lesions. (Zil-A-Rubab, Baig S, Siddiqui A et al. Human papilloma virus—Role in precancerous and cancerous oral lesions of tobacco chewers. *J Pak Med Assoc* 2013;63(10):1295–8.)

Langevin and coauthors did not control for other HPV serotypes, esophageal reflux, machining fluids, or other occupational exposures known to cause laryngeal cancer. The OR (the ratio of the proportion of a group experiencing an event or exposure to the proportion not experiencing an event or exposure) for an effect of asbestos exposure was 1.10 with a CI of 0.99–1.23. This means that any effect of asbestos exposure was not statistically significant or meaningful when considering the size of their study population. Epidemiologists would like to see an OR of at least 2.0 or greater, and a dose–response that strongly suggests that a causal relationship was important. The authors' claim that their study proves an association of asbestos with pharyngeal squamous cell cancer is contradicted by their own data, and demonstrates bias and lack of scientific objectivity. (Langevin SM, O'Sullivan MH, Valerio JL et al. Occupational asbestos exposure is associated with pharyngeal squamous cell carcinoma in men from the greater Boston area. *Occup Environ Med* 2013;70(12):858–63.)

Langevin and coworkers, published another study on other causes of head and neck cancers and investigated the relationship between occupational exposures to five types of dusts, including sawdust, concrete, leather, metal, chimney soot, and head and neck squamous cell carcinomas (HNSCCs) in the greater Boston area. They reported findings from a population-based case–control study involving 951 incident HNSCC cases, and 1193 controls, with frequency matched on age (±3 years), sex, and town/neighborhood of residence. Multivariable logistic regression was used to assess the association between occupational exposure to each type of dust, and HNSCC, both, overall and by primary tumor site. After adjusting for age, sex, race, smoking, alcohol consumption, education, and HPV 16 serology, laryngeal carcinoma risk increased for each decade of occupational exposure to sawdust (OR: 1.2; 95% CI: 1.0–1.3) and metal dust (OR: 1.2; 95% CI: 1.0–1.4), and HNSCC risk increased for each decade of occupational leather dust exposure (OR: 1.5; 95% CI: 1.2–1.9). They provided evidence for an association between occupational sawdust and metal dust, and laryngeal squamous cell carcinoma, and leather dust and HNSCC, with increasing risk with longer duration at the exposed occupation. (Langevin SM, McClean MD, Michaud DS et al. Occupational dust exposure and head and neck squamous cell carcinoma risk in a population-based case–control study conducted in the greater Boston area. *Cancer Med* 2013;2(6):978–86.)

There have been a variety of tissue and serological methods published to detect the presence of HPV 16 and 18. The discordant data from a variety of studies on the prevalence of HPV in oropharyngeal cancers, are in part due to methodologic reasons. The gold standard for the identification of patients with oropharyngeal tumors etiologically linked to HPV infection, is undoubtedly the detection of HPV 16 E6/E7 mRNA. The detection of a surrogate marker of active viral infection, p16ink4a, has a low sensitivity when used alone, and must therefore be combined with the detection of HPV DNA or HPV-specific antibodies. (Klozar J, Tachezy R. What are the implications of human papillomavirus status in oropharyngeal tumors for clinical practice? *Curr Opin Otolaryngol Head Neck Surg* 2014;22(2):90–4; Pytynia KB, Dahlstrom KR, Sturgis EM. Epidemiology of HPV-associated oropharyngeal cancer. *Oral Oncol* 2014;50(5):380–6.) Japanese investigators found that 20% of HPV DNA-positive tumors were negative for serological p16, with most of these tumors manifesting DNA methylation at the p16 gene promoter. (Kawakami H, Okamoto I, Terao K et al. Human papillomavirus DNA and p16 expression in Japanese patients with oropharyngeal squamous cell carcinoma. *Cancer Med* 2013;2(6):933–41.)

Tests, such as the measurement of HPV 16 in serum, have a variety of potential measurement errors, based on laboratory experience, methodology, reagents, equipment, and trained laboratory personnel. The results will vary from institution to institution. The specific institutional data must be verified by comparison to the gold standard of the detection of HPV 16 E6/E7 mRNA in tissue. The failure to verify the sensitivity and specificity of HPV detection techniques, in any institution reporting epidemiologic data on the causation of oropharyngeal cancer, makes that institution's data uninterpretable and lacking in acceptable statistical precision.

Recent results from the National Cancer Institute and National Institutes of Health are frightening. For example, HPV prevalence by Inno-LiPA increased from 16.3% during 1984–1989, to 71.7% during 2000–2004, and incidence for HPV-negative cancers declined by 50% (95% CI: 47–53%; from 2.0 per 100,000 to 1.0 per 100,000). Oral/pharyngeal cancer incidence has significantly increased during 1983–2002, predominantly in developed countries, and at younger ages. If recent incidence trends continue, the annual number of HPV-positive oropharyngeal cancers is expected to surpass the annual number of cervical cancers by the year 2020. (Chaturvedi AK, Engels EA, Pfeiffer RM et al. Human papillomavirus and rising oropharyngeal cancer incidence in the United States. *J Clin Oncol* 2011;29(32):4294–301; Chaturvedi AK, Anderson WF, Lortet-Tieulent J et al. Worldwide trends in incidence rates for oral cavity and oropharyngeal cancers. *Clin Oncol* 2013;31(36):4550–9.)

Many authors, mentioned earlier in this chapter, have found evidence of a variety of occupational exposures that are confounders to epidemiologic studies related to asbestos exposure. They include race, social class, diet, polycyclic aromatic hydrocarbons, rubber by-products, textile dust, engine exhaust, gastroesophageal reflux, cigarette smoke, alcohol, HPV, chewing tobacco, coal dust, formaldehyde, welding fumes, metal machining fluids, silica dust, blacksmithing by-products, plumber and pipefitter by-products, and genetic factors, to name a few of the purported causes of laryngeal cancer. The many different causes of laryngeal cancer make it very difficult to find a control population and avoid bias. Recent data from 2014 have demonstrated a synergistic effect between cigarette smoking and alcohol ingestion, and HPV coinfection. Confounding by other carcinogenic exposures is very important when differences between exposed and unexposed populations are small or nonexistent, as in laryngeal cancer. However, when the effect of asbestos is large, as in lung cancer, then confounding by other exposures that cause lung cancer, such as radon, has a smaller impact on the proof of causation. (Gan LL, Zhang H, Guo JH et al. Prevalence of human papillomavirus infection in oral squamous cell carcinoma: A case–control study in Wuhan, China. *Asian Pac J Cancer Prev* 2014;15(14):5861–5.)

The scientific community has carefully evaluated the possible association between oral/laryngeal cancer, and asbestos exposure, for many decades. My analysis indicates that no association/causation exists from asbestos exposure, after carefully reviewing the bias and confounding from the many other causes of oral/pharyngeal/laryngeal cancer, in the many published epidemiologic studies.

NON-HODGKIN'S LYMPHOMA AND ASBESTOS EXPOSURE

Lieben reviewed the records of 68 hospitalized patients with asbestosis, and noted an increased number of lymphoid tumors in this group, and this was published in her study in 1966. (Lieben J. Malignancies in asbestos workers. *Arch Environ Health* 1966;13:619–21.) Later, Gerber, in a study of a little bit more than 1300 autopsies, described four lymphomas among 35 patients with asbestosis. His study, entitled "Asbestosis and neoplastic diseases of the hematopoietic system," was published in the *American Journal of Clinical Pathology* 1970;53:204.

Elliott Kagan and coworkers, published an article in August 1979, in the *American Journal of Medicine* 1979;67:325–330, in which they described three patients with a history of heavy occupational exposure to asbestos, who had three different neoplasms, including chronic lymphocytic leukemia, and two cases of multiple myeloma. Two of the patients had asbestosis, and a third patient had a pleural mesothelioma. The authors hypothesized that these neoplasms were related to the asbestos exposure. (Kagan E, Jacobson RJ, Yeung KY et al. Asbestos-associated neoplasms of B cell lineage. *Am J Med* 1979;67(2):325–30.)

Irving Selikoff, and others, reviewed the data from 17,800 asbestos insulation workers in 1979 (*Ann NY Acad Sci* 1979;330:91–116), and again updated their data in 1991 and concluded that there was no association between asbestos exposure and lymphoma and leukemia. This is the largest study in the asbestos literature, and includes an observation time of 301,592.6 person-years. (Selikoff I, Seidman H. Asbestos associated deaths among insulation workers in the United States and Canada 1967–1987. *Ann NY Acad Sci* 1991;643:1–14.)

Another study was published by Ross and coworkers, from the Department of Pathology at the University of Southern California in Los Angeles, in the *Lancet* 1982;2:118. The authors noted 26 cases of non-Hodgkin's lymphoma of the large-cell type, and that these large-cell lymphomas were primarily of the GI tract and oral cavity. Ross and coworkers felt that there was an increased risk of non-Hodgkin's lymphoma of the GI tract associated with asbestos exposure. He also noted in the controlled population, an association with malaria, and the onset of lymphoma. (Ross R, Dworsky R, Nichols P et al. Asbestos exposure and lymphomas of the gastrointestinal tract and oral cavity. *Lancet* 1982;2(8308):1118–20.)

This provocative paper generated a lot of response, and in a letter to the editor of the journal *Lancet*, published on December 25, 1982, Bengtsson and others from Sweden, brought up the fact that of 109 cases of non-Hodgkin's lymphoma, 10% were reported to have exposure to asbestos, compared with 21, or 6.3%, of 335 controls. They noted that there was an association between non-Hodgkin's lymphoma and exposure to chlorophenols and phenoxy acids, or organic solvents. Bengtsson and coworkers hypothesized that exposure to other agents may occur in the same occupations where there is exposure to asbestos, and that this interaction had produced confounding. This means that asbestos exposure might simply be a marker of occupations, where there is also exposure to other carcinogenic agents, which are the real cause of the lymphoma rather than the asbestos. (Bengtsson NO, Hardell L, Eriksson M. Asbestos exposure and malignant lymphoma. *Lancet* 1982;2(8313):1463.)

This was followed up on January 23, 1983, with another letter to the editor by Richard Waxweiler and Cynthia Robinson from NIOSH. They pointed out in their study of 2722 males, working with asbestos textile friction and packaging products, in a facility in Pennsylvania that they noted seven deaths due to non-Hodgkin's lymphoma versus the 3.28 expected. On the death certificates, three of these cases were malignant lymphomas and four were lymphosarcomas. Among females, no lymphomas were reported. This is the same plant that had been studied by Lieben in 1966. (Waxweiler RJ, Beaumont JJ, Henry JA et al. A modified life-table analysis system for cohort studies. *J Occup Med* 1983;25(2):115–24.)

The authors point out that Bignon and coworkers had published a study on the translocation of asbestos fibers through the respiratory system, in the *Annals of the New York Academy of Sciences* 1979;330:745–50. Dr. Bignon noted the finding that the thoracic lymph nodes are important points in the clearance pathways of asbestos fibers in both animals and humans. What these authors did not comment on is that the previous studies had shown an increased number of GI lymphomas, and one would anticipate that if the irritating properties from asbestos fibers were the cause of lymphomas, then the site of the lymphoma would usually be in the mediastinum of humans, where the greatest concentration of asbestos fibers are present in the lymph nodes. (Bignon J, Monchaux G, Sebastien P et al. Human and experimental data on translocation of asbestos fibers through the respiratory system. *Ann NY Acad Sci* 1979;330:745–50.)

In a letter to the editor of *The Lancet*, on January 22, 1983, Spanedda and co-workers from Italy reported two other cases, one with multiple myeloma, and one with a chronic B-cell lymphocytic leukemia. (Spanedda R, La Corte R, Minisci S et al. Exposure to asbestos and lymphoid neoplasms. *Med Lav* 1983;74(4):295–301.) Olsson and Brandt responded to Ross's paper, in a letter to the editor of *The Lancet* on March 12, 1983, in which they reviewed 169 cases of men with a recent diagnosis of non-Hodgkin's lymphoma, admitted to the hospital between 1979 and 1982. All occupations were recorded up to the day of diagnosis. They found 11 patients with histiocytic lymphomas of the oral cavity and GI tract, and another six patients with histiocytic lymphomas in the oral cavity and GI tract at other sites, for a total of 17 patients. None of these had been exposed to asbestos for any significant length of time. They went on to state

> Thus our data does not support a relation between asbestos exposure and histiocytic lymphoma presenting in the oral cavity or gastrointestinal tract. There is evidence that exposure to several exogenous factors may promote the development of non-Hodgkin's lymphoma [e.g. irradiation or exposure to organic solvents, chlorophenols, phenoxy acids, and Epstein–Barr virus]. (Olsson H, Brandt L. Asbestos exposure and non-Hodgkin's lymphoma. *Lancet* 1983;1(8324):588.)

Elliott Kagan and Robert Jacobson published another paper entitled "Lymphoid and plasma cell malignancies: Asbestos-related disorders of long latency" in the *American Journal of Clinical Pathology* 1983;80(1):14–20. They identified 13 asbestos workers with lymphoplasmocytic neoplasms, six of which had chronic lymphocytic leukemia, four had IgG myeloma, two had IgA myeloma, and one had histiocytic lymphoma. All had experienced protracted asbestos exposure. Dr. Kagan felt that lymphoid neoplasia may be the result of persistent immunologic stimulation, in a milieu deprived of normal immunoregulatory influences. He concluded this paper by stating that "although our observations are based on selected case material, they clearly underscore the need for large-scale epidemiologic studies to determine whether asbestos exposure can definitely be linked causally to lymphoma and plasma cell dyscrasias." (Kagan E, Jacobson RJ. Lymphoid and plasma cell malignancies: Asbestos-related disorders of long latency. *Am J Clin Pathol* 1983;80(1):14–20.)

This paper resulted in a response by Paul Silcocks, a pathologist and clinical epidemiologist at St. George's Hospital in London. He stated

> The recent article by Kagan and Jacobson, supporting the view that lymphoplasmocytic neoplasms are associated with asbestos exposure, should not go unchallenged: since most of the cases

were chosen on the basis of existing asbestos-associated disease, it is hardly surprising that a positive history of occupational exposure was obtained. This study is also based on small numbers, which would result in a lack of statistical power, where any control group available for comparison [without which it is hard to see what, if any, valid conclusions could be drawn].

He went on to say, "Amongst studies cited, Lieben's suffers from selection bias, being the comparison of mortality from cancer amongst a heterogeneously selected group of asbestos cases with the general population." He also stated that Gerber's article suffered from selection bias, and mentioned Robinson's study, which detected only a nonsignificantly raised SMR for malignant lymphoma, with the SMR being 213 with a 95% confidence limit being between 82 and 405. He criticized the work of Ross and coauthors on the basis of a survivorship bias. He concluded his paper by stating, "No single criteria is sufficient to adduce a causal relationship, but among those suggested, it is consistency with other knowledge. Other asbestos-exposed occupational cohorts have shown no excess of lymphoid neoplasms." (Silcocks P. Asbestos link to lymphoid neoplasms still just a hypothesis. *Am J Clin Pathol* 1984;81(3):41.)

This study was followed up in 1985 with a paper by Efremidis and coworkers from the Mt. Sinai School of Medicine in New York City. The authors reported two lymphocytic neoplasms in the form of a chronic lymphocytic leukemia and a poorly differentiated lymphoma, and felt that these reports suggested a possible association. They went on to mention that "it has been estimated that during the years 1940 to 1945 in the U.S., 4.5 million men and women worked in shipyards where asbestos exposure was intensive. Over 3 million of these individuals are alive today." (Efremidis AP, Waxman JS, Chahinian AP. Association of lympho-cytic neoplasia and mesothelioma. *Cancer* 1985;55(5):1056–9.)

Richard Doll and Julian Peto reviewed the literature of asbestos-related neoplasms, and reported this in the book *Asbestos-Related Malignancy* in 1987, where on page 93 it mentions the positive case reports and goes on to say

The association is not supported by experience in Sweden nor by Selikoff's massive study of insulation workers in North America, but the latter grouped all lymphomas together and large-cell lympho-mas limited primarily to the oral cavity and gastrointestinal tract accounted for only five percent of the total. On these data it is not possible to reach any conclusion, but the possibility that these rare tumors can be produced by exposure to asbestos has to be kept in mind. (Doll R, Peto J. *Asbestos-Related Malignancy*. In: Antman K, Aisner J. (Eds.), New York: Grune & Stratton, 1987.)

A large study investigating this issue was done in North Carolina by Mary Catherine Schumacher and Elizabeth Delzell, entitled "A death certificate case–controlled study of non-Hodgkin's lymphoma and occupation in men in North Carolina," published in the *American Journal of Industrial Medicine*

988;13:317–30. They found 501 men who died of non-Hodgkin's lymphoma, and looked at the occupations and industries of those with lymphoma. There was an increased risk for men in professional, technical, and managerial occupations, as compared with others, and an increased risk was detected for black painters while not for whites. There was no association found between non-Hodgkin's lymphoma and employment in the following areas: the textile industry, farming, and laborers with occupations with exposure to asbestos or benzene. The OR for exposure to asbestos was 0.78 for whites and 1.16 for blacks controlling for age, and the year of death. (Schumacher MC, Delzell E. A death certificate case–controlled study of non-Hodgkin's lymphoma and occupation in men in North Carolina. *Am J Ind Med* 1988;13:317–30.)

In a letter to the editor of the *New England Journal of Medicine*, E Peter Garbor of UCLA, commented on a case discussion of a 65-year-old ex-shipyard worker with pulmonary infiltrates and an axillary mass. Garbor stated that he was disappointed that there was no mention of the relationship between a large-cell lymphoma and prior asbestos exposure. Richard Kardin of the Massachusetts General Hospital replied to Dr. Garbor's letter to the editor as follows:

Dr. Garbor's letter correctly suggests there may be an association between exposure to asbestos and the development of certain lymphoproliferative disorders. However, the association has not been firmly established. Specifically, a large number of reports have indicated the possible association between exposure to asbestos and chronic lymphocytic leukemia, large-cell lymphoma of the gastrointestinal tract and oral cavity, and multiple myeloma. Ross and coworkers performed an epidemiologic case control study of patients with non-Hodgkin's lymphoma and included that exposure to asbestos was statistically associated with the development of lymphoma. In contrast, Olsson and colleagues using a similar approach were unable to confirm such a relation. For these reasons, I purposely avoided discussion of this topic during my clinical–pathological conference. (Garbor EP. Case 28-1989: Pulmonary infiltrates and an axillary mass. *N Engl J Med* 1990;322:131, reply to Garbor's letter by Richard Kradin, *N Engl J Med* 1990;322:131.)

Greenberg and Roggli summarized the literature as of 1992, in the textbook *Pathology of Asbestos-Related Diseases* as follows: "Overall, in the authors' opinion, the balance of the evidence available at present does not support an association between asbestos exposure and lymphoma or leukemia." (Roggli VL, Greenberg SD, Pratt PC. *Pathology of Asbestos-Related Diseases.* Boston: Little Brown, 1992, p. 218.)

In a comment on a paper published by Tondini and colleagues in *Thorax* 1994;49:1269–70, Hughes and McGavin report, in a letter to the editor of *Thorax,* that "lymphoproliferative disorders are not recognized as prescribed asbestos-related diseases, although their case and others attempt to make this relationship." They added a case of a man with a mesothelioma who had a lymphocytic lymphoma of the stomach. They went on to state that "further study into the relationship between lymphoma and asbestos should be conducted." (Hughes P, McGavin CR. Pleural mesothelioma with non-Hodgkin's lymphoma. *Thorax* 1995;50(8):915.)

In a paper published in the *International Journal of Occupational Medicine and Environmental Health* 1996;9:309–321, Bodil Persson published a paper entitled "Occupational exposure and malignant lymphoma." He looked at the issue of which occupational exposures are most likely to be associated with lymphoma. In his review of the literature, he mentioned that "several subsequent studies have dealt with malignant lymphoma amongst woodworkers and pulp and paper mill workers pointing to excessive risks. Exposure to phenoxy herbicides has provided reasonable evidence to be connected with an increased risk of non-Hodgkin's lymphoma." He went on to mention that several Swedish studies showed a relationship between solvent exposure and malignant lymphoma, and an excess risk of Hodgkin's disease and non-Hodgkin's lymphoma among drycleaners. Wood preservatives, including a high-grade exposure to chlorophenols, had yielded a ninefold increase in the risk of non-Hodgkin's lymphoma, and a sixfold increase in Hodgkin's disease in one study. (Persson B. Occupational exposure and malignant lymphoma. *Int J Occup Environ Health* 1996;9:309–21.)

Persson also looked at welding and related occupations, and it is mentioned that there was a study done in British Columbia that found increased mortality due to Hodgkin's disease among welders, but in a large study of 11,092 male welders in nine European countries, there was a slight increased risk of lymphosarcoma, but not Hodgkin's disease. He went on to mention that "exposure to asbestos has been common amongst welders, plumbers, and pipe fitters, and has been implicated as a cause of large-cell non-Hodgkin's lymphoma, primarily of the gastrointestinal tract and oral cavity." He went on to mention that in the Swedish study of non-Hodgkin's lymphoma, only a slight increased risk in workers exposed to asbestos was found, when chlorophenols were taken into account, referring to the paper by Bengtsson and coworkers, published in *The Lancet* in 1982. (Bengtsson NO, Hardell L, Eriksson M. Asbestos exposure and malignant lymphoma. *Lancet* 1982;2(8313):1463.)

Two good meta-analysis studies were done in 1999 and 2001. The first was performed by Goodman et al. (Goodman M, Morgan RW, Ray R, Malloy CD, Zhao K. Cancer in asbestos-exposed occupational cohorts: A meta-analysis. *Cancer Causes Control* 1999;10:453–65.) A second review was performed in 2001 by Becker et al. (Becker N, Berger J, Bolm-Audorff U. Asbestos exposure and malignant lymphomas—A review of the epidemiological literature. *Int Occup Environ Health* 2001;74:459–69.) These authors were unable to find any correlation between asbestos exposure and lymphoma after reviewing 16 studies.

In 2002, Dennis Weisenburger and Brian Chiu from the University of Nebraska rereviewed the world's literature available as of 2002 (Weisenburger DD, Chiu BC. Does asbestos exposure cause non-Hodgkin's Lymphoma or related hematolymphoid cancers? A review of the epidemiologic literature. *Clin Lymphoma* 2002;3(1):36–40). The authors again pointed out that 32 out of 35 epidemiologic studies of asbestos exposure and lymphoma were negative for an association with non-Hodgkin's lymphoma and other hematolymphoid cancers. Also, the authors noted that studies in animals had not shown an increased risk of non-Hodgkin's lymphoma associated with asbestos exposure.

More recently, Treggiari and Weiss, from the Department of Epidemiology, School of Public Health and Community Medicine, University of Washington in Seattle, published a study in the *Annuals of Epidemiology* entitled "Occupational asbestos exposure and the incidence of non-Hodgkin's lymphoma of the gastrointestinal tract: An ecologic study." They noted,

> A previous case–control study (Ross study 1982) observed a strong association between occupational exposure to asbestos and the incidence of non-Hodgkin lymphoma of the gastrointestinal tract (GINHL). To test this hypothesis, they sought to determine whether the geographic pattern of the incidence of GINHL in the US has paralleled that of mesothelioma. Using data obtained from the nine US regions participating in the National Cancer Institute's Surveillance, Epidemiology and End Results program, they examined the incidence of malignancies among men ages 50 to 84 years between 1973 and 1984. The rates of mesothelioma, but not of GINHL, were about two times higher in the areas of Seattle and San Francisco, than in the other regions. Overall, there was no correlation between the rates of mesothelioma and of GIHNL. (Pearson correlation coefficient-0.12, p = 0.77). This ecologic study finds no support for the hypothesis that occupational asbestos exposure is related to the subsequent incidence of GINHL. (Treggiari MM, Weiss NS. Occupational asbestos exposure and the incidence of non-Hodgkin lymphoma of the gastrointestinal tract: An ecologic study. *Ann Epidemiol* 2004;14:168–71.)

There is an association between lymphoma treatment by radiation and an increased risk of mesothelioma, but this is not related to asbestos exposure. De Bruin and others recently reported an increased risk of mesothelioma as a result of radiation, in the medical journal *Blood* in February 2009. They concluded that "malignant mesothelioma is a relatively uncommon malignancy. Recently, increased risks for second primary mesothelioma following radiation for lymphoma have been reported. The risk was almost 30-fold increased in Hodgkin's lymphoma patients treated with irradiation compared to the general population." It is important to remember that an association between two diseases does not necessarily prove causation. If one examines all mesothelioma cases, there will be an increased incidence of lymphomas in patients with mesothelioma as a result of radiation treatment. Radiation treatment is an independent cause of mesothelioma unrelated to asbestos exposure. (De Bruin ML, Burgers JA, Baas P. Malignant mesothelioma after radiation treatment for Hodgkin's lymphoma. *Blood* 2009;113(16):3679–81; Chirieac LR, Barletta JA, Yeap BY et al. Clinicopathologic characteristics of malignant mesotheliomas arising in patients with a history of radiation for Hodgkin's and non-Hodgkin's lymphoma. *J Clin Oncol* 2013;31(36):4544–9.)

In summary, my review of the literature finds no scientific basis to conclude that asbestos exposure predisposes to non-Hodgkin's lymphoma. The data were evaluated using the proposed criteria of Sir Bradford Hill in 1965. (Bradford-Hill A. The environment and disease: Association or causation? *Proc R Soc Med* 1965;58:295–300.) The animal studies are negative for experimental evidence of asbestos exposure and lymphoma, yet there is strong animal experimental evidence for asbestos exposure, and lung cancer and mesothelioma. There is a lack of consistency in the various studies in the published literature. In addition, the strength of association was poor in the various epidemiologic studies, as was the lack of specificity, temporality, or dose–response. Finally, there is a lack of biologic plausibility and coherence. My conclusion that there is no scientific evidence of causation between asbestos exposure and lymphoma is strongly backed by a review of the world's scientific literature and the epidemiologic evidence. (Seidler A, Becker N, Nieters A et al. Asbestos exposure and malignant lymphoma: A multicenter case–control study in Germany and Italy. *Int Arch Occup Environ Health* 2010;83(5):563–70; Treggiari MM, Weiss NS. Occupational asbestos exposure and the incidence of non-Hodgkin's lymphoma of the gastrointestinal tract: An ecologic study. *Ann Epidemiol* 2004;14(3):168–71; Weisenburger DD, Chiu BC. Does asbestos exposure cause non-Hodgkin's lymphoma or related hematolymphoid cancers? A review of the epidemiologic literature. *Clin Lymphoma* 2002;3(1):36–40.)

OVARIAN CANCER AND ASBESTOS EXPOSURE

The issue about ovarian cancer and its relationship with asbestos exposure is very difficult to resolve, because of the difficulty in separating a variety of other intra-abdominal neoplasms from ovarian cancer. Several studies have reported an increased mortality from ovarian cancer in women exposed to amphibole asbestos, but because of large uncertainty about the diagnosis, the question remains unresolved. Keal, in 1960, reported on a series of women with pulmonary asbestosis, who had suffered ovarian cancers. There were 23 women with a diagnosis of asbestosis, of which 15 had died and nine had intra-abdominal neoplasms. One was thought to be an ovarian cancer and four had peritoneal growths, possibly of ovarian origin. Newhouse performed a case–control study of carcinoma of the ovary and asbestos exposure in 1977, which was negative. An increased mortality from cancer of the ovary was observed by Wignall and Fox and Acheson et al. in 1982, in very heavily exposed women. Differentiating peritoneal mesothelioma, primary peritoneal serous papillary adenocarcinoma, metastatic carcinoma from other sites (carcinomatosis peritonei), and other rare tumors from ovarian cancer, is challenging to pathologists of varying experience and ability. This lack of certainty of the diagnosis, makes the interpretation of epidemiologic studies relying of death certificates for a certain diagnosis of ovarian cancer, uncertain and speculative. It is very difficult to draw conclusions on subsequent studies of the relationship between ovarian cancer and asbestos exposure because of the lack of certainty that the pathologic diagnosis is correct. (Keal EE. Asbestosis and abdominal neoplasms. *Lancet* 1960;3:1211–6; Newhouse ML, Pearson RM, Fullerton JM et al. A case–control study of carcinoma of the ovary. *Br J Prev Soc Med* 1977;31(3):148–53; Acheson ED, Gardner MJ et al. Mortality of two groups of women who manufactured gasmasks from chrysotile and crocidolite asbestos: A 40-year follow-up. *Br J Ind Med* 1982;39:344–8; Wignall BK, Fox AJ. Mortality of female gas-mask assemblers. *Br J Ind Med* 1982;39:34–8.)

I am not going to discuss the many studies that have purported a relationship between asbestos exposure and ovarian cancer, other than to say that I find the information uninterpretable because of the lack of agreement between experts as to whether an abdominal neoplasm is truly of ovarian origin, or related to a mesothelioma. There is no question that asbestos exposure in women will cause an increase in peritoneal mesotheliomas if the exposure is sufficiently high, as it was in the Keal study, where all of the afflicted individuals had asbestosis. Most women today have lower dose exposures, such as para-occupational exposures, and develop pleural mesotheliomas. Perhaps the largest and best study was done by Reid and colleagues of the Australian blue asbestos industry in Northwest Australia, in which the SIR for women was 1.27. The mortality rate was much higher in an Italian study of 631 women who worked in the textile industry, and had been compensated for asbestosis, in which the SMR for ovarian cancer was 526, suggesting a diagnosis bias. (Reid A, Heyworth J, de Klerk N et al. The mortality of women exposed environmentally and domestically to blue asbestos at Wittenoom, Western Australia. *Occup Environ Med* 2008;65:743–9; Reid A, Segal A, Heyworth JS et al. Gynecologic and breast cancers in women after exposure to blue asbestos at Wittenoom. *Cancer Epidemiol Biomarkers Prev* 2009;18:140–7; Germani D, Belli S, Bruno C et al. Cohort mortality study of women compensated for asbestosis in Italy. *Am J Ind Med* 1999;36:129–34.)

In the past, there was concern about commercial talc as a cause of ovarian cancer and mesothelioma in women. Many talc deposits are contaminated with asbestos cleavage fragments and asbestiform fibers. However, these fibers usually are not Stanton pathogenic fibers (<0.2 μm in diameter and >8 μm long). Again, I must reiterate that not all asbestos is pathogenic, but must meet certain fiber diameter and length qualifications, as well as sufficient respiratory fiber exposures or doses, to be pathogenic. (Heller DS, Gordon RE, Katz N. Correlation of asbestos fiber burdens in fallopian tubes and ovarian tissue. *Am J Obstet Gynecol* 1999;181(2):346–7; Rohl A, Langer A. Consumer talcum's and powders: Mineral and chemical characteristics. *J Toxicol Environ Health* 1976;2:255–84; Gordon RE, Fitzgerald S, Millette J. Asbestos in commercial cosmetic talcum powder as a cause of mesothelioma in women. *Int J Occup Environ Health* 2014;20(4):318–32.)

Samuel Hammar and coauthors (Hammar SP, Lemen RA, Henderson DW, Leigh J. Asbestos and other cancers. In: R Dodson, SP Hammar (Eds.), *Asbestos: Risk Assessment, Epidemiology, and Health Effects*, 2nd Edition. Boca Raton: CRC Press, 2011, p. 435) stated,

It has been difficult to draw conclusions on the basis of epidemiologic studies of ovarian cancers because, histologically, their distinction between peritoneal mesothelioma and carcinomatous peritonei (including primary peritoneal serous papillary adenocarcinoma) is difficult. Ovarian tumors tend to grow by extension and uncommonly metastasize through the bloodstream, which is similar to tumors of mesothelial origin according to Longo and Young. (Longo DL, Young RC. Cosmetic talc and ovarian cancer. *Lancet* 1979;2:349–51.)

In conclusion, the lack of certainty of the pathologic diagnosis of ovarian cancer versus a peritoneal mesothelioma in epidemiologic studies, has made any conclusions of asbestos causation of ovarian cancer uninterpretable.

I have taken time to provide a thorough evaluation of the literature on the health effects of asbestos and my conclusions do not support the conclusions of the Institute of Medicine's 2006 report or the IARC's 2009 reports, which concluded that there was sufficient evidence that asbestos caused cancer of the larynx and ovary, and that there was limited evidence that asbestos caused colorectal, pharyngeal, and stomach cancers. (Straif K, Benbrahim-Tallaa L, Baan R et al. A review of human carcinogens—Part C: Metals, arsenic, dusts, and fibres. *Lancet Oncol* 2009;10(5):453–4.)

AUTOIMMUNE DISEASE

Jean Pfau and others reviewed the literature on the association of asbestos exposure and autoimmune disease and concluded,

> Despite a body of evidence supporting an association between asbestos exposure and autoantibodies indicative of systemic autoimmunity, such as antinuclear antibodies (ANA), a strong epidemiological link has never been made to specific autoimmune diseases. This is in contrast with another silicate dust, crystalline silica, for which there is considerable evidence linking exposure to diseases such as systemic lupus erythematosus, systemic sclerosis, and rheumatoid arthritis. Instead, the asbestos literature is heavily focused on cancer, including mesothelioma and pulmonary carcinoma. Possible contributing factors to the absence of a stronger epidemiological association between asbestos and autoimmune disease include: a lack of statistical power due to relatively small or diffuse exposure cohorts, exposure misclassification, latency of clinical disease, mild or subclinical entities that remain undetected or masked by other pathologies, or effects that are specific to certain fiber types, so that analyses on mixed exposures do not reach statistical significance.

Their review summarizes epidemiological, animal model, and *in vitro* data related to asbestos exposures and autoimmunity. Their combined data help build toward a better understanding of the fiber-associated factors contributing to immune dysfunction that may raise the risk of autoimmunity, and the possible contribution to asbestos-related pulmonary disease. The important issue, of course, is whether the association between asbestos exposure and autoimmunity produces clinically significant disease. There is a need for more studies to demonstrate a dose–response or biological gradient, the strength of the association, consistency, and specificity or single effect, according to Bradford Hill. (Hill AB. The environment and disease: Association or causation? *Proc R Society Med* 1965;58:295–300.)

The authors concluded that, nevertheless

...the data summarized here provide compelling evidence of an association between asbestos exposure and autoimmunity, including a possible contribution of autoantibodies to the fibrotic disease process. It will be critical for future studies to carefully examine immune dysfunction following specific types of asbestos since there are important clues already suggesting unique pathologic mechanisms with chrysotile compared to amphibole. Such studies will need to include asbestos-like fibers such as erionite and nanofibers, which could significantly expand the potential public health impacts of environmental autoimmunity if such fibers induce similar immune dysfunction. Importantly, if there is an autoimmune component to asbestos-related lung diseases, specifically targeting the adaptive immune system may provide better therapeutic approaches for fibrotic processes, leading to far better health outcomes. (Pfau JC, Serve KM, Noonan CW. Autoimmunity and asbestos exposure. *Autoimmune Dis* 2014;2014:782045.)

12

Asbestos exposure and mesothelioma

Mesothelioma is a rare tumor that primarily affects the lining of the chest cavity or pleura, or the lining of the abdominal cavity, the peritoneum. It rarely can primarily involve the tunica vaginalis of the testicle, the pericardium, and other areas. The most common cause of mesothelioma is heavy amphibole asbestos exposure. The U.S. rate of mesothelioma has been fairly constant since 1994, while it is increasing in some European nations that imported crocidolite asbestos. The rate for malignant mesothelioma in women has been remarkably stable for several decades in the United States. (Erdogan S, Acikalin A, Zeren H et al. Well-differentiated papillary mesothelioma of the tunica vaginalis: A case study and review of the literature. *Korean J Pathol* 2014;48(3):225–8; Mery É, Hommell-Fontaine J, Capovilla M et al. Peritoneal malignant mesothelioma: Review and recent data. *Ann Pathol* 2014;34(1):26–3.)

The total number of mesothelioma cases in the United States is unknown, since only 70% of all cancers are reported to the National Cancer Database. Between 2000 and 2010, 26,605 cases of mesothelioma have been reported to the National Cancer Database, averaging 2660 cases reported each year. Of those cases reported between 2000 and 2010, 89% were Caucasian, 78% were male, and 60% were over the age of 70 years. Unfortunately, mesothelioma has a very poor prognosis. The life expectancy of an average of around 12 months has shown little change in the last 20 years, in spite of intensive chemotherapy, radiation, and extrapleural pneumonectomy (EPP). (Skammeritz E, Omland LH, Johansen JP, Omland O. Asbestos exposure and survival in malignant mesothelioma: A description of 122 consecutive cases at an occupational clinic. *Int J Occup Environ Med* 2011;2(4):224–36.)

Suzuki reviewed 1517 mesothelioma deaths in asbestos insulators, and noted that 77% were pleural mesotheliomas, 0.3% were pericardial, and the rest were peritoneal mesotheliomas. However, the risk of peritoneal mesothelioma was 2.6 times greater in heavily exposed insulators. (Suzuki Y. Pathology of human malignant mesothelioma—Preliminary analysis of 1517 mesothelioma cases. *Ind Health* 2001;39:183–5.) Victor Roggli and coworkers confirmed that a much greater exposure to asbestos is necessary to develop a peritoneal mesothelioma. (Roggli VL, Sharma A, Butnor KJ, Sporn T, Vollmer RT. Malignant mesothelioma and occupational exposure to asbestos: A clinicopathological correlation of 1445 cases. *Ultrastruct Pathol* 2002;26(2):55–65.)

The small increase in survival seen in some recent series, may be due to earlier detection with the advent of computed tomography (CT) and positron emission tomography scanning. (Helland A, Solberg S, Brustugun OT. Incidence and survival of malignant pleural mesothelioma in Norway: A population-based study of 1686 cases. *J Thorac Oncol* 2012;12:1858–61.) Attempts at early detection via blood tests and pleural effusion analysis, have been largely unsuccessful, but continued attempts to find suitable biomarkers, such as mesothelin, osteopontin, and more recently fibulin-3, look promising. (Pass HI, Levin SM, Harbut MR et al. Fibulin-3 as a blood and effusion biomarker for pleural mesothelioma. *N Engl J Med* 2012;367:1417–27.) The most recent epidemiological studies from the Centers for Disease Control, reveal that the incidence of mesothelioma is falling in men and is remaining stable in women. (Henley SJ, Larson TC, Wu M et al. Mesothelioma incidence in 50 states and the District of Columbia, United States, 2003–2008. *Int J Occup Environ Health* 2013;19(1):1–10.)

Mesotheliomas have been associated with a variety of different causative agents besides amphibole asbestos, including other fibrous mineral fibers, radiation, viruses, metals, chemicals, and genetics. The common denominator seems to be an inflammatory response to pleural injury, such as from tuberculosis or radiation from Hodgkin's disease. A variety of thin, fibrous, needle-like materials, present in the environment, have caused mesotheliomas. The most common fibrous material to cause mesothelioma is amphibole asbestos. Both pleural and peritoneal types of mesotheliomas have been associated with amphibole asbestos exposure.

Mesotheliomas have been known for centuries. The story of the discovery of this rare tumor, and the subsequent controversies that arose around its causation by specific forms of commercial asbestos, is a long and complex story that could fill an entire book. This chapter will focus on the early history of the discovery (1767–1900), histologic controversies (1900–1942), diagnostic controversies, and the role of asbestos from 1960 to 1973. The period from 1972 to the early 1980s could be characterized by advances in industrial hygiene assessment of exposures, case–control studies, and other major epidemiologic studies, concerning health effects in asbestos end-product users, para-occupational exposures, household exposures, school and building exposures, and the role of specific asbestos fiber types. The period from the 1980s to the 1990s was also the age of the discovery of the role of environmental exposure to erionite, tremolite, ceramic fibers, and a molecular and cellular biological focus on the characteristics of fiber carcinogenicity. The final period is the late 1990s until the present, during where the focus has been more on the viral contribution to pathogenesis of mesothelioma, such as simian virus-40, as well as human genetics, biomarkers, and treatment strategies.

EARLY DISCOVERY: 1767–1900

The history of the term *mesothelioma* is one of more than 100 years of controversy. The earliest mention of a possible tumor of the chest wall was by Joseph Lieutaud (Lieutaud J. *Historia Anatomico-Medica, etc.* Paris, 1767;ii:86), generally regarded as the founder of pathologic anatomy in France, according to Wolf (Wolf. *Die Lehre von der Krebskrank,* 1911;ii:834), as quoted by Robertson. (Robertson HE. Endothelioma of the pleura. *J Cancer Res* 1924;8:317–75.) Lieutaud published a study of 3000 autopsies, among which were two cases of "pleural tumors." The published account mentions a boy who suffered from marked dyspnea following trauma, who at postmortem showed fleshy masses adherent to the pleura and the ribs. Laennec, in 1819, is also said by Robertson to have suggested that there was an entity of primary malignancy of the pleura, based on the epithelial nature of these pleural cells. (Laennec R. *Traite de l'Auscultaton Medicale,* 1819;ii:368.) In 1843, von Rokitansky (von Rokitansky C. *Lehrbuch der pathol. anatomie,* 1843;iii) actively opposed the idea of primary cancer of the pleura, and states in effect that pleural cancer was always secondary to a primary focus elsewhere. Ironically, in 1854, von Rokitansky described what were called primary tumors of the peritoneum, which he called "colloid cancer," which most likely were peritoneal mesotheliomas. (von Rokitansky C. *Manual of Pathological Anatomy.* London: Sydenham So. Trans., 1854, p. 265.) This strong opinion on the metastatic origin of pleural mesotheliomas by the German pathologist, was to remain the opinions of many pathologists up through the mid-twentieth century, as stated by Willis. (Willis RA. *Pathology of Tumors,* 4th Edition. London: Butterworth, 1967.) There were further reports in the early nineteenth century of what could be considered pleural-based cancers. It was Wagner, in 1870, who first described a lesion, which he classified as *Das Tuberkelähnliche Lymphadenom.* He felt that this was a primary malignancy of the pleura in a 69-year-old woman in whom an epithelial-based malignancy was found. Wagner had described lymph channels filled with tumors. The tumor was called an endothelial carcinoma, or an endothelioma arising from the lymph vessels, and it was not until 1891 that Engelbach first raised the question of whether these tumors arose from the endothelium of the lymph vessels, or from the surrounding serosal surfaces. (Engelbach. *Ein Beitrag Zur Differential Diagnose Pleuritischer Exudate Und Neubildungen Der Pleur Im Anschluss Daren Ein Fall Von Endothelcarinom Der Pleur.* Freburg: Inaug-Diss, 1891.)

During the end of the nineteenth century and early twentieth century, there was general acceptance that some sarcomas arose from the pleura when there was no evidence of a primary elsewhere, and it was generally accepted that the only tumor that might be primary to the pleura, or the subpleura, was a primary sarcoma. This was generally the Italian view as summarized by De Renzi. (De Renzi. *La Riforma Med.* 1893;ix(1):188.) In 1890, Biggs was the first American to report two cases of "endothelioma of the pleura" at the New York Pathological Society (Biggs H. *Proc NY Pathol Soc* 1890:119.) Generally speaking, during this period, primary fibrous sarcomas of the pleura were generally accepted as arising from the fibroblast, but not the pleural tissue itself. The fact that the pleural lining was capable of producing tumors that were both epithelial, and of connective tissue origin, was first pointed out by Paltauf (Paltauf R. Ueber Geschwülsten Der Glandula Carotica, *Beitr Z Path Anat U Z Allg Path* 1892;11:277), Borst (Borst M. *Dielehre von Den Geschwülsten.* Wiesbaden: J. F. Bergmann, 1902;I:287), and Kaufmann (Kaufmann E. *Spezielle Pathologische Anatomy.* Berlin: W. de Gruyter and Co., 1922;I:385).

HISTOLOGIC CONTROVERSY: 1900–1942

Miller and Wynn were the first to advance the opinion that a peritoneal neoplasm was able to present both epithelial and fibroblastic characteristics, because of the embryologic relationship of these cells to the mesoderm. (Miller J, Wynn WH. A malignant tumor arising from the endothelium of the peritoneum and provoking a mucoid acidic fluid. *J Pathol Bacteriol* 1908;12:267.) Later, Maximow was able to demonstrate, via tissue culture, direct transitions from the mesothelioma cell to fibroblast. (Maximow A. Ueber Das Mesothelium, (Deckzellen Der Serösen Haute) Und Die Zellen Der Serösen Exudate. *Arch F Exper Zelforsch* 1927;4:1.)

In 1924, Robertson's review of the subject of "endothelioma of the pleura" was probably the most thorough review of the literature that had been done up until that time. (Robertson HE. Endothelioma of the pleura. *J Cancer Res* 1924;8:317–75.) At the time of that publication, endotheliomas or primary pleural malignancies were certainly rare, in that Clarkson in 1914 stated that out of 10,829 postmortem examinations performed in Munich, Germany, there were only two cases of primary endothelioma of the pleura, although he could find records of only 41 cases. (Clarkson: *Canad. M. A. J.* 1940;iv:192.) Later, Robertson quoted Keilty, who reviewed the records of the pathology department at the University of Pennsylvania, and found nine cases of primary endothelioma of the pleura in 5000 postmortem examinations. (Keilty: *Am J Med Soc* 197 cliii, 888.)

Bayne-Jones described a 16-year-old boy with a pleural-based malignancy, which he felt was a primary neoplasm of the lining cells of the pleura, and an epithelial tumor, which was described as a carcinoma of the pleura. This, he felt, was not an endothelioma, and did not arise from the endothelium of the lymphatics, but from the mesothelial cells. (Bayne-Jones: *John Hopkins Hospital Rep.* 1919;xviii:213.) It was in the following years that Du Bray and Rosson proposed the term primary mesothelioma of the pleura. They felt the terms pleural carcinoma or endothelioma were not appropriate, and that the term mesothelioma was most appropriate. (Du Bray, Rosson. *Arch Intern Med* 1920;xxvi:715.) Zeckwer also used the term mesothelioma in his report of 1928. (Zeckwer IT. Mesothelioma of the pleura. *Arch Intern Med* 1928;34:191.) The issue as to whether there was such a thing as a primary endothelial malignancy arising from the pleura, was carefully discussed by Robertson in his seminal paper that rejected the idea that these tumors were primary tumors of the mesothelioma, and that these tumors were most likely metastatic tumors of some other origin. Robertson felt that only sarcomas could be classified as primary malignant tumors, and that all other types of growth were secondary tumors, with implementations or metastasis from unrecognized, latent primary malignancies elsewhere.

In 1931, Paul Klemperer and Coleman Rabin published a report of five cases from Mt. Sinai Hospital in New York City, and they reported a case with both epithelial and mesenchymal characteristics. They felt that diffuse neoplasms of the pleura arose from the surface lining cells, the mesothelium, and should be designated mesothelioma as previously suggested by others. (Klemperer P, Rabin C. Primary neoplasms of the pleura. *Arch Pathol* 1931;11:385–412.)

In 1933, SR Gloyne reviewed his series of asbestosis cases, and mentioned "of the complications unrelated to the asbestosis the following have been noted: (a) abdominal carcinoma; (b) mitral stenosis; (c) cerebral hemorrhage; and (d) cholelithiasis. There has been one case of squamous carcinoma of the pleura. There is no evidence at the moment that this was in any way related to asbestosis." (Gloyne SR. The morbid anatomy and histology of asbestosis. *Tubercle* 1933;14:550–8.) It is of course easy to speculate as to whether these were the earliest cases of mesotheliomas in asbestos-exposed workers!

In 1940, Ewing raised the question of the influence of chronic irritation or trauma, and low grades of inflammation, as causing connective tissue changes in the pleura, and wondered whether some of the cases of pleural malignancy were connected with tuberculosis. Many of the previously reported cases had evidence of coexistent tuberculosis, in that several attacks of pleurisy on the involved side were reported. His observation would be important 20 years later, when Wagner would report a large number of mesotheliomas from a tuberculosis hospital in South Africa. The subject of trauma and chronic inflammation, as to the cause of pleural transformation, were reviewed by Ewing in his book. (Ewing J. *Neoplastic Diseases*, 4th Edition. Philadelphia: W.B. Saunders, 1940, pp. 355–9.)

Ewing's comments were amplified by a wonderful review of the literature by Andrea Saccone and Aaron Coblenz, from New York City, in 1943. (Saccone A, Coblenz A. Endothelioma of the pleura. *Am J Clin Pathol* 1943;13:186–207.) The authors were able to identify 41 cases in seven published series between 1910 and 1938, for a total of 46,000 autopsies, or 0.09% mesotheliomas. They concluded from their review of the case reports that some of these tumors were misdiagnosed and were metastatic from other sites. Certainly the confusion in making the pathological diagnosis would continue for many years. From 1960 to 1968, only half of Canadian mesothelioma cases on death certificates could be confirmed by an expert panel. (Ducic S. L'exactacttitude des cases de dececes. Une comparison avec les diagnostics àl'autopsie dans une serie de mesotheliomas et autres tumeurs malignes du poumon. *Can J Pub Health* 1971;62:395–402.)

Further support for the idea that these tumors arose from the mesothelium, rather than the endothelium, was supported by Stout and Murray of New York City in 1942. (Stout AP, Murray MR. Localized pleural mesothelioma. *Arch Pathol* 1942;34:951–64.) It was Murray and Stout who used their studies on tissue cultures to support the idea that malignant cells arose primarily from the mesothelial cell. Their concept of histogenesis was so controversial at that time that their Department of Pathology chairman required them to publish a statement of his disbelief in their paper. Stout was later to become Professor of Pathology at

Columbia University in New York City. He was able to accumulate pathological material on 156 mesotheliomas between July 1919 and June 1964. This was the largest series from a single institution in the world, in 1964, and yet he later commented that, in retrospect, he was unaware of a single case associated with asbestosis. (Stout AP. Comments. In: IJ Selikoff, J Churg (Eds.), Biological Effects of Asbestos. *Annals of the New York Academy of Sciences*, 1965;132:680.)

Further support for Stout's theory of histogenesis came from Canada, in a paper by Postoloff, entitled "Mesothelioma of the pleura," in which he concluded that, indeed, the mesothelioma is capable of transforming into both an epithelioid malignancy and a sarcomatous malignancy. He emphasized the importance of an osteoid matrix in the histologic features of mesothelioma. He also mentioned that they found only seven mesotheliomas out of 7878 consecutive autopsies (0.088%) covering a 20-year period between 1923 and 1942. (Postoloff AV. Mesothelioma of the pleura. *Arch Pathol* 1944;37:286–9.)

By 1946, Arnold Piatt, a radiologist at the Newark Hospital, reviewed the radiologic aspects of primary mesothelioma, or endothelioma of the pleura. (Piatt AD. Primary mesothelioma (endothelioma) of the pleura: Case report. *AJR Am J Roentgenol* 1946;55:173–80.) By then, over 200 authors had discussed and offered opinions on the entity, at that time called primary mesothelioma, or endothelioma of the pleura. Piatt pointed out that it was a very difficult diagnostic problem for pathologists, who argued amongst themselves, as to the type and histologic origin of the neoplasm. By then, there were as many as 30 different terms used to describe this clinical entity, including terms such as endothelioma, mesothelioma, endothelial carcinoma, pleural carcinoma, primary papillary endothelioma of the pleura, adenoendothelioma, sarcoendothelioma, pleural sarcoma, sarcomatous malignancy of the pleura, malignant tumor of the pleura, mesothelial carcinoma, perithelioma, endothelioma carcinomatodes, lymphangio-endothelioma, fibro-endotheliosis of the pleura, lymphangitis proliferans, pleuroma, abdominal colloid tumor, and tubercle-like lymphadenoma.

DEFINITION AND SUSPICION: 1943–1960

In the state of confusion as to whether mesothelioma was truly a separate clinical entity, there were four different opinions as to the source of the tumor. One was that there was an aberrant nest of lung epithelium that became malignant, and was within the lining of the pleura. The second was that the endothelial lining of the subpleural lymphatics was the source of the tumor, hence the name endothelioma. The third was the concept that the tumor might arise from the pleural endothelium, or endothelial lining of the subpleural lymphatics, or both. Finally, the fourth opinion was that it arose from the endothelium lining of the pleura itself, or was a mesothelial-derived tumor, or a mesothelioma. It is because of the differences in opinion as to the origin of the tumor that such a large number of terms was used to describe the same process. It is in this setting of much confusion that early reports began to filter out of an association between patients with asbestosis, who developed an unusual form of pleural malignancy. The first report was by Wedler, who reported the results of 30 autopsies on asbestos workers in Germany. They excluded one case, and of the 29 remaining autopsies, four had bronchial cancers, and two others had a malignant pleural growth. He then not only commented about his own impression that the incidence of cancer, which was 20% for malignant tumors in this population, was much too high to be by chance, but also that the lung cancer was due to the asbestos exposure.

He reviewed all of the known literature at that time, and pointed out that the first mention of a lung cancer associated with asbestosis, was made in 1933 by Gloyne, who stated "there has also been one case of squamous cancer of the pleura. There is no evidence at the moment this was in any way related to asbestosis." (Gloyne SR. The morbid anatomy and histology of asbestosis. *Tubercle* 1933;14:550–8.) Later, in 1935, Gloyne was able to report two additional patients with lung cancer and asbestosis. (Gloyne SR. *Tubercle* 1935;17:5.) Wedler did not discuss whether the pleural cancers he found were true mesotheliomas, or related to an underlying lung cancer, in that he simply reported these findings and called them pleural growths of epithelial origin.

His conclusion was that lung cancer was the most common complication encountered in cases of asbestosis. (Wedler HW. Lung cancer in asbestosis patients. *Dtsch Arch Klin Med* 1943;191:189–209.) While the report of Wedler was readily accepted in Germany, most of the world apparently yawned, and the information was generally ignored. In 1947, a patient with a mesothelioma of the pleura and pericardium, who worked with asbestos, cutting insulation board, was reported as a clinical pathological conference (CPC) of the Massachusetts General Hospital, but the association with the asbestos exposure was not made. (Mallory PB, Castleman B, Parris EE. Mesothelioma of the pleura and pericardium. *N Engl J Med* 1947;236:407.)

In 1952, Cartier reported in a scientific meeting, via an abstract of a discussion of a paper by WE Smith (Cartier P. In discussion of paper entitled Smith WE, Survey of some current British and European studies of occupational tumor problems. *Arch Ind Hyg Occup Med* 1952;5:262–63) seven cases of respiratory cancer in 4000 asbestos workers working in the Quebec chrysotile mining and milling industry. Included in the cohort were two cases of pleural mesothelioma (0.05%). He felt that since the two mesothelioma cases did not have asbestosis, causation from asbestos exposure could not be made. The details of these cases were never published. The issue about mesothelioma occurring in the population of workers from the Thedford mines in Quebec, was further evaluated by Dr. McDonald and colleagues, who in 1970, released a national survey of mesothelioma cases in Canada between 1960 and 1968, and found only a small proportion of mesothelioma cases, mostly in insulators or workers in asbestos products manufacturing. (McDonald AD, Harper A, El Attar OA et al. Epidemiology of primary malignant mesothelial tumors in Canada. *Cancer* 1970;26:109–12.) A follow-up paper in 1973 discovered that when a panel of pathologists reviewed the cases, diagnostic agreement was found in 50% of cases. (McDonald AD, Magner D, Eyssen G. Primary malignant mesotheliomas in Canada, 1960–1968. A pathological review by the mesothelioma panel of Canadian Tumor Reference Center. *Cancer* 1973;31:869–76.) It is impossible to know whether these tumors reported by Cartier were true mesotheliomas.

In 1953, Weiss added a third case to the two malignant tumors of the pleura, described by Wedler, of a man with asbestosis and pleural mesothelioma, who had done insulation work in a naval dockyard from 1920 until 1935. He felt that the association between asbestosis and pleural mesothelioma was strong, and therefore he recommended the German government accept this as a work-related condition. (Weiss A. Pleurakrebs Bei Lungenaspestose, *In Vivo* Morphologish Gesichert. *Medizinische* 1953;3:93.)

von Rokitansky, in 1854, described what were called primary tumors of the peritoneum, which he called "colloid cancer." (von Rokitansky C. *Manual of Pathological Anatomy*. London: Sydenham So. Trans., 1854, p. 265.) While this tumor was mentioned in the English literature, first by Miller and Wynn in 1908 (Miller J, Wynn WH. A malignant tumor arising from the endothelium of the peritoneum and producing mucoid ascitic fluid. *J Pathol* 1908;12:267), the association between peritoneal tumors and possible asbestos exposure was not made until 1954, when another German, Leichner, described an autopsy done 2 years earlier on a 53-year-old man, who worked in an asbestos factory between 1929 and 1951, primarily as a spinner. He reported that the patient had asbestosis and tuberculosis, but had what appeared to be an incidental finding of a peritoneal mesothelioma. Leichner found evidence of asbestos fibers in the tumor, and felt that this peritoneal mesothelioma was again work related. (Leichner F. Primary mesothelial-cell tumor of the peritoneum in asbestosis. *Arch Gewerbepathol Gewerbehyg* 1954;13:382.) A short time later in 1955, Bonser, Faulds, and Stewart, reported 72 autopsies of patients with asbestosis, in which four cases were found to have abdominal neoplasms consistent with a peritoneal mesothelioma, but the authors never made the association or connection that these were asbestos-induced peritoneal mesotheliomas. (Bonser GM, Faulds JS, Stewart MJ. Occupational cancer of the urinary bladder in dyestuffs operatives and of the lung in asbestos textile workers and iron ore miners. *Am J Clin Pathol* 1955;25:126–33.)

In 1956, Ackerman wrote that it was the majority opinion that primary mesotheliomas were rare but do exist. (Acherman LV. *Atlas of Tumor Pathology*. Washington DC: Armed Forces Institute of Pathology, 1956. Section 6, Part 23, p. 100.) A year later in 1957, Godwin wrote a very important paper that laid down strict diagnostic criteria for the diagnosis of pleural mesotheliomas. (Godwin MC. Diffuse mesotheliomas with comment in their relation to localized fibrous mesotheliomas. *Cancer* 1957;10:298–319.) In 1958, Van der Schoot reported two mesotheliomas in insulation workers. (Van der Schoot HCM. Asbestosis en pleuragezwellen. *Ned Tijdchr Geneeskd* 1958;102:1125.) In 1958, McCaughey from Belfast, Ireland, reported 11 diffuse and two localized pleural mesotheliomas. He felt that there was strong evidence to support the belief that diffuse pleural mesothelioma was a clinical entity, in spite of opposition to this idea. (McCaughey WTE. Primary tumors of the pleura. *J Pathol Bacteriol* 1958;66:517–29.) At that time, McCaughey did not make the association in this group of mesotheliomas with asbestos exposure as a cause of mesothelioma, but he would do so in retrospect a few years later. (McCaughey WTE, Wade OL, Elmes PC. Exposure to asbestos dust and diffuse pleural mesotheliomas. *Br Med*

J 1962:1397.) His paper was basically a response to an article published by Smart and Hinson of the London Chest Hospital, who reported 24 cases of pleural neoplasm, and concluded that the occurrence of a true neoplasm of pleura could not really be denied, but the lesion is produced from known primaries, and there was no need to postulate an origin from that site. (Smart J, Hinson KFW. Pleural neoplasms. *Br J Tuberculosis* 1957;51:319–30; Willis RA. *Pathology of Tumors.* Washington DC: Butterworth Inc., 1960, p. 185.) In 1956, HB Eisenstadt, of Port Arthur, Texas, reported a patient who worked in a refinery, who developed what appeared to be a malignant mesothelioma of the pleura. He again pointed out the fact that very experienced pathologists denied the existence of such a tumor, but felt compelled to report the case anyway. (Eisenstadt HB. Malignant mesothelioma of the pleura. *Dis Chest* 1956;30:549–56.)

A good example of the problems of the ambiguity as to what to do with the diagnosis of mesothelioma, is the treatment of the condition by Sir Richard Doll in his classic study of the association between lung cancer and asbestosis in 1955. In Table II of the article, he describes 15 patients with asbestosis and some type of lung cancer, but only uses 11 of the 15 in his analysis. Two of the patients are recorded as having either an endothelioma of the pleura, or epithelial carcinoma. Three additional patients with lung cancer were found, but they did not have asbestosis. The association between the asbestos exposure and the endothelioma of the pleura was not made, and evidently was excluded from this statistical analysis.

1960 is really the seminal year for making the association between asbestos exposure and mesothelioma. The seminal paper, of course, is the paper by Wagner, Sleggs, and Marchand. (Wagner JC, Sleggs CA, Marchand P. Diffuse pleural mesothelioma and asbestos exposure in northwestern Cape providence. *Br J Ind Med* 1960;17:260–71.) The paper by Wagner et al. was very controversial because it described 33 cases of diffuse pleural mesothelioma with exposure to only one type of asbestos, so-called "Cape Blue" asbestos, mined in the asbestos hills west of Kimberly in the northwest Cape providence of South Africa. Wagner said the tumor was rarely seen elsewhere in South Africa. This meant the tumor seemed to be rather specific to a certain geographical area, and a specific type of crocidolite asbestos. The data were considered suspect by many pathologists, in that only four of the patients had full autopsies, the rest having had simple pleural biopsies. The other problem was that previously reported patients had heavy industrial exposure, and usually asbestosis, while the majority of his cohort did not have asbestosis or heavy industrial exposure. The general consensus at that time, of course, was that a true mesothelioma diagnosis could not be made unless there was a complete autopsy excluding some primary tumor elsewhere in the body that had metastasized to the pleura, and there also was concomitant asbestosis.

The initial response was muted because of—as so eloquently stated by Elliott McCaughey—"the lack of experimental animal evidence, rejection or lack of knowledge of science conducted outside of the United States, and reluctance of individual writers to change their minds." (McCaughey WTE. Asbestos and cancer, 1934–1965. *Am J Ind Med* 1993;23:503–4.) In an editorial written in South Africa in 1968, the relationship between crocidolite exposure and mesothelioma was still felt to be unproven. (Van Die Redaksie. Editorial: Asbestos and neoplasia. *S Afr Med J* 1968;6:325.)

In 1960, Eisenstadt and Wilson published a paper describing two patients with pleural mesothelioma. The second case had a long-term history of exposure to asbestos, and there were asbestos bodies in the lung biopsy specimen. The authors felt that there was an association between the asbestos exposure and the subsequent development of this unusual pleural malignancy. (Eisenstadt HB, Wilson FW. Primary malignant mesothelioma of the pleura. *J Lancet* 1960;80:511–4.) Unfortunately, Eisenstaedt's paper was not accepted by a major medical journal, and was published in an obscure medical society journal called *Lancet*, which was the published by the North Dakota State Medical Association, the South Dakota State Medical Association, and the Montana State Medical Association. *Lancet* had no affiliation with the well-respected British medical journal *The Lancet,* and was not widely circulated.

ASSOCIATION AND CAUSATION: 1960–1973

Also, in 1960, Keal reviewed the records of an English hospital and found the records of 23 women with asbestosis. Four had carcinomatosis of the peritoneum without a known primary, one had ovarian cancer, and four others had peritoneal malignancy, possibly of ovarian origin. (Keal EE. Asbestosis and abdominal neoplasms. *Lancet* 1960;2:1211–6.) The association with asbestosis is glaring in this study of Keal, but the connection between asbestos exposure and peritoneal malignancy was not strongly suggested until 4 years later. Winslow and Taylor published a series of 12 cases of peritoneal mesothelioma in 1960, and also reviewed 13 previously reported cases found in the world's literature. No association with asbestos exposure was mentioned in their paper. (Winslow DJ, Taylor HB. Malignant peritoneal mesotheliomas. A clinico–pathological analysis of 12 fatal cases. *Cancer* 1960;13:127.) However, the association between asbestos exposure and diffuse abdominal tumors was established in the English literature, by the paper of Enticknap and Smither in 1964 (Enticap JB, Smither WJ. Peritoneal tumors in asbestosis. *Br J Ind Med* 1964;21:20), and here again, the Germans made the association between asbestos exposure and this rare tumor earlier than other investigators. While attempts to define the tumor mesothelioma were made by earlier investigators such as Klemperer and Rabin in 1931, there was no general agreement amongst pathologists that such an entity really existed. In 1957, Godwin published strict criteria for the diagnosis of pleural mesotheliomas that placed the pathological identification on a more firm scientific footing (Godwin MC. Diffuse mesotheliomas—With comment on their relation to localized fibrous mesotheliomas. *Cancer* 1957;10:298), and it was not until 1960 that Winslow and Taylor did the same thing for peritoneal mesothelioma tumors.

After Wagner's discovery of the association between Cape Blue crocidolite asbestos and the increased risk of mesothelioma in South Africa, the question arose as to whether this was a unique problem limited to South Africa, or whether this was a problem occurring in the United States. The American

Medical Association Council on Occupational Health published an article on pneumoconiosis. (*Arch Environ Health* 1963;7:14–55.) In this article, in a section on asbestosis the panel of experts concluded that

> The relationship between cancer of the lung and asbestosis constitutes a problem of great current interest. There is no doubt that the two diseases appear in the same lung. Whether that occurrence is one of mere coincidence, or of direct cause–effect relationship cannot be resolved on the basis of a single case. The total body of evidence favors a relationship, especially as it involves certain kinds of asbestos and possibly only those, which contain specific chemical substances having the capacity to cause cancer. Attention is invited to experiences in the union of South Africa where pleural mesotheliomas have been discovered in appreciable numbers of persons exposed to the inhalation of crocidolite–amosite asbestos. Certainly detailed epidemiologic clinical and experimental studies are required for the ultimate resolution of the problem.

In 1962, Wagner was able to produce mesothelial tumors of the pleura by direct implantation of asbestos dusts in laboratory animals. (Wagner JC. Experimental production of mesothelial tumors of the pleura by implantation of dusts in laboratory animals. *Nature* 1962;196:180.) By 1963, Wagner reported, at the 14th International Congress of Occupational Health, on 120 cases of mesothelioma, but curiously less than half of the patients directly worked with asbestos, and rather simply lived in an area where there was environmental exposure. The question at that time was whether this was a localized group of mesothelioma patients, or the forerunner of an international epidemic. This question was answered at the International Meeting on "Biological Effects of Asbestos" at the New York Academy of Sciences in New York City, in October 1964, but not published until December 31, 1965. (Selikoff IJ, Churg J. (Eds.). Biological effects of asbestos. *Ann NY Acad Sci* 1965;132:1–766.) Reports from Newhouse and Thompson in London, Elmes and Wade from Ireland, Jacob and Anspach from Germany, Hammond, Selikoff, and Churg from the United States, and Vigliani and coworkers from Italy, at the New York meeting confirmed the global extent of the problem.

Initially, there was much uncertainty about Wagner's 1960 study, but Dr. Wagner quickly discovered more cases and developed an animal model for the production of mesotheliomas, which greatly improved the confidence in his discovery. In 1965, when he reported his updated series of cases at the New York Academy of Sciences, there was general consensus that this indeed was a unique observation, and that there was an association between a specific type of Cape Blue crocidolite asbestos and mesothelioma. (Wagner JC. Epidemiology of diffuse mesothelioma tumors: Evidence of an association from studies in South Africa and United Kingdom. *Ann NY Acad Sci* 1965;132:575–8.)

Dr. Wagner moved from South Africa, to the English Pneumoconiosis Research Unit in Wales, to carry on his research on the health effects of asbestos.

He published in 1963, a review of the prior literature on asbestosis in experimental animals, and added his own observations. He concluded that it appeared that chrysotile asbestos was less fibrogenic than amosite asbestos in rats. (*Br J Ind Med* 1963;20:1–12; *Nature* 1962;196:180–1; *Ann NY Acad Sci* 1965;132:77–86.)

In 1962, Wagner began experimental animal studies by injecting asbestos into the pleural cavity of rats. This was a brilliant stoke because previous inhalation studies had failed to produce mesotheliomas in animals. Laboratory rats have a short life expectancy, which because of the long latency of mesotheliomas, does not allow time for the tumor to develop. Wagner later began to use pathogen-free rats, which are rats born by Cesarean section into a sterile environment in which they remain for the rest of their lives. The rats are protected from infections, and their life expectancy is sufficiently prolonged to develop mesotheliomas by inhalation exposure. Wagner and Skidmore reported their pleural asbestos implantation in 1965, at which time they had demonstrated that chrysotile, crocidolite, and silicon dioxide powder, produces mesotheliomas and to a lesser extent, amosite in guinea pigs. (Wagner JC, Skidmore JW. Asbestos dust deposition and retention in rats. *Ann NY Acad Sci* 1965;132:77–86.)

The discovery by Wagner, Pott, and later Stanton, Davis, and others that non-mesothelioma-producing dusts by inhalation, such as silicon dioxide powder and fiberglass, produced mesotheliomas by direct injection into the pleura, was a huge breakthrough in science. This was critically important in the understanding of the basic pathogenesis of mesothelioma via irritation of mesothelial cells, and the release of damaging chemicals and free radicals that alter crucial signaling pathways, and cause genetic and epigenetic events that lead to cell transformation. (Stanton MF, Wrench C. Mechanisms of mesothelioma induction with asbestos and fibrous glass. *J Natl Cancer Inst* 1972;48(3):797–821; Stanton M, Layard M, Tegeris A et al. Relation of particle dimension to carcinogenicity in amphibole asbestos and other fibrous minerals. *J Natl Cancer Inst* 1981;67:965–75; Pott F. Some aspects on the dosimetry of the carcinogenic potency of asbestos and other fibrous dusts. *Staub Reinhalt Luft* 1978;38:486–90; Davis JM. The use of animal models for studies on asbestos bioeffects. *Ann NY Acad Sci* 1979;330:795–8.) More recently, others have produced mesotheliomas in rats by the intra-peritoneal injection of slag wool fibers, ceramic fibers, and carbon nanotube fibers, as well as by inhalation studies of potassium titanate whiskers. (Magnani C, Fubini B, Mirabelli D et al. Pleural mesothelioma: Epidemiological and public health issues. Report from the Second Italian Consensus Conference on Pleural Mesothelioma. *Med Lav* 2013;104(3):191–202.)

This explains why any cause of chronic inflammation in the pleural space such as tuberculosis, radiation damage, familial Mediterranean fever, and a variety of noncommercial fibrous minerals, may cause mesothelioma. (Mossman BT, Shukla A, Heintz NH, Verschraegen CF, Thomas A, Hassan R. New insights into understanding the mechanisms, pathogenesis, and management of malignant mesotheliomas. *Am J Pathol* 2013;182(4):1065–77.)

After Wagner's discovery of the association between crocidolite asbestos and the increased risk of mesothelioma in South Africa, the question arose as to whether this was a unique problem limited to South Africa, or whether this was a problem also occurring in the United States. The American Medical Association Council on Occupational Health published an article on pneumoconiosis. (*Arch Environ Health* 1963;7:14–55.) In this article, there is a section on asbestosis, and the panel of experts concluded that

> It is believed there may be an association between bronchogenic carcinoma and asbestosis in workers with well-established asbestosis, particularly among those with long exposures. When carcinoma supervenes in asbestosis, it is usually squamous cell type and it is frequently located in the lower lung field where the fibrosis is usually the most extensive. An increased incidence or risk of lung cancer in other pneumoconioses probably does not exist.

They go on to say on page 37 of their article that

> The relationship between cancer of the lung and asbestosis constitutes a problem of great current interest. There is no doubt that the two diseases appear in the same lung. Whether that occurrence is one of mere coincidence, or of direct cause–effect relationship cannot be resolved on the basis of a single case. The total body of evidence favors a relationship, especially as it involves certain kinds of asbestos and possibly only those, which contain specific chemical substances having the capacity to cause cancer. Attention is invited to experiences in the union of South Africa where pleural mesotheliomas have been discovered in appreciable numbers of persons exposed to the inhalation of crocidolite–amosite asbestos. Certainly detailed epidemiologic clinical and experimental studies are required for the ultimate resolution of the problem.

The question about the risk to end users of asbestos products was raised by Thompson, Kaschula, and MacDonald in 1963. They wrote

> The enormously increased world consumption of asbestos, from 300,000 tons in 1934 to 2,400,000 tons in 1961, is used in a variety of industrial products, from obvious ones such as asbestos roofing, roof tiles, ceilings, floor tiles, pipe insulation, and electrical insulation, to less obvious ones where asbestos is added to all sorts of materials, cement, etc. It is possible for those manufacturing, selling, and using these products to inhale asbestos fibers, although their occupations are in general not labeled or recognized as ones in which asbestos as a hazard to be anticipated. (Thomson JG, Kaschula RO, MacDonald RR. Asbestos as a modern urban hazard. *S Afr Med J* 1963;37:77–81.)

Selikoff, Churg, and Hammond reported their experience of the relationship between asbestos exposure and mesothelioma in the *New England Journal of*

Medicine in 1965, further cementing the relationship between asbestos exposure and mesothelioma, and raising the question as to whether others types of asbestos might also cause mesotheliomas. (Selikoff I, Churg J, Hammond E. Relation between exposure to asbestos and mesothelioma. *N Engl J Med* 1965;272:560–5.)

Even while there was growing information amongst other workers that they were finding increased incidences of this rare tumor, other workers were still unimpressed. Part of the controversy was generated by the fact that when Sluis-Cremer and others looked at other areas of South Africa, they only found an increased incidence of mesothelioma in the areas of the Northwest Cape, where Cape Blue asbestos was mined. They looked for increased incidence of mesothelioma in the amosite mining area, and the area of the Transvaal, where another form of crocidolite was mined, and were unable to find an increased incidence. This caused a lot of confusion since it suggested that mesothelioma was just related to an exposure to one certain type of asbestos. Ian Webster, the brother-in-law of Dr. JC Wagner, still felt that there were unsolved problems in the relationship between asbestos and malignancy, in a paper he published in February 1973. (Webster I. Asbestos and malignancy. *S Afr Med J* 1973;47:165–71.)

Selikoff, Churg, and Hammond reported their experience of the relationship between asbestos exposure and mesothelioma in the *New England Journal of Medicine* in 1965, further cementing the relationship between asbestos exposure and mesothelioma, and raising the question as to whether others types of asbestos might also cause mesotheliomas. The authors did not believe that American workers had significant exposure to crocidolite. They felt that the emergence of mesotheliomas in their cohort of asbestos insulators represented mainly exposure to chrysotile and amosite. All patients had heavy exposure and asbestosis. (Selikoff I, Churg J, Hammond E. Relation between exposure to asbestos and mesothelioma. *N Engl J Med* 1965;272:560–5.) This article was followed by an editorial in the *New England Journal of Medicine* on March 18, 1965. (Collins RN, Nadel MS. Asbestosis and malignant disease. *N Engl J Med* 1965;272:590–1.) The editorial mentions, "amosite, the third commercially used form of asbestos, has yet to be incriminated, but there are no definitive studies to date to confirm or deny such a connection."

Dr. Sluis-Cremer of the Miner's Medical Bureau in Johannesburg, South Africa, gave a report to the New York Academy of Science that was published in 1965. (Sluis-Cremer GK. Asbestosis in South Africa—Certain geographical and environmental considerations. *Ann NY Acad Sci* 1965;132(1):215–34.) Dr. Sluis-Cremer in his discussion of mesotheliomas pointed out that his epidemiologic studies found mesotheliomas only in the Northwest Cape area of South Africa. The Transvaal amosite deposits had been actively developed for longer than this period, and he mentions that in the 1940s, amosite was in fact at three times the level of production of the northwest crocidolite, yet no mesotheliomas were seen in the northwest area related to amosite exposure.

It seems that every advance in science has its nay-sayers that are pulled along screaming and kicking. Garrett Schepers, then working as an American pathologist, originally from South Africa, related his own experience at the New York Academy of Sciences meeting and stated,

> As a boy, I lived not far from Kuruman for a number of years. One could not imagine a more healthy territory. However, there is a particular irritating type of grass in the area (Klitsgras), whose seeds burrow into every garment they cling to, as these seeds are armed with fine barbs. Surely, when the wind blows, as often it does in Kuruman, some of these minute barbs may be inhaled. I wonder whether some of these fiber structures reported in the lungs of persons in that area may not represent reactions to grass barbles. I offer this Klitsgras theory of Kuruman mesotheliomatosis in order to clear the hurdle created by the discovery of this rare disease in such abundance in persons with such little meaningful exposure to asbestos. Perhaps the South African pathologists will now have their turn to make mincemeat of my theory. (Schepers GWH. Comments at New York Academy of Sciences meeting October 1964. *Ann NY Acad Sci* 1965;132:599.)

Also at that meeting Dr. Schepers stated,

> My first impression is that there is now less certainty that asbestos inhalation is associated with pulmonary neoplasia than there was 10 or 20 years ago. Perhaps this is due to greatly reduced dust exposures. Asbestos may after all prove to be carcinogenic only in overwhelming dosage. Thus, the high prevalence of neoplasia which was reported several decades ago may be a function of the severity of exposure rather than an indication of high carcinogenic potency. I suspect that in the final analysis that the carcinogenicity of asbestos will be rated as of low order. Perhaps carcinogenicity will prove to be a correlate of asbestosis rather than a specific biological function of the mineral asbestos. This may be the crux of the matter in all cases of asbestos-associated lung cancer, which I have personally studied (the theory now exceeds two dozen); there invariably was well-established asbestosis. Not only was the asbestosis of marked degree in the areas where the cancer arose, but there generally was evidence from serial chest X-rays that asbestosis had been present in the lungs for a protracted period. (Schepers GWH. Comments at New York Academy of Sciences meeting October 1964. *Ann NY Acad Sci* 1965;132:595.)

Of particular interest was the case–control study of Newhouse and Thompson. (Newhouse ML, Thompson H. Mesothelioma of pleura and peritoneum following exposure to asbestos in the London area. *Br J Ind Med* 1965;22:261–9.) They diagnosed 83 patients—41 men and 42 women—with mesothelioma in association with a Cape Blue asbestos factory that opened in London in 1913. There were

27 peritoneal tumors and 56 pleural tumors. The factory used Cape crocidolite exclusively until 1926, then small amounts of amosite and chrysotile were added. Eighteen cases were persons who had been employed in the asbestos factory and eight as insulators and laggers. An additional nine cases were in persons who lived in the same house as an asbestos worker. Particularly distressing was the discovery of 36 patients with no known work or domestic exposure to asbestos. Eleven of these patients lived within a half mile of the asbestos factory, suggesting neighborhood exposure.

This case–control study and one by Elmes et al. (Elmes PC, McCaughey WT, Wade OL. Diffuse mesothelioma of the pleura and asbestos. *Br Med J* 1965;1:350–3) were the first two case–control studies to confirm the earlier report of Wagner from South Africa. The concern about neighborhood exposure was echoed by Jan Lieben of the Pennsylvania Health Department, who reported that, of 42 cases of mesothelioma, only 20 had occupational exposure, eight lived within the vicinity of an asbestos plant, and three had family exposure. (Lieben J, Pistawka H. Mesothelioma and asbestos exposure. *Arch Envrion Health* 1967;14:559–63.)

The relationship between peritoneal tumors and asbestosis was discussed in an article in the *British Journal of Industrial Medicine* in 1964 by Enticknap and Smither. (Enticknap J, Smither W. Peritoneal tumours in asbestosis. *Br J Ind Med* 1964;21:20–31.) They stated,

> There are three commercially important types of asbestos: chrysotile, crocidolite, and amosite. The latter two are grouped as amphibole asbestos. They differ in geological formation, in chemical composition, in crystalline form, in fiber size, and in many other aspects. Wagner et al. (1960) have reported primary mesothelioma of tumors associated with exposure to crocidolite. In North America, primarily peritoneal tumors have been reported by Cartier (personal communication) and by Mancuso and Colter (1963) (Mancuso, Coulter. Methodology in Industrial Health Studies. *Arch. Envir. Health*, 1963;6:210–66) and (personal communication) in workers thought to be exposed to chrysotile (actually crocidolite was also present). So far there have been no cases reported where the exposure was only to amosite.

Bonser, Faulds, and Stewart, found four cases of peritoneal mesothelioma among 72 postmortem autopsies of workers with asbestosis in 1955. However, the causal association of asbestos exposure with mesothelioma was not made by these investigators. (Bonser GM, Faulds JS, Stewart MJ. Occupational cancer of urinary bladder in dyestuffs operatives and of lung cancer in asbestos textile workers and iron ore miners. *Am J Clin Pathol* 1955;25:126–34.)

The British government held an advisory panel on problems arising from the use of asbestos in 1967. This was stimulated by the publication of an article in October 1965, in the *British Journal of Industrial Medicine,* by Dr. Newhouse and Thomson, on the association between asbestos exposure and mesothelioma. The panel's statement on page 7 was

The first suggestions that asbestosis might be complicated by the development of carcinoma of the lung followed within a few years, but an association was not generally accepted until the 1950's. In recent years, there has been concern over the occurrence of mesothelial tumors of the pleura or peritoneum, which appear in many instances to be causally related to asbestos exposure. There is also evidence suggesting that these mesothelial tumors, at one time considered to be pathological rarities, are becoming commoner and that where asbestos exposure has occurred, that a variety known as crocidolite or blue asbestos is of particular significance. (British Advisory Panel on Asbestos 1967; Department of Employment and Productivity: HM Factory Inspectorate. *Problems Arising From the Use of Asbestos.* London: HMSO, 1968.)

Furthermore, the panel pointed out on page 14 that Merewether, summing up in 1930 in his *Report on Effects of Asbestos Dust on the Lungs and Dust Suppression in the Asbestos Industry*, expressed the view that "in the space of a decade, or thereabouts, the effects of energetic application of preventive measures should be apparent in a great reduction in the incidence of asbestosis." (Mereweather ERA, Price CW. *Report on Effects of Asbestos Dust on the Lungs and Dust Suppression in the Asbestos Industry.* London: HMSO, 1930.) This hopeful prediction that dust suppression by engineering controls would prevent future development of asbestosis unfortunately was not fulfilled. McVittie has reported that "of 247 new cases of asbestosis diagnosed between 1955 and 1963 by four pneumoconiosis medical panels, no fewer than 165 or 67%, had entered the industry in 1933 [by which time the asbestos industry regulations were fully operative] or at a later date." They further pointed out that "although the survey by the inspector indicates that many, probably a large majority, of the workers using asbestos come within the scope of these regulations, laggers, the total of whom is not known with any accuracy, tend to be excluded." (McVittie JC. Asbestos in Great Britain. *Ann NY Acad Sci* 1965;132:121–7.)

The panel goes on, in pages 15 and 16, to discuss the relationship between asbestosis and cancer of the lung. They point out that the British experience was that asbestosis was always present when lung cancer was present. However, they point out that Selikoff's data suggested that lung cancer could be caused by asbestos exposure without asbestosis. They further report on page 16 that the results of Dr. Knox suggest that when asbestosis is prevented, there is no increased incidence of lung cancer. (Report and Recommendations of the Working Group on Asbestos and Cancer. *Br J Ind Med* 1965;22:165–71 and *Ann NY Acad Sci* 1965;132:706–21 (Appendix 2); Gilson JC. Wyers memorial lecture, 1965 Health Hazards of Asbestos: Recent studies on its biological effects. *Trans Soc Occup Med* 1966;16:62–74.)

On page 18 of the report, they point out that Gloyne, in 1933, reported the complications of pulmonary asbestosis, and reported one case of abdominal cancer, and another with cancer of the pleura, without attributing either to asbestos exposure. Furthermore, on page 18 of this report, they point out that based on the New York Academy of Sciences symposium in New York, the Minister of Social

Security had prescribed on August 22, 1966, that malignant mesothelioma was related to certain occupations involving exposure to asbestos. The report on page 20, suggests that the evidence indirectly suggests that mesothelioma was related to a specific form of asbestos, namely crocidolite. They go on to point out that very few cases had been reported in asbestos workers in Quebec, and none in southern Rhodesia, where chrysotile was mined. It was highlighted that amosite had not been associated with any mesotheliomas in South Africa, its only commercial source of supply. Furthermore, it was pointed out in rats that all forms of asbestos caused mesothelioma in experimental animals. Their conclusion was a restatement of the Working Group on Asbestos and Cancer, published in the proceedings of the New York Academy of Sciences, on the biological effects of asbestos in 1964. They requoted the statement from this group as follows:

In the case of mesotheliomas evidenced from certain countries suggests that exposure to crocidolite may be of particular importance, but it cannot be concluded that only this type of fiber is concerned with these tumors, and further investigations of this problem is needed.

Furthermore, they state,

In the light of present knowledge, we must record our opinion that where asbestos, particularly crocidolite is used, some risk of mesothelioma will have to be accepted. At this time we do not know the level of exposure below which the risk will be negligible. It seems quite possible that those mesotheliomas, which appear to be related to environmental and home exposures were in people who had quite an appreciable dose of asbestos. There is also some evidence relating to past exposures, which supports the view that, if occupational exposures are reduced to the levels indicated in the above paragraph, the risk of developing mesothelioma is greatly reduced. The latent period between first exposure to asbestos and the development of mesothelioma is very long, in some cases up to 30 to 40 years or more.

The conclusions of the advisory panel were on page 23 as follows:

1. There is little evidence of asbestosis occurring apart from in those industries in which asbestos is extensively used.
2. British evidence points to bronchial carcinoma being a complication of asbestosis rather than asbestos exposure. Further work is desirable before this can be proved. There is no British evidence to support American claims of a high incidence of gastrointestinal cancer in asbestos workers, but further investigations are required.
3. There is strong evidence linking asbestos exposure with the development of many mesothelial tumors of the pleura and peritoneum.

4. The evidence suggesting that crocidolite had a special significance in relation to mesothelial tumors is discussed and some conflicting observations are noted. (Report and Recommendations of the Working Group on Asbestos and Cancer. *Br J Ind Med* 1965;22:165–71 and *Ann NY Acad Sci* 1965;132:706–21 (Appendix 2).)

Drs. Selikoff, Churg, and Hammond, produced a paper entitled "Asbestos exposure and neoplasia" in 1964, which pointed out a significant incidence of asbestosis in individuals with heavy asbestos exposure, as well as an increased risk of lung cancer. In 1965, Dr. Hammond, who was the head epidemiologist for the American Cancer Society, stated,

I believe there was hardly anyone a few years ago who would have suspected there was a lung cancer risk in this group of insulation workers. These men were not asbestos weavers nor asbestos miners, and nobody at the time had suggested an increased risk at all for insulation workers. So certainly, in so far as the deaths that occurred in the early part of this study are concerned from 1943 to 1962, before we began to investigate this group of men, I do not think it is a tenable hypothesis that lung cancer was looked for more carefully. (*Ann NY Acad Sci* 1965;132:600.)

Earlier American investigators were uncertain as to what the relationship was between asbestos and lung cancer. Mayer and a group of contributors published in 1963 (The pneumoconioses. *Arch Environ Health* 1963,7:14–55), a statement in which it was stated that "there may be an association between asbestos exposure and lung cancer."

One of the issues, of course, is why American and other Western physicians failed to heed the warnings of German researchers. The German works of Wedler in 1943 on asbestosis and lung cancer, Weiss in 1953 on asbestosis and mesothelioma, and Leischer in 1954 on asbestosis and peritoneal mesothelioma, failed to really provoke much interest in the global community. The Nazis had such an aggressive anti-cancer program that held that the environment was the main source of lung cancer. This question of why American scientists ignored German research cannot be answered simply, but I do want to refer the reader to a relatively short article published by Robert Proctor. (Proctor R. Why did the Nazis have the world's most aggressive anti-cancer campaign. *Endeavor* 1999;23:76–9.) His statements here are related to a larger work that he has authored. (Proctor R. *The Nazi War on Cancer*. Princeton: Princeton University Press, 1999, pp. 111–3.) Part of the root of the Nazi anti-cancer campaign was related to a type of medical moralism, which is perhaps why the world remained asleep and tended to ignore a lot of the information published by these Nazi doctors. Proctor often points out the symbiotic relationship between science and politics.

The Nazi agenda stressed racial hygiene and racial purity. The Nazis viewed tobacco, and any possible environmental carcinogen, as a threat to the purity of the German race. The relationship between tobacco and lip cancer had been suggested as early as the eighteenth century. German physicians in the 1920s became increasingly concerned about the health effects of tobacco, and first published a paper on the statistical relationship between cigarette smoking and lung cancer in 1929. One of the most scholarly indictments on the health effects of cigarette smoking and lung cancer was published in 1935 by Lickint and contained many references. (Lickint F. Der Bronchialkrebs der Raucher. *Munch Med Wochenschr* 1935;2:1232–4.)

The British were not convinced about the health effects of cigarette smoking until the publication of a paper examining the risk of lung cancer in British doctors was published in 1954. (Doll R, Hill AB. The mortality of doctors in relation to their smoking habits: A preliminary report. 1954. Republished in *BMJ* 2004;328(7455):1529–33.) Meanwhile, Americans remained unconvinced until the seminal work of Hammond and others in the early 1960s. (Hammond EC, Horn D. Smoking and death rates: A report of 44 months of follow-up of 187,783 men. II Death rates by cause. *JAMA* 1958;166:1294–368.) The Surgeon General did not warn about the adverse health effects, and lung cancer risk, until 1964. It is quite remarkable how long it took to establish the link between cigarette smoking and lung cancer, when you consider that Peto et al estimated that the long-term risk of lung cancer in those living to 75 years of age to be 16% for men, and 9.5% for women. (Peto R, Darby S, Deo H, Silcocks P, Whitley E, Doll R. Smoking, smoking cessation, and lung cancer in the UK since 1950: Combination of national statistics with two case-control studies. *BMJ* 2000;321(7270):1225.)

There are always those who will argue that we should have known about the risk of cancer associated with asbestosis, based on the Nazi work about these adverse health effects of asbestos. I think all experts will agree that, while the basic assumptions that were made were correct, there was not enough scientific evidence, based on the way we evaluate scientific evidence today, to draw the conclusions they made at that time. The mere association of two independent variables such as asbestosis and lung cancer is not sufficient evidence for scientific proof of causality. Case reports suggest a possible association between two variables, but are not scientific evidence of a cause-and-effect relationship, such as the reports by Wagner in 1960 of mesotheliomas in South Africa. No population-based epidemiological studies of the correlation between end users of asbestos, and risk of mesothelioma, were performed until 1965, with the first scientific epidemiologic study by Selikoff, Churg, and Hammond, published in the *New England Journal of Medicine,* of ten cases of mesothelioma found in 307 insulators. (Selikoff IJ, Churg J, Hammond EC. Relation between exposure to asbestos and mesothelioma *N Engl J Med* 1965;272:560–5.)

Commenting on exposure levels and disease, Dr. Selikoff states,

> Thus, amongst the insulation workers in New York, I have yet to see a mesothelioma in a man who began work after 1930 or a case of lung cancer in an asbestos worker who had worked in that industry less than 20 years. Our concern is with the future. (Selikoff IJ. Asbestos. *Environment* 1969;11:3–7.)

In a letter to the editor of the *Journal of the American Medical Association* on March 25, 1968, Drs. de Treville, Gross, and Davis wrote

This asbestos scare has ignored some of the facts on mesotheliomas not all of which can be taken at face value. First, asbestos is not a single mineral. Wagner's mesothelioma cases were associated with crocidolite areas and not with amosite or chrysotile. In other countries attempts to demonstrate that exposure to dust other than crocidolite could produce mesotheliomas have so far been almost completely unsuccessful. The mesothelioma problem is, therefore, not one that involves the whole asbestos industry, but only users of crocidolite, and this mineral represents a relatively small proportion of total consumption.

In 1969, Dr. George W Wright, a very well-qualified expert on the health effects of asbestos, presented a review of the health effects on asbestos. This was published in the same year in the *American Review of Respiratory Disease*. (Wright GW. Asbestos and health in 1969. *Am Rev Respir Dis* 1969;100(4):467–79.) Dr. Wright was very cautious in his comments on mesothelioma, pointing out

There is a lively controversy amongst pathologists regarding the requirements for establishing the diagnosis of primary mesothelioma. Not only is there a question with respect to the histologic criteria, but even more important the necessity for establishing by autopsy whether the tumor is primary or secondary. It is apparent that the overwhelming number of cases thus far being related to asbestos are diagnosed on the basis of biopsy alone. Further study will be needed to demonstrate whether the mesothelioma is being over or under diagnosed.

Dr. Wright went on to comment further and pointed out

The contention that crocidolite *per se* causes mesothelioma becomes difficult to accept. Sluis-Cremmer pointed out this paradox in 1964. Webster in his current report on asbestos exposures in South Africa likewise calls attention to this disparity. It is of equal interest that only three cases of mesothelioma have been reported as originating from the Transvaal, these being from the amosite asbestos mines.

He goes on to say that "something other than or in addition to asbestos plays a role in mesothelioma formation seems inescapable." He further goes on to state,

If one postulates there are respirable fibers of asbestos in ambient air breathed by the general public, the strikingly rare occurrence of mesothelioma not related to occupation strongly suggests there is a tolerable level of airborne asbestos fiber which does not cause an undue risk of development of mesothelioma. The findings of Newhouse and McDonald and associates, which indicate that genuine occupational exposures to asbestos has been tolerated without evidence of an increased risk of developing a mesothelioma, suggests that the tolerable level is substantial. The evidence strongly favors the concept that the causal relationship of the general public has not exceeded such a level in the past. (Wright GW. Asbestos and health in 1969. *Am Rev Respir Dis* 1969;100(4):467–79.)

The general medical community had believed that if asbestosis could be avoided by reducing exposure to friable asbestos, then asbestos-related malignancy would also be avoided. The early mesothelioma cases were generally heavily exposed in the early 1900s prior to the promulgation of dust control measures. Selikoff mentions in 1969, "I have yet to see a mesothelioma in a man who began work after 1930 or a case of lung cancer in an asbestos worker who had worked in that industry less than twenty years." (Selikoff IJ. Asbestos. *Environment* 1969;11:3–7.)

However, the data of Wagner, Newhouse, and Thompson, and Lieben and others challenged this paradigm. Thompson reported in 1963 asbestos bodies in the lungs of people who were not asbestos workers and called it a modern urban hazard. (Thomson JG. Exposure to asbestos dust and diffuse pleural mesotheliomas. *Br Med J* 1963;1:123; Thomson JG, Kaschula O, MacDonald RR. Asbestos as a modern urban hazard. *S Afr Med J* 1963;37:77–81.) In 1968, Utidjian, Gross, and de Treville reported that almost 100% of urban dwellers had asbestos bodies in their lungs. (Utidjian MD, Gross P, de Treville R. Ferruginous bodies in human lungs. *Arch Environ Health* 1968;17:327.)

By 1970, Thompson's original observations were widely confirmed in Montreal, Milan, London, Newcastle, Glasgow, Belfast, Dresden, Pittsburgh, Miami, and New York. (Selikoff IJ. Asbestos. *Environment* 1969;11:3–7.) A paradigm shift had occurred; by 1970, it was generally accepted that low-level exposure to Northwest Cape Blue crocidolite was capable of causing mesothelioma. The question remained as to how much exposure was too much. The next 30 years would be focused on the role of other types of commercial asbestos and noncommercial asbestiform materials. By 1969, Wagner and Berry had perfected an animal model that would help answer many of these questions. (Wagner JC, Berry G. Mesotheliomas in rats following inoculation with asbestos. *Br J Cancer* 1969;23:567–81.)

The acceptance of new ideas moved slowly. In 1988, Selikoff and coworkers opined, "Nevertheless, only during the past 25 years (i.e., 1963) has malignant mesothelioma been widely accepted as an independent diagnostic entity." (Ribak J, Lilis R, Suzuki Y, Penner L, Selikoff IJ. Malignant mesothelioma in a cohort of asbestos insulation workers: Clinical presentation, diagnosis, and causes of death. *Br J Ind Med* 1988;45:182–7.)

It seems ironic that 100 years earlier in 1870, the distinct pathological entity of pleural mesothelioma was postulated by one Wagner and then, 100 years later, greatly advanced by another physician named Wagner whose contributions have propelled science into the next millennium.

Ian Webster, who was JC Wagner's brother-in-law, still felt that there were unsolved problems in the relationship between asbestos and malignancy in a paper he published in February 1973 in the *South African Medical Journal*. (Webster I. Asbestos and malignancy. *S Afr Med J* 1973;47:165–71.) Dr. Webster remained skeptical as to why this previously rare tumor only seemed to be found primarily in direct relationship to crocidolite exposure. He stated, "Furthermore it is difficult to conceive of amosite in the intermediate group of asbestos fibers causing malignancy, as suggested by Wagner et al. when there are so few cases in the employees of the amosite mines." He went on to say

> The production of amosite far exceeded that of Cape Blue asbestos. It is suggested that more attention should be paid to the determination of the nature of the substance of the Cape Blue areas and not in the Transvaal Blue, and apparently limited to the areas where amosite is mined.

Dr. JS Harington wrote a chapter on mesothelioma in the book *The Prevention of Cancer* by Raven and Rowe in 1967. He states that "the results of animal experimentation so far available suggests that crocidolite and chrysotile may be more active in inducing mesotheliomas than amosite" (Harrington and Rowe, 1965). If the present trend is confirmed, substitution in mining and industry of amosite (e.g., for the more dangerous types of asbestos when they cannot be safely used) may be a practical and important preventive measure.

In an unsigned editorial in *The Lancet* published on March 5, 1966, the author stated,

> A possible important clue to prevention was just uncovered by Wagner in South Africa, where after showing association between mesothelial tumors and exposure to crocidolite form of asbestos, he and his colleagues were unable to find any tumors in those exposed only to the amosite or chrysotile-types of fiber. The position in South Africa remains the same, despite continuing intensive search in the amosite and chrysotile mining areas.

The author goes on to say

> Mesothelioma tumors have been seen in a few individuals apparently exposed only to chrysotile in the United States and Canada, and other populations either industrial or residential exposed only to one type of fiber must now be investigated. This can be achieved only by international cooperation, because such exposures are almost entirely limited to those engaged in mining and milling of the fiber, which is done in the countries where the different types of asbestos are found.

Selikoff, Hammond, and Churg reviewed the results of a study of an asbestos insulation manufacturing plant in Paterson, New Jersey, and published their results in the *Archives of Environmental Health* in September 1972. (Selikoff I, Hammond E, Churg J. Carcinogenicity of amosite asbestos. *Arch Environ Health* 1972;25:183–6.) In this paper, they pointed out that "few data exist concerning the comparative neoplastic potential in man of the several kinds of asbestos, and particularly there has been no evidence concerning whether amosite variety is carcinogenic." In 1972, they went on to say

Whether or not amosite is carcinogenic is of some practical importance. Because this variety of asbestos has not been reported to cause cancer, there has been a tendency in Great Britain for example to substitute it for other types of asbestos, especially crocidolite.

Dr. Selikoff and coworkers went on to report an increased incidence of lung cancer and mesothelioma in this plant because it was thought to be just pure exposure to amosite asbestos.

While it was generally accepted in the United States that pure amosite caused a high incidence of mesotheliomas and lung cancers, the paper by Selikoff and coworkers was not well accepted abroad. McCullagh published a paper in the *Journal of Society of Occupational Medicine* in 1980 on "Amosite as a cause of lung cancer and mesothelioma in humans." (McCullagh S. Amosite as a cause of lung cancer and mesothelioma in humans. *J Soc Occup Med* 1980;30:153–6.) He pointed out that many of the Paterson, New Jersey, cohorts studied by Selikoff had previous exposure to asbestos. He felt that rather than 1/50th of the group, it seemed more likely that one-third of the group or 300 members of the Paterson cohort had been occupationally exposed to asbestos before entering the cohort. This is of import since crocidolite was being used in large quantities in asbestos factories in the same area. Dr. Selikoff had felt that very little crocidolite had been used in the shipyards and in the United States, and therefore if a mesothelioma developed, it was most likely related to amosite since, there was very little crocidolite exposure. In fact, the monthly trade journal *Asbestos* mentions the use of crocidolite and amosite asbestos in July 1919.

Drs. John Harington and Neil McGlashan reviewed the destination of South African exports of crocidolite and amosite asbestos as well as chrysotile from 1959 until 1993, and the studies indicate that the United States received considerable amounts of crocidolite asbestos right up until 1992. This study and others have suggested there was actually more crocidolite asbestos used in the United States than had been previously recognized, and that the use of crocidolite asbestos is a major reason as to why there was an increased risk of mesothelioma. (Harington JS, McGlashan ND. South African asbestos: Production, exports, and destinations, 1959–1993. *Am J Ind Med* 1998;33:321–6.)

The issue of any other fiber other than crocidolite as a cause of mesothelioma remained controversial, and in February 1973, Ian Webster published an article in the *South African Medical Journal* entitled "Asbestos and malignancy."

He looked at exposure to asbestos and the association with 232 cases of pleural mesothelioma. Almost all of the individuals had been exposed to Cape Blue asbestos and only two miners had been exposed to amosite as far as could be discerned. Thirty-two cases occurred in which there was no evidence of any asbestos exposure, presumably having environmental exposure. Therefore, there were only two cases related to exposure to amosite out of 232 confirmed cases of mesotheliomas.

Dr. JC Wagner recapitulated his overview of the association between blue asbestos and mesotheliomas in 1991. (Wagner J. The discovery of the association between blue asbestos and mesotheliomas and the aftermath. *Br J Ind Med* 1991;48:399–403.) Wagner reviewed his story of the discovery of the association between asbestos and mesothelioma, and concluded that there was evidence that all types of commercial asbestos except anthophyllite may be responsible for a mesothelioma. He went on to state, "The risk is greatest with crocidolite, less with amosite, and apparently less with chrysotile. With both amosite and chrysotile there appears to be a higher risk in the manufacturing than in mining and milling." He further stated, "There is overwhelming evidence that crocidolite is a main fiber associated with mesotheliomas." This has primarily been the British view, and Raymond Parkes, in the second edition of his classic book *Occupational Lung Disorders* (1982), stated, "Crocidolite is apparently the type of asbestos, which is overwhelmingly if not exclusively causally related to mesotheliomas in man."

The most recent article relating to the historical crocidolite exposure issue in the United States was "Asbestos in the lungs of persons exposed in the USA" (Langer and Nolan, *Monaldi Archives of Chest Disease,* 1998). In their appendix of crocidolite consumption in the United States, they pointed out that blue asbestos for boiler and steam coverings for locomotives were advertised in trade journals, such as *The Engine,* as early as 1897. The data from the U.S. Department of Commerce reveal significant crocidolite importation in the 1920s and 1930s, and this included the spraying of crocidolite in the form of Limpet up until 1966. The paper goes on to mention that all three major fiber types were permanently used on ships and crocidolite was extensively applied among warships in the United Kingdom. Some international investigators outside the United States have interpreted this to mean that crocidolite was also used aboard American ships, and if mesotheliomas occurred amongst American insulation workers who worked in military shipyards, this would be indirect evidence of crocidolite exposure. They went on to state, "Still other investigators suggested that British ships were re-outfitted in U.S.A. ports during the war, and they have been the source of crocidolite exposure to American shipyard workers. This most certainly occurred and citations in the literature support this."

Dr. Selikoff in hindsight also reviewed the literature on mesothelioma and states,

During the 1950s there were several reports of deaths in asbestos workers caused by these diffuse tumors of the mesothelial surfaces. These isolated cases would have received little notice had it not been for the fact that the tumor has always been considered extraordinarily rare. It is no longer rare amongst asbestos workers. Indeed, it is so common a cause of death amongst them now. While still rare amongst individuals not known to be exposed to asbestos—it almost constituted tumor specific to asbestos exposure.

Furthermore, writing in 1988, Dr. Selikoff and coworkers state, "Nevertheless only in the past 25 years has malignant mesothelioma been widely accepted as an independent diagnostic entity." These workers found 175 deaths from mesothelioma occurred among 2221 men who died between 1967 and 1976 and 181 more deaths in the next 8 years for a total of 356 deaths from mesothelioma out a total of 3500 deaths from all causes by 1984 (134 of these were pleural and 222 were peritoneal mesotheliomas). (Ribak J, Lilis R, Suzuki Y, Penner L, Selikoff IJ. Malignant mesothelioma in a cohort of asbestos insulation workers: Clinical presentation, diagnosis, and causes of death. *Br J Ind Med* 1988;45:182–7.)

The history of the early years of mesothelioma discovery is an example of how slowly the medical community accepts new discoveries. Acceptance was in part retarded by the lack of specific mesothelial cell markers such as are available today, and experts disagreed among themselves as to the proper diagnosis. As the frequency of these tumors increased, pathologists made the diagnosis with more confidence, and as noted by Selikoff, there was not only general acceptance of the criteria for diagnosis, but also a clear association with asbestos exposure by 1973. Early studies showed poor pathologic diagnostic accuracy. Iwatsubo and colleagues noted that in different studies the true incidence of pathologically confirmed diagnoses varied from 26% to 96%. (Iwatsubo Y, Pairon JC, Archambault de Beaune C, Chamming's S, Bignon J, Brochard P. Pleural mesothelioma: A descriptive analysis based on a case–control study and mortality data in Ile de France, 1987–1990. *Am J Ind Med* 1994;26:77–88.) During 1967–1968, there were 413 cases of mesothelioma reported in the United Kingdom based on their national register. After careful review, 246 cases were accepted as definite mesotheliomas. (Greenberg M, Davies TA. Mesothelioma register 1967–68. *Br J Ind Med* 1974;31(2):91–104.)

The misdiagnosis rate has remained at about 20% in more recent studies. (Cambridge DR, Stockton DL, Bain M. Factors affecting the mesothelioma detection rate within national and international epidemiologic studies: Insights from Scottish Linked Cancer Registry—Mortality data. *Br J Cancer* 2006;95:649–52.) In a 1991 report of the United States and Canadian Mesothelioma Panel, only 70.5% of 200 cases had a three-quarter majority agreement for the diagnosis of mesothelioma from this panel of North American experts (Cagle PT, Churg A. Differential diagnosis of benign and malignant mesothelial proliferations on pleural biopsies. *Arch Pathol Lab Med* 2005;129:1421–7) and agreement between benign versus malignant was 78% for a group of 217 cases. Some cancers metastasize to the pleura from other sites and appear to be mesotheliomas but are actually pseudomesotheliomas, further confusing the pathologic certainty of the diagnoses. (Dodson RF, Hammar SP. Analysis of asbestos concentration in 20 cases of pseudomesotheliomatous lung cancer. *Ultrastruct*

Pathol 2015;39(1):13–22.) Kerger and colleagues have suggested guidelines for starting a genetics-based tumor registry for tumors that mimic asbestos-related mesotheliomas. (Kerger BD, James RC, Galbraith DA. Tumors that mimic asbestos-related mesothelioma: Time to consider a genetics-based tumor registry? *Front Genet* 2014;5:151.)

The most recent guidelines for the pathologic diagnosis of mesothelioma were published as a consensus statement of the International Mesothelioma Interest Group (*Arch Pathol Lab Med* 2012) and discuss the pitfalls in the diagnosis of malignant mesothelioma, including

1. Lack of experience of the laboratory.
2. Lack of standardization of immunohistochemical procedures.
3. Problems caused by small-needle biopsies resulting in false-positive immunostaining.
4. Variation as to what is positive calretinin staining—nuclear versus cytoplasmic.
5. Putting too much emphasis on weak or focal staining.
6. False invasion of surrounding structures.
7. Failure to understand that none of the immunohistochemical marker stains are 100% specific.
8. The diagnosis is based on clinical, radiologic, and ultimately pathologic features. The issue of asbestos exposure is irrelevant.

DW Henderson and coworkers from South Australia have also been concerned about the diagnosis of mesothelioma by cytology alone: "The detection of neoplastic invasion remains the linchpin for a clear diagnosis of malignant mesothelioma. Cytology-only diagnosis of epithelioid mesothelioma on aspirated effusion fluid remains controversial." Cytology, according to the authors, has poor sensitivity and specificity. (Henderson DW, Reid G, Kao SC, van Zandwijk N, Klebe S. Challenges and controversies in the diagnosis of mesothelioma: Part 1. Cytology-only diagnosis, biopsies, immunohistochemistry, discrimination between mesothelioma and reactive mesothelial hyperplasia, and biomarkers. *J Clin Pathol* 2013;66(10):847–53; Henderson DW, Reid G, Kao SC, van Zandwijk N, Klebe S. Challenges and controversies in the diagnosis of malignant mesothelioma: Part 2. Malignant mesothelioma subtypes, pleural synovial sarcoma, molecular and prognostic aspects of mesothelioma, BAP1, aquaporin-1 and micro RNA. *J Clin Pathol* 2013;66(10):854–61.)

The advent of a large battery of immunochemical markers has provided better tools for the diagnosis of mesothelioma; however, immunostaining can often be misleading or inconsistent, as mentioned by Henderson. A report by Oczypok and Oury highlights the lasting utility of electron microscopy in the diagnosis of mesothelioma. (Oczypok EA, Oury TD. Electron microscopy remains the gold standard for the diagnosis of epithelial malignant mesothelioma: A case study. *Ultrastruct Pathol* 2015:39(2):153–7.)

One of the great mysteries in understanding mesothelioma carcinogenesis has been the lack of association between cigarette smoking and mesothelioma across multiple epidemiologic studies. Cigarette smoking slows cilia function and fiber removal by the mucociliary blanket. This increases fiber retention by at least twofold, yet has not been associated with any increased risk of mesothelioma. Cigarette smoking decreases life expectancy by about 7 years due to increased risk of lung cancer, cardiovascular disease, and other disorders. This means that there is a population of smokers who would normally develop a mesothelioma later in life, but die prematurely prior to the discovery of a mesothelioma, due to its very long latency. (Berry G, Newhouse ML, Antonis P. Combined effect of asbestos and smoking on mortality from lung cancer and mesothelioma in factory worker. *Br J Ind Med* 1985;42(1):12–8; Muscat JE, Wynder EL. Cigarette smoking, asbestos exposure, and malignant mesothelioma. *Cancer Res* 1991;51(9):2263–7; Tagnon I, Blot WJ, Stroube RB et al. Mesothelioma associated with the shipbuilding industry in coastal Virginia. *Cancer Res* 1980;40(11):3875–9.)

Mesothelioma treatment

A malignant mesothelioma is an aggressive tumor, which in the past had an average life expectancy of 13–15 months. Mesotheliomas are classified into three main groups as epithelial, biphasic, and sarcomatoid tumors. The life expectancy averages about 18 months for epithelial, 11 months for biphasic, and 8 months for sarcomatoid tumors. Approximately 70% of mesotheliomas are epithelial. Several recent studies have been performed to evaluate new treatment strategies and their effects on prognosis. New patients with pleural mesotheliomas are staged with a variety of imaging techniques that may include lymph node sampling, and they are then separated into four groups: no treatment, chemotherapy alone, EPP with the removal of the entire lung, diaphragm, and pericardium, or pleural decortication (PD). PD is a less invasive lung-sparing surgery since it removes only the parietal/visceral pleura. In comparison with EPP, PD is associated with less perioperative mortality/morbidity and less postoperative deterioration of cardiopulmonary function. These surgical procedures are usually followed by or preceded by radiation and chemotherapy. Survival with early-stage treatment is higher with PD then EPP, but for late-stage disease, survival is better with EPP in some studies, but is associated with a higher operative and perioperative mortality. This may simply reflect differences in patient selection bias (i.e., those patients with the best survival chances get the most aggressive surgery). The Society of Thoracic Surgeons reviewed the data on 225 surgical cases and found that EPP was associated with greater morbidity and mortality with an odds ratio of 6.51 compared with PD when performed by participating surgeons of the Society of Thoracic Surgery. (Burt BM, Cameron RB, Mollberg NM et al. Malignant pleural mesothelioma and the Society of Thoracic Surgeons Database: An analysis of surgical morbidity and mortality. *J Thorac Cardiovasc Surg* 2014;48(1):30–5; Spaggiari L, Marulli G, Bovolato P et al. Extrapleural pneumonectomy for malignant mesothelioma: An Italian multicenter retrospective study. *Ann Thorac Surg* 2014;97(6):1859–65; Becklake MR, Bagatin E, Neder JA. Asbestos-related diseases of the lungs and pleura: Uses, trends and management over the last century. *Int J Tuberc Lung Dis* 2007;11(4):356–69; Taioli E, Wolf AS, Flores RM. Meta-analysis of survival after pleurectomy decortication versus extrapleural pneumonectomy in mesothelioma. *Ann Thorac Surg* 2015;99(2):472–80.)

Appropriate surgical management has been questioned by others outside of the United States, since radical surgery is currently abandoned in many centers in Europe, whereas debulking or cyto-reduction surgery has been proposed within a multimodality approach that also includes adjuvant chemotherapy and radiotherapy in the United States. A large European study of 1365 patients concluded that patients with good prognostic factors had a similar survival whether they received medical therapy only, PD, or EPP. The modest benefit observed after surgery during medical treatment will require further investigation, and a large, multicenter randomized trial, testing PD after induction chemotherapy versus chemotherapy alone in malignant pleural mesothelioma (MPM) patients with good prognostic factors, is needed. (Bovolato P, Casadio C, Billè A et al. Does surgery improve survival of patients with malignant pleural mesothelioma? A multicenter retrospective analysis of 1365 consecutive patients. *J Thorac Oncol* 2014;9(3):390–6.)

There still is a need for more prospective trials. Pemetrexed and cisplatin-based chemotherapy remains the reference treatment, which has proved to have some efficacy on overall survival in mesothelioma in randomized trials, with a 13 to 15-month median overall survival. (Campbell K, Brosseau S, Reviron-Rabec L et al. Malignant pleural mesothelioma: 2013 state of the art. *Bull Cancer* 2013;100(12):1283–93; Cao C, Tian D, Park J et al. A systematic review and meta-analysis of surgical treatments for malignant pleural mesothelioma. *Lung Cancer* 2014;83(2):240–5; van Zandwijk N. Clinical practice guidelines for malignant pleural mesothelioma. *J Thorac Dis* 2013;5(6):724–5; Treasure T, Dusmet M, Fiorentino F et al. Surgery for malignant pleural mesothelioma: Why we need controlled trials. *Eur J Cardiothorac Surg* 2014;45(4):591–2; Flores RM, Pass HI, Seshan VE et al. Extrapleural pneumonectomy versus pleurectomy/decortication in the surgical management of malignant pleural mesothelioma: Results in 663 patients. *J Thorac Cardiovasc Surg* 2008;135(3):620–6; Papaspyros S, Papaspyros S. Surgical management of malignant pleural mesothelioma: Impact of surgery on survival and quality of life-relation to chemotherapy, radiotherapy, and alternative therapies. *ISRN Surg* 2014;2014:817203; Hasegawa S. Extrapleural pneumonectomy or pleurectomy/decortication for malignant pleural mesothelioma. *Gen Thorac Cardiovasc Surg* 2014;62(9):516–21.)

Patients with an epithelial histology survive longer than patients with a sarcomatous or mixed histology. Women survive longer than men, which is thought to be related to the effects of estrogen on tumor biology. Patients with no history of smoking or asbestos exposure, women under 50 years of age, and patients with left-sided tumors have longer survival, which now approaches 30–35 months if surgical removal of the macroscopic tumor is successful. Survival is 13 months if macroscopic tumor removal is unsuccessful. Women with pleural mesotheliomas have an average survival that is three times greater than men for unknown reasons. Patents over the age of 75 years have a worse prognosis. Nonepithelioid histology, age >75 years, advanced International Mesothelioma Interest Group stage, and presence of comorbidities according to the Charleston Comorbidity Index were significant prognostic factors in elderly patients with malignant pleural mesothelioma. Median survival was 11.4 months. Treatment with pemetrexed-based chemotherapy was feasible in this setting, but comorbidities became increasingly important in this age group. (Ceresoli GL, Grosso F, Zucali PA et al. Prognostic factors in elderly patients with malignant pleural mesothelioma: Results of a multicenter survey. *Br J Cancer* 2014;111(2):220–6; Lim JY, Wolf AS, Flores RM. The use of surgery in mesothelioma. *Lancet Respir Med* 2013;1:184–6.) A good general review of mesothelioma management was published in the *Journal of Thoracic Diseases* from Greece. (Porpodis K, Zarogoulidis P, Boutsikou E et al. Malignant pleural mesothelioma: Current and future perspectives. *J Thorac Dis* 2013;5(Suppl. 4):S397–406; Taioli E, Wolf AS, Camacho-Rivera M, Flores RM. Women with malignant pleural mesothelioma have a threefold better survival rate than men. *Ann Thorac Surg* 2014;98(3):1020–4.)

Patients with advanced disease who are not surgical candidates can be treated with a talc pleurodesis. A British group undertook an open-label, parallel-group, randomized controlled trial with any subtype of confirmed or suspected mesothelioma with pleural effusion recruited from 12 hospitals in the United Kingdon. Eligible patients were randomly assigned (1:1) to either video-assisted thoracoscopic partial pleurectomy (VAT-PP) or talc pleurodesis. Overall survival at 1 year was 52% (95% CI: 41–62) in the VAT-PP group and 57% (95% CI: 46–66) in the talc pleurodesis group. The authors concluded that VAT-PP is not recommended for improving overall survival in patients with pleural effusion due to malignant pleural mesothelioma, and talc pleurodesis might be preferable considering the fewer complications and shorter hospital stay associated with this treatment. (Rintoul RC, Ritchie AJ, Edwards JG et al. Efficacy and cost of video-assisted thoracoscopic partial pleurectomy versus talc pleurodesis in patients with malignant pleural mesothelioma (MesoVATS): An open-label, randomised, controlled trial. *Lancet* 2014;384:1118–27.)

The fiber burden in peritoneal mesotheliomas related to asbestos exposure is generally much higher than that in pleural mesotheliomas. Low fiber counts suggest spontaneous peritoneal mesotheliomas (Figure 12.1). (Roggli VL, Oury TD, Sporn TA. *Pathology of Asbestos-Associated Diseases*, 2nd Edition. New York: Springer-Verlag, 2004.)

Advances have been made in the treatment of peritoneal mesotheliomas, namely intraperitoneal chemotherapy, cytoreductive surgery, and hyperthermic intraperitoneal chemotherapy. Intraperitoneal chemotherapy, involving the administration of certain chemotherapeutic agents directly to the intraperitoneal cavity, was developed as a novel therapeutic strategy early in the 1950s. Intraperitoneal administration of chemotherapy results in higher intraperitoneal concentrations of the cytotoxic medications, particularly when heated, resulting in minimal systemic exposure compared with intravenous administration, which in turn may increase the efficacy of these agents with a substantial reduction in systemic toxicity. Intraperitoneal chemotherapy was used successfully in peritoneal surface malignancies, including malignant peritoneal mesothelioma, pseudomyxoma peritonei, malignant ascites, sarcomatosis, and peritoneal carcinomatosis from gastrointestinal and ovarian cancers. The advent

---

Peritoneal mesothelioma is not the same disease as pleural mesothelioma-II

Fiber burden data from Roggli 2004 (as medians)

- Pleural mesothelioma
  - With asbestosis: 14,900 bodies/77,800 uncoated fibers
  - With plaques: 900 bodies/24,900 uncoated fibers
- Peritoneal mesothelioma
  - With asbestosis: 140,000 bodies/380,000 uncoated fibers
  - With plaques: 1450 bodies/122,000 uncoated fibers
- Asbestosis alone (n = 170 cases)
  - Asbestos bodies: 17,100 uncoated fibers: 152,000

Figure 12.1   Peritoneal mesotheliomas require much higher exposures than pleural mesothelioma or asbestosis. (With kind permission from Springer Science+Business Media: *Pathology of Asbestos-Associated Diseases*, 2004, Roggli VL, Oury TD, Sporn TA, New York: Springer-Verlag.)

of cytoreduction with hyperthermic intraperitoneal chemotherapy has dramatically improved survival outcomes, with wide median survival estimates of between 2.5 and 9 years. (Elias D, Goéré D, Dumont F et al. Role of hyperthermic intraoperative peritoneal chemotherapy in the management of peritoneal metastases. *Eur J Cancer* 2014;50(2):332–40; Raza A, Huang WC, Takabe K. Advances in the management of peritoneal mesothelioma. *World J Gastroenterol* 2014;20(33):11700–12.)

The results of the treatment of mesotheliomas have generally been poor. Great efforts have been made to make an early diagnosis with the hope that early treatment will extend life expectancy. A variety of serum markers have been used for diagnostic and prognostic purposes, but not enough information is available to recommend their use routinely. (Tabata C, Shibata E, Tabata R et al. Serum HMGB1 as a prognostic marker for malignant pleural mesothelioma. *BMC Cancer* 2013;13:205; Hollevoet K, Reitsma JB, Creaney J et al. Serum mesothelin for diagnosing malignant pleural mesothelioma: An individual patient data meta-analysis. *J Clin Oncol* 2012;30(13):1541–9; Creaney J, Sneddon S, Dick IM et al. Comparison of the diagnostic accuracy of the MSLN gene products, mesothelin and megakaryocyte potentiating factor, as biomarkers for mesothelioma in pleural effusions and serum. *Dis Markers* 2013;35(2):119–27.)

13

The many causes of mesothelioma

Mesothelioma causation is related to a variety of causes, but the most common cause is mineral fibers, of which asbestos is the most common fibrous mineral known to cause mesothelioma. Despite asbestos being identified as the single most important cause of malignant mesothelioma, the tumor is known to occur in only 10%–20% of heavily exposed individuals. In a Canadian series, 25% of cases in Ontario had exposure in their country of origin. (Finkelstein MM. Mortality among employees of an Ontario asbestos cement factory. *Am Rev Respir Dis* 1984;129:754–61.) In addition, about 20%–80%+ of the patients in different published series, have no history of asbestos exposure, even after detailed assessment. Fiber burden studies have provided further evidence that some mesotheliomas are not associated with asbestos. Mesotheliomas in children occur with such a short latency that the evidence suggests that these mesotheliomas in children are genetic in origin. (Jasani B, Gibbs A. Mesothelioma not associated with asbestos exposure. *Arch Pathol Lab Med* 2012;136(3):262–7.)

The molecular pathogenesis of malignant mesothelioma has not been entirely defined. Unlike most carcinomas, malignant mesothelioma is not associated with a mutation in the gene encoding tumor-suppressor P53. Chromosomal deletions are common but no specific pattern has been observed. Abnormalities in the apoptosis- pathway genes *BCL2* and *BAX* and in the tumor-suppressor gene *NF2* have been described. (Fennel DA. Genetics and molecular biology of mesothelioma. In: A Tannaphel (Ed.), *Malignant Mesothelioma*. Berlin: Springer-Verlag, 2011, pp. 149–67.)

Some authors have emphasized that pleural hyaline plaques, or even parenchymal asbestosis, must be present in order to consider asbestos to be a cause of malignant mesothelioma. However, the pathogenesis of pleural plaques and asbestosis is entirely different from the pathogenesis of mesothelioma; any association of pleural plaques and parenchymal asbestosis with mesothelioma is variable in the literature. Pleural plaques and asbestosis are signatures of asbestos exposure, but are not necessary to prove causation. (Kradin RL. A man chest pain and a pleural effusion. Case records of the Massachusetts General Hospital. *N Engl J Med*

2014;370:2132.) Other investigators have focused on T-cell activity. T-cells play an important role in anti-tumor immunity, and Japanese investigators have demonstrated that malignant mesothelioma patients have characteristics of impairment in stimulation-induced cytotoxicity of peripheral blood CD8$^+$ lymphocytes, and that pleural plaque and malignant mesothelioma patients have a common character of functional alteration in those lymphocytes, namely an increase in memory cells, possibly related to exposure to asbestos. (Kumagai-Takei N, Nishimura Y, Maeda M et al. Functional properties of CD8$^+$ lymphocytes in patients with pleural plaque and malignant mesothelioma. *J Immunol Res* 2014;2014:670140.)

Therefore, there has been speculation for some time that asbestos alone may not be sufficient to cause mesothelioma, and that other factors may be involved either as cocarcinogens, or as independent mechanisms of cancer causation. The predominant cause of mesothelioma is largely confined to amphibole asbestos. (Hodgson and Darnton 2000; Berman DW, Crump KS. A meta-analysis of asbestos-related cancer risk that addresses fiber size and mineral type. *Crit Rev Toxicol* 2008;38(Suppl. 1):49–73; Berman DW, Crump KS. Update of potency factors for asbestos-related lung cancer and mesothelioma. *Crit Rev Toxicol* 2008;38(Suppl. 1):1–47; McDonald JC. Epidemiology of malignant mesothelioma—An outline. *Ann Occup Hyg* 2010;54:851–7.) While amphibole asbestos is the most important cause of mesothelioma, genetic factors have become increasingly important. (Kalogeraki A, Tamiolakis DJ, Lagoudaki ED et al. Familial mesothelioma in first degree relatives. *Diagn Cytopathol* 2013;41(7):654–7.)

Fiber research has focused on chemical composition, charge or release of free electrons, crystalline structure, fiber shape and dimension, and fiber length, as well as fiber bio-persistence. A series of epidemiologic studies from North and South Carolina textile plants that used predominately chrysotile asbestos, has demonstrated that long, thin fibers are the predominant cause of asbestos-related lung cancer. The thin (<0.25 μm) and long fibers (Stanton fibers) are not visible by standard phase-contrast microscopy (PCM), which raises serious questions about correlations made by standard fiber counting techniques and epidemiologic studies about asbestos fiber counting and lung cancer. (Elliott L, Loomis D, Dement J et al. Lung cancer mortality in North Carolina and South Carolina chrysotile asbestos textile workers. *Occup Environ Med* 2012;69:385–90.)

PCM has several limitations in counting long, thin fibers, as well as the inability to count very thin fibers, including the inability to distinguish fiber type. More recently, suggestions have been made for counting rules for estimating long asbestos fibers. (Crump KS, Berman DW. Counting rules for estimating concentrations of long asbestos fibers. *Ann Occup Hyg* 2011;55:723–35.)

KNOWN NATURALLY OCCURRING MESOTHELIOGENIC MINERAL FIBERS

1. Amosite asbestos
2. Crocidolite asbestos
3. Tremolite asbestos

4. Anthophyllite asbestos
5. Actinolite asbestos
6. Winchite/richterite (contaminants of Libby, Montana, vermiculite)
7. Balangeroite
8. Fluoro-edenite
9. Erionite
10. Ophiolites
11. Antigorite
12. Swift Creek Sumas Mountain fiber, Whatcom County, Washington
13. Silicate-contaminated sugar cane
14. Taconite mining

Other noncommercial fibrous silicates, not considered to be asbestos or regulated, including winchite, richterite, actinolite, erionite, and low-level tremolite (contaminants of vermiculite from Libby, Montana), have been associated with mesothelioma pathogenesis. (Dunning KK, Adjei S, Levin L et al. Mesothelioma associated with commercial use of vermiculite containing Libby amphibole. *J Occup Environ Med* 2012;54(11):1359–63; Anato VC, Larson TC, Horton DK. Libby vermiculite exposure and risk of developing asbestos-related lung and pleural diseases. *Curr Opin Pulm Med* 2012;18:161–7.)

The Libby vermiculite revelation of new types of hazardous amphiboles, has awakened the medical community concerning environmental, nonoccupational amphibole asbestiform mineral exposure, as a cause of mesothelioma. (Goldberg. Health effects of non-occupational exposure to asbestos. *Asbestos Health Conference*. Environmental Protection Agency (EPA) May 2001, www.epa.gov/swerrims/ahec/)

Balangeroite, a newly implicated iron-rich asbestiform fiber, has been implicated in Italy as a cause of mesothelioma. (Turci F, Tomatis M, Comagnoni R, Fubini B. Role of associated mineral fibers in chrysotile asbestos health effects: The case of balangeroite. *Ann Occup Hyg* 2009;53:491–7.) It is a fibrous magnesium–iron silicate, consisting of brown, rigid, and brittle xyloid fibers, with a complex structure similar to gageite, and usually inter-grown with chrysotile. It is very similar to other amphiboles morphologically and has bio-durability similar to crocidolite.

Fluoro-edenite, a newly discovered fibrous amphibole silicate, found on the slopes of Mt. Etna near the rural municipality of Biancavilla, has also been associated with mesotheliomas in these volcanic areas of Italy. (Comba P, Gianfaga A, Paoletti L. Pleural mesothelioma cases in Biancavilla are related to a new fluoro-edenite fibrous amphibole. *Arch Environ Health* 2003;58:229–32.) It is currently unclear where else this volcanic fiber may be found. Many of the cases in Italy were from a nearby stone quarry. (Biggeri A, Pasetto R, Belli S et al. Mortality from chronic obstructive pulmonary disease and pleural mesothelioma in an area contaminated by natural fiber (fluoro-edenite). *Scand J Work Environ Health* 2004;30:249–52; Fazzo L, Minelli G, De Santis M et al. Mesothelioma mortality experience and asbestos exposure in Italy. *Ann Ist Super Sanita* 2012;48:300–10; Ballan G, Del Brocco A, Loizzo S et al. Mode of action of fibrous amphiboles: The case of Biancavilla (Sicily, Italy). *Ann 1st Super Sanita* 2014;50(2):133–8; Conti S, Minelli G, Manno V et al. Health impact of the exposure to fibres with fluoro-edenite composition on the residents in Biancavilla (Sicily, Italy): Mortality and hospitalization from current data. *Ann 1st Super Sanita* 2014;50(2):127–32.)

Erionite, a fibrous zeolite, is the most mesotheliogenic, noncommercial fiber yet discovered. Natural zeolites are used in animal feed, pet litter, odor control, water purification, fertilizer, oil absorbent, and many other uses. Erionite may contaminate commercial deposits of zeolites mined in Arizona, Idaho, California, Oregon, Washington, Nevada, New Mexico, North Dakota, Texas, and Mexico. How many of these zeolite products are contaminated with erionite is unclear at this time, but the potential is quite large. Erionite exposure was thought initially to be a problem limited to Turkey (Baris YI, Sahin AA, Ozesmi M et al. An outbreak of plural mesothelioma and chronic fibrosing pleurisy in the village of Karain/Urgup in Anatolia. *Thorax* 1978;33:181–92), but it is present in most of the Western United States and Mexico, and has been implicated in mesothelioma causation in Dunn County, North Dakota. (Michele C et al. *Proc Natl Acad Sci USA* 2011;108:13618–23; Kliment CR, Clemens K, Oury TD. North American erionite-associated mesothelioma with pleural plaques and pulmonary fibrosis: A case report. *Int J Clin Exp Pathol* 2009;2(4):407–10; Ortega-Guerrero MA, Carrasco-Núñez G, Barragán-Campos H, Ortega MR. High incidence of lung cancer and malignant mesothelioma linked to erionite fibre exposure in a rural community in Central Mexico. *Occup Environ Med* 2015;72(3):216–8; Dogan AU, Dogan M, Hoskins JA. Erionite series minerals: Mineralogical and carcinogenic properties. *Environ Geochem Health* 2008;30(4):367–81; Carbone M, Yang H. Molecular pathways: Targeting mechanisms of asbestos and erionite carcinogenesis in mesothelioma. *Clin Cancer Res* 2012;18(3):598–604; Carbone M, Ly BH, Dodson RF et al. Malignant mesothelioma: Facts, myths, and hypotheses. *J Cell Physiol* 2012;227(1):44–58; Van Gosen BS, Blitz TA, Plumlee GS et al. Geologic occurrences of erionite in the United States: An emerging national public health concern for respiratory disease. *Environ Geochem Health* 2013;35(4):419–30.)

Organic fiber exposure in sugarcane workers, who were also potentially exposed to crystalline silica, has been implicated in the causation of mesothelioma. (Newman RH. Fine biogenic silica fibres in sugar cane: A possible hazard. *Ann Occup Hyg* 1986;30:365–70.)

Environmental exposure to the amphibole tremolite asbestos is a common source of mesothelioma in certain parts of the world such as Turkey and Greece. It was used in a tremolite-containing whitewash called "luto" and a high incidence of mesothelioma was reported in 1987. (Gogli A, Manda-Stachouli, Nitzani EE et al. Malignant mesothelioma in Metsovo, Greece, from domestic use of asbestos: 30 years later. *Eur Respir J* 2012;39:217–8.) A recent evaluation of tremolite asbestos exposures associated with the use of commercial products such as brakes, clutches, gaskets, drywall products, and other chrysotile products was performed. (Finley BL, Pierce JS, Phelka AD et al. Evaluation of tremolite asbestos exposures associated with the use of commercial products. *Crit Rev Toxicol* 2012;42:119–46.)

Tremolite asbestos is a common environmental contaminant in the Western United States, along the Cascade and Sierra mountain ranges, particularly the El Dorado hills of California, and its role as an environmental cause of mesothelioma in the United States is being investigated. (Pan X, Day HW, Wang W, Beckett LA, Schenker MB. Residential proximity to naturally occurring asbestos and mesothelioma risk in California. *Am J Respir Crit Care Med* 2005;172:1019–25.) Recently, there has been interest in an increased risk of mesothelioma in Southern Nevada. (O'Hanlon LH. Researchers explore possible link between mesothelioma and dust emissions in Southern Nevada. *J Natl Cancer Inst* 2013;105(5):312–4.)

Ophiolites are special geologic green-colored rocks, and are a source of naturally occurring asbestos, usually chrysotile and tremolite. They are found in Mediterranean countries including Corsica, Cyprus, Greece, Italy, and Turkey, as well as New Caledonia and California. Ophiolites are associated with pleural plaques and mesothelioma. (Bayram M, Dongel I, Bakan ND et al. High risk of malignant mesothelioma and pleural plaques in subjects born close to ophiolites. *Chest* 2013;143(1):164–71; Döngel I, Bayram M, Bakan ND, Yalçın H, Gültürk S. Is living close to ophiolites related to asbestos related diseases? Cross-sectional study. *Respir Med* 2013;107(6):870–4.)

Recently, in Whatcom County, Washington, a deposit of a chrysotile-like fiber has been discovered along Swift Creek/Sumas Mountain, just below the toe of the Sumas Mountain landslide due east of Everson, Washington. Animal bioassay has suggested that this type of fiber of chrysotile was uniquely more pathogenic in rats than standard amphibole fibers, for reasons unknown to date. (Cyphert J, Nyska A, Mahoney RK et al. Sumas mountain chrysotile induces greater lung fibrosis in Fisher 344 rats than Libby amphibole, El Dorado Tremolite, and Ontario ferroactinolite. *Toxicol Sci* 2012;130(2):405–15.)

Antigorite, a different type of serpentine mineral, has been implicated in the causation of mesothelioma in New Caledonia. Antigorite can exhibit a fibrous morphology. (Baumann F, Maurizot P, Mangeas M et al. Pleural mesothelioma in New Caledonia: Associations with environmental risk factors. *Environ Health Perspect* 2011;119:695–700.) Antigorite and chrysotile asbestos fibers are released in serpentine quarries and stone-processing facilities, but the level of exposure usually remains below the permissible exposure limit. (Cattaneo A, Somiglianna A, Gemmi M et al. Airborne concentrations of chrysotile asbestos in serpentine quarries and stone processing facilities in Valmalenco, Italy. *Ann Occup Hyg* 2012;56:671–83.) Mining other types of nonasbestiform minerals, such as nephite or jade in Taiwan, can be associated with pulmonary fibrosis from exposure to nonasbestiform tremolite asbestos. (Yang HY, Shie RH, Chen PC. Pulmonary fibrosis in workers exposed to non-asbestiform tremolite asbestos minerals. *Epidemiology* 2013;24:143–9.)

Allen and coworkers evaluated a cohort of 31,067 taconite workers with at least 1 year of documented employment. Among those, there were 9094 deaths, of which 949 were from lung cancer, and 30 from mesothelioma. Mortality from lung cancer and mesothelioma was higher than expected, with standard mortality ratios (SMRs) of 1.16 for lung cancer (95% confidence interval [CI]: 1.09–1.23) and 2.77 for mesothelioma (95% CI: 1.87–3.96). There is evidence that taconite workers may be at increased risk for mortality from lung cancer, mesothelioma, and some cardiovascular diseases. Occupational exposures during taconite mining operations may be associated with these increased risks, but nonoccupational exposures may also be important contributors. (Allen EM, Alexander BH, Maclehose RF et al. Mortality experience among Minnesota taconite mining industry workers. *Occup Environ Med* 2014;71(11):744–9.)

There has been concern about the mesotheliogenic effects of rock or slag wool. The epidemiological evidence is sufficient to conclude that there has been no mesothelioma risk to workers producing or using glass wool, rock wool, or slag wool. The epidemiological studies have been large and powerful, and they show no evidence of a cause–effect relationship between lung cancer and exposure to glass wool, rock wool, or slag wool fibers. There is some evidence of a small cancer hazard attached to the manufacturing process in slag wool plants 20–50 years ago, when asbestos was used in some products and other carcinogenic substances were present. However, this hazard is not associated with any index of exposure to slag wool itself. Animal inhalation studies of ordinary insulation wools also show that there is no evidence of hazard associated with exposure to these relatively coarse, soluble fibers. The evidence of carcinogenicity is limited to experiments with special-purpose fine durable glass fibers or experimental fibers, and only when these fibers are injected directly into the pleural or peritoneal cavity. Multiple chronic inhalation studies of these same special-purpose fine glass fibers, have not produced evidence of carcinogenicity. It is suggested that the present IARC evaluation of the carcinogenic risk of insulation wools should be revised to Category 3: not classifiable as to carcinogenicity to humans. (Brown RC, Davis JM, Douglas D et al. Carcinogenicity of the insulation wools: Reassessment of the IARC evaluation. *Regul Toxicol Pharmacol* 1991;14(1):12–23.)

While mineral wool may not be a primary cause of mesothelioma, French investigators have shown that occupational coexposure to asbestos and other fibers or particles could modify the carcinogenicity of asbestos with regards to pleural mesothelioma. Their results are in favor of an increased risk of pleural mesothelioma for subjects exposed to both asbestos and mineral wool and asbestos and silica. (Lacourt A, Gramond C, Audignon S et al. Pleural mesothelioma and occupational coexposure to asbestos, mineral wool, and silica. *Am J Respir Crit Care Med* 2013;187:977–82.)

Smoking a Kent filtered cigarette is an obscure cause of mesothelioma. The original version of the Kent Micronite cigarette filter used crocidolite asbestos from 1952 until at least mid-1956. One filter contained approximately 10 mg of crocidolite. A person smoking a pack of these cigarettes each day would take in more than 131 million crocidolite structures longer than 5 µm in 1 year. (Longo WE, Rigler MW, Slade J. Crocidolite asbestos fibers in smoke from original Kent cigarettes. *Cancer Res* 1995;55(11):2232–5; Talcott JA, Thurber WA, Kantor AF et al. Asbestos-associated diseases in a cohort of cigarette-filter workers. *N Engl J Med* 1989;321:1220–3.)

In summary, there are many naturally occurring exposures to other fibrous minerals like asbestos. Remember, the word asbestos is not a mineralogical term, but simply a term for commercially useful fibrous minerals of an asbestiform nature. It is clear that naturally occurring asbestiform, or asbestos-like, noncommercial minerals, are present in many areas of the world and pose a significant risk for the development of mesothelioma. The general population is not generally aware that they have been exposed to dangerous nonindustrial asbestos-like materials in the general environment.

The toxicity of asbestos, and asbestiform minerals, depends primarily on six factors.

1. Dose
2. Fiber size, shape, width, length, and aerodynamics
3. Bio-durability
4. Surface reactivity
5. Genetic factors in the host
6. Iron content

There are many good, detailed reviews available on the molecular basis of asbestos-induced lung disease. The most recent is by Liu et al. (Liu G, Cheresh P, Kamp D. Molecular basis of asbestos-induced lung disease. *Ann Rev Pathol Mech Dis* 2013;8:161–87.)

14

Other causes of mesothelioma not related to asbestiform mineral fibers

This list of causes of mesothelioma, not related to asbestos or asbestiform minerals, is complete up to 2014, but it is likely that other causes of mesothelioma will be found in the future.

1. Carbon nanotubes?
2. Ceramic fibers?
3. Nickel
4. Beryllium
5. Simian virus-40 (SV40)
6. Familial Mediterranean fever
7. Tuberculosis
8. Familial mesothelioma (genetic predisposition)
9. Diet?
10. Thorium dioxide
11. Paraffin oil
12. Radiation
13. Drugs and chemicals: Isoniazide (INH), ethylene oxide, polyurethane, polysilicone, and ethylene dibromide
14. Genetics
15. Pulmonary alveolar microlithiasis

Although asbestos is the predominant cause of mesothelioma, exposure to other elements that also induce cell necrosis, inflammation, proliferation, or DNA damage, such as ionizing radiation, particularly in conjunction with asbestos exposure, may contribute to the development of mesothelioma.

Firstly, genetic susceptibility plays a significant role because there is a constant background level of mesothelioma. Secondly, various studies have shown that only 20%–80%+ of individuals with mesothelioma have a history of asbestos exposure. (Spirtas R, Heineman E, Bernstein L et al. Malignant mesothelioma: Attributable risk of asbestos exposure. *Occup Environ Med* 1994;51:804–11; Shepherd KE, Oliver LC, Kazemi H. Diffuse malignant pleural mesothelioma in an urban hospital: Clinical spectrum and trend in incidence over time. *Am J Ind Med* 1989;16(4):373–83.) Thirdly, mesotheliomas have been found historically in populations with mesotheliomas prior to the industrial use of asbestos.

In Cappadocia, Turkey, an unprecedented mesothelioma epidemic caused 50% of all deaths in three small villages. This was linked solely to the exposure to the fibrous mineral erionite. Studies by scientists from Turkey and the United States have shown that erionite causes mesothelioma mostly in families that are genetically predisposed to mineral fiber carcinogenesis. (Roushdy-Hammady I, Siegel J, Emri S, Testa JR, Carbone M. Genetic-susceptibility factor and malignant mesothelioma in the Cappadocian region of Turkey. *Lancet* 2001;357(9254):444–5; Carbone M, Emri S, Dogan AU et al. A mesothelioma epidemic in Cappadocia: Scientific developments and unexpected social outcomes. *Nat Rev Cancer* 2007;7(2):147–54.)

Italian investigators studied the occurrence of mesothelioma among blood relatives of confirmed mesothelioma cases. So-called familial mesothelioma, may point to genetic susceptibility or shared exposures. The burden of the familial disease is unknown. The aims of their study were to assess, at a population level, the proportion of familial mesotheliomas among all mesotheliomas, and to investigate the family history of cancer among relatives of mesothelioma cases. They actively searched familial clusters based on a mesothelioma registry from central Italy (5.5 million people, 10% of the Italian population) of the National Mesothelioma Register Network, as well as a pathology-based archive. Among 997 incident mesotheliomas recorded in a 32-year period (1980–2012), they detected 13 clusters and 34 familial cases, accounting for 3.4% of all mesotheliomas. The most common clusters of mesothelioma cases where those with affected siblings and unaffected parents (Figure 14.1). (Ascoli V, Romeo E, Carnovale

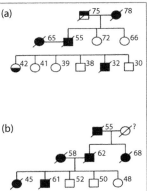

Malignant pleural mesothelioma (MPM)
in Cappadocia—Genetic studies: Genetic mapping study

- Analysis of a six-generation extended pedigree of 526 individuals showed that malignant mesothelioma (MM) was genetically transmitted.

- It was suggested that vertical transmission of MM occurs probably in an autosomal dominant way.

- Studies are in progress to identify the gene(s), which increase(s) the susceptibility to erionite and asbestos.

Figure 14.1 Genetic factors in erionite asbestos-induced mesothelioma. (From Hammady-Roushdy et al. *Lancet* 2001;357:444–445.)

Scalzo C et al. Familial malignant mesothelioma: A population-based study in Central Italy (1980–2012). *Cancer Epidemiol* 2014;38(3):273–8.)

Bruce Robinson and coworkers in Western Australia have identified some suggestive genomic traits that would explain why a small percentage of heavily exposed workers develop mesothelioma. (Cadby G, Mukherjee S, Musk AW et al. A genome-wide association study for malignant mesothelioma risk. *Lung Cancer* 2013;82(1):1–8; Robinson BW, Lake RA. Advances in malignant mesothelioma. *N Engl J Med* 2005;353:1591–603; Powers A, Carbone M. The role of environmental carcinogens, viruses, and genetic predisposition in the pathogenesis of mesothelioma. *Cancer Biol Ther* 2002;1:348–53; Bianchi C, Brollo A, Ramani L, Bianchi T, Giarelli L. Familial mesothelioma of the pleura—A report of 40 cases. *Ind Health* 2004;42(2):235–9.)

Only 2%–17% of individuals heavily exposed to amphibole asbestos develop a mesothelioma. Ribak and co workers found 17 mesotheliomas in 820 short-term amosite asbestos workers, or about 2% of exposed workers. (Ribak J, Seidman H, Selikoff IJ. Amosite mesothelioma in a cohort of asbestos workers. *Scand J Work Environ Health* 1989;15(2):106–10.) This suggests a significant influence of genetic factors that affect susceptibility to the cancer-causing effects of asbestos and other mineral fibers as a promoter of malignant change in human mesothelial cells. (Matullo G, Guarrera S, Betti M et al. Genetic variants associated with increased risk of malignant pleural mesothelioma: A genome-wide association study. *PLoS One* 2013;8(4):e61253.)

The incidence of mesothelioma was studied in 17,800 members of the International Association of Heat and Frost Insulators and Asbestos Workers in the United States and Canada between 1967 and 1984 and 356 deaths from mesothelioma out of 3500 deaths were found, or about 10% of all deaths in heavily exposed workers. The majority of mesothelioma deaths were from peritoneal mesothelioma (134 pleural and 222 peritoneal) in this heavily exposed cohort. The duration of exposure was 33.8 years for pleural mesothelioma and 36.4 years in the peritoneal mesothelioma cases. The remarkable fact in this study of heavily exposed workers, is that only 10% of workers developed a mesothelioma, suggesting that the majority of workers were not susceptible to mesothelioma on a genetic basis. (Ribak J, Lilis R, Suzuki Y, Penner L, Selikoff IJ. Malignant mesothelioma in a cohort of asbestos insulation workers: Clinical presentation, diagnosis, and causes of death. *Br J Ind Med* 1988;45(3):182–7.)

A similar incidence of mesothelioma (10% or 65/640) was found in a group of mainly women, who worked in the assembly of gas mask filters that were comprised of 20% crocidolite asbestos, during World War II from 1940 to 1944. (McDonald JC, Harris JM, Berry G. Sixty-years on: The price of assembling military gas masks in 1940. *Occup Environ Med* 2006;63:852–5.) The incidence of mesothelioma is much lower if workers with heavy exposure, such as insulation workers, are excluded. The incidence in a Dutch shipyard with secondary exposure was 0.68%, or 21 out of 3102. (Stumphius J. The epidemiology of mesothelioma on Walcheren Island. *Br J Ind Med* 1971;28:59–66.)

The Mt. Sinai Selikoff group investigated an amosite insulation plant in Paterson, New Jersey. From 1941 to 1945, 933 men worked there for short periods during World War II. The employees tended to be older and many may have worked elsewhere in New Jersey in the asbestos products industry. By 1986, 820 were available for follow-up and 740 were dead. There were 17 mesothelioma cases (eight pleural and nine peritoneal), comprising 2.3% of the deaths. A similar plant operated in Tyler, Texas, from 1954 until 1971. The exposures were extremely high, ranging from 15.9 to 19.4 fibers/cc. In 1998, Levin et al. found six mesothelioma cases in 315 deaths out of 1130 former workers, for an incidence of 1.9%. (Seidman H, Selikoff I, Gelb S. Mortality experience of amosite asbestos factory workers: Dose–response relationships 5–40 years after onset of short-term work exposure. *Am J Ind Med* 1986;10:479–51; Levin JL, McLarty JW, Hurst GA, Smith AN, Frank AL. Tyler asbestos workers: Mortality experience in a cohort exposed to amosite. *Occup Environ Med* 1998;55:155–60.)

The data from the medical literature have showed that other nonfibrous materials have been associated with mesothelioma production, such as nickel and beryllium. Chronic radiation and thorotrast exposure are also important.

Viruses such as SV40 and MC29 avian leukosis virus are important cofactors in mesothelioma production. SV-40 inactivates tumor-suppressor genes and has demonstrated oncogenic potential in animal models. It has a predilection for human epithelial cells, but its actual role in mesothelioma carcinogenesis is likely as a promoter with mineral fibers such as asbestos, rather than a primary cause of human mesothelioma. An estimated 62% of 92 million U.S. residents received the potentially SV40-contaminated Salk polio vaccine for the 8 years it was used (1955–1963); of these, at least one-fifth may have received live, infectious SV40-containing vaccine. In addition, although efforts were made to exclude SV40 from polio vaccines, the testing done was not rigorous enough to totally ensure that all cohorts born after 1963 were given SV40-free polio vaccines. For example, a major Eastern European manufacturer used a procedure that did not fully inactivate SV40 in oral poliovirus vaccine; these SV40-contaminated vaccines were produced from the early 1960s to about 1978 and were used throughout the world. (Comar M, Zancotta N, Pesel G et al. Asbestos and SV40 in malignant pleural mesothelioma from a hyperendemic area of North-Eastern Italy. *Tumori* 2012;98:210–4; Cleaver AL, Bhamidipaty K, Wylie B et al. Long-term exposure of mesothelial cells to SV40 and asbestos leads to malignant transformation and chemotherapy resistance. *Carcinogenesis* 2014;35(2):407–14.)

Any cause of chronic chest or abdominal serosal inflammation, such as tuberculosis or familial Mediterranean fever, may also cause a mesothelioma. (Jasani B, Gibbs A. Mesothelioma not associated with asbestos exposure. *Arch Pathol Lab Med* 2012;136:262–7.)

Various drugs have been implicated as possible causes of mesothelioma, including INH, ethylene oxide, polyurethane, polysilicone, and ethylene dibromide. (Pelnar P. Development of knowledge on health effects of asbestos and of some other minerals and mineral fibres, particularly in Canada—Development up to 1966. In: G Scherr (Ed.), *J Environ Pathol, Toxicol Oncol.* Park Forest: Chem-Orbital, 1988, Vol I; Pelnar PV. Further evidence of non-asbestos-related mesothelioma: A review of the literature. *J Work Environ Health* 1988;14:141–4.)

There has been concern about workers exposed to synthetic vitreous fibers (SVFs) among those employed in the production of rock/slag wool, glass wool, or continuous glass filament in the United States, Canada, and Europe. A systematic review of this population has not found a significant increased risk of mesothelioma. The toxicology review of SVFs suggested that they present a low hazard, mostly due to their low bio-persistence, typically with a half-life in rat studies of tens days compared to amphibole asbestos, which has a half-life of 400–500 days. (Boffetta P, Donaldson K, Moolgavkar S, Mandel JS. A systematic review of occupational exposure to synthetic vitreous fibers and mesothelioma. *Crit Rev Toxicol* 2014;44(5):436–49.)

Nanoparticles can assume a fibrous shape (carbon nanotubes) and the fear has been as to whether high-aspect nanoparticles may be sufficiently fibrogenic to cause lung cancer and/or mesothelioma. Ceramic fibers, and other man-made mineral fiber exposures, are being monitored carefully since ceramic fibers can produce mesotheliomas in animals and pleural plaques in humans. Ceramic fiber exposure may be synergistic with asbestos exposure, producing a greater risk of mesothelioma than from asbestos exposure alone. (Lacourt A, Rinaldo M, Gramond C et al. Co-exposure to refractory ceramic fibres and asbestos and risk of pleural mesothelioma. *Eur Respir J* 2014;44(3):725–33; Utell MJ, Maxim LD. Refractory ceramic fiber (RCF) toxicity and epidemiology: A review. *Inhal Toxicol* 2010;22(6):500–21.) This question of the hazards of man-made fibers is of great concern but has not been answered. (Donaldson K, Poland CA. Inhaled nanoparticles and lung cancer—What we can learn from conventional particle toxicology. *Swiss Med Wkly* 2012;142:1–9; Donaldson K, Poland CA, Murphy FA, Macfarlane M, Chernova T, Schinwald A. Pulmonary toxicity of carbon nanotubes and asbestos—Similarities and differences. *Adv Drug Deliv Rev* 2013;65(15):2078–86; Xu J, Alexander DB, Futakuchi M et al. Size- and shape-dependent pleural translocation, deposition, fibrogenesis and mesothelial proliferation by multiwalled carbon nanotubes. *Cancer Sci* 2014;105(7):763–9.)

Nanofibers can be manufactured to specific lengths. While the pleural effects of fibers depend on fiber length, the key threshold length beyond which adverse effects occur had not been identified until now, because all asbestos and vitreous fiber samples are heterogeneously distributed in their lengths. Nanotechnology advantageously allows for highly defined length distribution assessment of synthetically engineered fibers that enables in-depth investigation of this threshold length. Schinwald and others have shown a clear threshold effect for pleural inflammation, demonstrating that fibers beyond 4 μm in length are pathogenic to the pleura in mice. The identification of the threshold length for nanofiber-induced pathogenicity in the pleura has important implications for understanding the structure–toxicity relationship for asbestos-induced mesothelioma and consequent risk assessment. (Schinwald A, Murphy FA, Prina-Mello A et al. The threshold length for fiber-induced acute pleural inflammation: Shedding light on the early events in asbestos-induced mesothelioma. *Toxicol Sci* 2012;128(2):461–70.)

In another paper, it was hypothesized that long fibers elicit an inflammatory response in the pleural cavity via frustrated phagocytosis in pleural macrophages. The activated macrophages then stimulate an amplified pro-inflammatory cytokine response from the adjacent pleural mesothelial cells. This mechanism for producing a pro-inflammatory environment in the pleural space exposed to long carbon nanotubes, has implications for the general understanding of fiber-related pleural disease. (Murphy FA, Schinwald A, Poland CA, Donaldson K. The mechanism of pleural inflammation by long carbon nanotubes: Interaction of long fibres with macrophages stimulates them to amplify pro-inflammatory responses in mesothelial cells. *Part Fibre Toxicol* 2012;9(8):1–15.)

The relationship between cumulative external radiation dose and the proximal mortality ratio (PMR) for mesothelioma, suggests that external radiation at nuclear facilities is associated with an increased risk of mesothelioma. (Gibb H, Fulcher K, Nagarajan S et al. Analyses of radiation and mesothelioma in the US transuranium and uranium registries. *Am J Public Health* 2013;103(4):710–6.) Thorium dioxide has been implicated as a cause of mesothelioma. (Maurer R, Egloff B. Malignant peritoneal mesothelioma after cholangiography with thorotrast. *Cancer* 1975;36(4):1381–5.)

David Sugarbaker's group in Boston has reviewed the characteristics of 22 patients with Hodgkin's and non-Hodgkin's lymphoma and postradiation mesothelioma, and concluded that patients with lymphoma-associated pleural diffuse malignant mesothelioma (PDMM) postradiation are likely to have unusual histologic features, are significantly younger, and seem to have a longer overall survival compared with patients with asbestos-associated PDMM. (Chirieac LR, Barletta JA, Yeap BY et al. Clinicopathologic characteristics of malignant mesotheliomas arising in patients with a history of radiation for Hodgkin's and non-Hodgkin's lymphoma. *J Clin Oncol* 2013;31(36):4544–9.)

Paraffin oil has been mentioned by Peterson and colleagues as a chemical cause of mesothelioma and they postulated, as had others, that other chemical agents could possibly be implicated based on animal studies. (Peterson JT Jr, Greenberg SD, Buffler PA. Non-asbestos-related malignant mesothelioma. A review. *Cancer* 1984;54(5):951–60; Paterour MJ, Bignon J, Jaurand M. *In vitro* transformation of rat pleural mesothelial cells by chrysotile fibres and/or benzo[a]pyrene. *Carcinogenesis* 1985;6(4):523–9.)

A rare cause of pleural plaques with calcification and lung fibrosis is pulmonary alveolar microlithiasis. (Malhotra B, Sabharwal R, Singh M, Singh A. Pulmonary alveolar microlithiasis with calcified pleural plaques. *Lung India* 2010;27(4):250–2.)

The role of diet in the causation of mesothelioma is unclear, but acrylamide, a water-soluble contaminant in baked and fried starchy foods, has recently been found to cause mesothelioma in male rats. (National Toxicology Program. Toxicology and carcinogenesis studies of acrylamide (CASRN 79-06-1) in F344/N rats and B6C3F1 mice (feed and drinking water studies). *Natl Toxicol Program Tech Rep Ser* 2012;575:1–234.)

15

Mesothelioma and asbestos fiber type

Review of the literature specific to mesothelioma reveals that there was much confusion as to whether a primary tumor of the mesothelium (lining of the chest cavity) existed.

By 1946, Arnold Piatt, a radiologist at the Newark Hospital, reviewed the radiologic aspects of primary mesothelioma or endothelioma of the pleura. (Piatt AD. Primary mesothelioma (endothelioma) of the pleura, Case Report. *AJR Am J Roentgenol* 1946;55:173–80.) By then, over 200 authors had discussed and offered opinions on the entity at that time called primary mesothelioma, or endothelioma of the pleura. Piatt points out that it was a very difficult diagnostic problem for pathologists who argued amongst themselves as to the type and histologic origin of the neoplasm. By then, there were as many as 30 different terms used to describe this clinical entity, including terms such as endothelioma, mesothelioma, endothelial carcinoma, pleural carcinoma, primary papillary endothelioma of the pleura, adenoendothelioma, sarcoendothelioma, pleural sarcoma, sarcomatous malignancy of the pleura, malignant tumor of the pleura, mesothelial carcinoma, perithelioma, endothelioma carcinomatodes, lymphangio-endothelioma, fibro-endotheliosis of the pleura, lymphangitis proliferans, pleuroma, abdominal colloid tumor, and tubercle-like lymphadenoma.

In 1957, Godwin published criteria for the diagnosis of pleural mesotheliomas, and it was not until 1960 that Winslow and Taylor did the same thing for peritoneal mesothelioma tumors. Once relatively good criteria for the diagnosis of mesothelioma were established, epidemiologic studies could be performed. The criteria for the "pathologic diagnosis and staging of mesothelioma" have undergone many revisions over the years since 1960, and were last revived in 2012. (Hussain AN, Colby T, Ordonez N et al. Guidelines for pathologic diagnosis of malignant mesothelioma: 2012 Update of the consensus statement from the International Mesothelioma Interest Group. *Arch Pathol Lab Med* 2013;137:647–67.)

The case for the association with asbestos exposure and diffuse pleural mesothelioma was really best made by a seminal paper published in the *British Journal of Industrial Medicine* by a young pathologist (Wagner JC, Sleggs CA, Marchand

P. Diffuse pleural mesothelioma and asbestos exposure in the North Western Cape Province. 1960;17:260–71). Wagner studied 33 individuals who had various types of exposure to Cape Blue asbestos. He showed that people who had only environmental exposures, and had not worked directly with asbestos, had developed this rare type of tumor called a mesothelioma. This was a very controversial paper because only two of the 33 individuals actually had thorough autopsies. Only a quarter of these cases had a history of working with asbestos. The majority denied having worked with asbestos at all. Their occupations were diverse, including housewives, domestic servants, cattle herders, farmers, a water-bailiff, an accountant, and an international goal-keeper. According to Professor J Gough of Cardiff, UK, the editorial board of the *British Journal of Industrial Medicine* was about to reject the paper because the senior pathologist did not accept the existence of mesotheliomas, but Gough persuaded the editorial board to accept the paper. (Wagner JC. Mesothelioma and exposure to asbestos in South Africa: 1956–62. In: BW Robinson, AP Chahinian (Eds.), *Mesothelioma*. Kent: Matin Dunnitz Ltd, 2002, Chapter 4, pp. 87–91.)

Earlier, it was mentioned that Robertson denied the existence of a primary tumor of the mesothelium, and he felt that all of these tumors were metastatic tumors from a primary elsewhere, commonly the lung. Willis, a world-respected British pathologist, and others, published criteria that no patient could have a diagnosis of a mesothelioma unless they had had a thorough autopsy, and another primary elsewhere had been excluded. It was felt that since a primary tumor elsewhere is very difficult to disprove, this made the diagnosis of a primary tumor of the mesothelium unlikely. Therefore, there was a lot of controversy as to whether this paper should have even been published in 1960.

After Wagner's discovery of the association between crocidolite asbestos and the increased risk of mesothelioma in South Africa, the question arose as to whether this was a unique problem limited to South Africa, or whether this was a problem occurring in the United States. The American Medical Association Council on Occupational Health published an article on pneumoconioses in the *Archives of Environmental Health* (1963;7:14–55). In this article, there is a section on asbestosis, and the panel of experts concluded that

It is believed there may be an association between bronchogenic carcinoma and asbestosis in workers with well-established asbestosis, particularly among those with long exposures. When carcinoma supervenes in asbestosis, it is usually squamous cell type and it is frequently located in the lower lung field where the fibrosis is usually the most extensive. An increased incidence or risk of lung cancer in other pneumoconioses probably does not exist.

They go on to say on page 37 of their article:

The relationship between cancer of the lung and asbestosis constitutes a problem of great current interest. There is no doubt that the two diseases appear in the same lung. Whether that occurrence is one of mere coincidence, or of direct cause–effect relationship cannot be resolved on the basis of a single case. The total body of evidence favors a relationship, especially as it involves certain kinds of asbestos and possibly only those, which contain specific chemical substances having the capacity to cause cancer. Attention is invited to experiences in the union of South Africa where pleural mesotheliomas have been discovered in appreciable number of persons exposed to the inhalation of crocidolite–amosite asbestos. Certainly detailed epidemiologic clinical and experimental studies are required for the ultimate resolution of the problem.

The question about the risk to end users of asbestos products was raised by Thompson, Kaschula, and MacDonald in 1963. They wrote

The enormously increased world consumption of asbestos, from 300,000 tons in 1934 to 2,400,000 tons in 1961, is used in a variety of industrial products, from obvious ones such as asbestos roofing, roof tiles, ceilings, floor tiles, pipe insulation, and electrical insulation, to less obvious ones where asbestos is added to all sorts of materials, cement, etc. It is possible for those manufacturing, selling, and using these products to inhale asbestos fibers, although their occupations are in general not labeled or recognized as ones in which asbestos as a hazard to be anticipated. (Thomson JG, Kaschula RO, MacDonald RR. Asbestos as a modern urban hazard. *S Afr Med J* 1963;37:77–81.)

Meanwhile, JC Wagner moved from South Africa to the Pneumoconiosis Research Unit in Wales, to carry on his research on the health effects of asbestos. He published, in 1963, a review of the prior literature on asbestosis in experimental animals, and added his own observations. He concluded that it appeared that chrysotile asbestos was less fibrogenic than amosite asbestos. (Wagner JC. Asbestosis in experimental animals. *Br J Ind Med* 1963;20:1–12.)

Selikoff, Churg, and Hammond reported their experience of the relationship between asbestos exposure and mesothelioma in the *New England Journal of Medicine* in 1965. This was an important paper in that it was the first U.S. retrospective analysis of 632 men employed before 1942 as pipe fitters/insulators. There were 307 deaths, of which ten were from mesothelioma. This further cemented the possible relationship between asbestos exposure and mesothelioma while raising the question as to whether other types of asbestos might also cause mesotheliomas. Even while there was growing information among other workers, that they were finding increased incidences of this rare tumor, other workers were still unimpressed. Part of the controversy was generated by the fact that when Sluis-Cremer and others looked at other areas of South Africa, they only found an increased incidence of mesothelioma in the areas of the Northwest Cape, where Cape Blue asbestos was mined. They looked for increased incidences of mesothelioma in the amosite mining area, and the area of the Transvaal where another form of crocidolite was mined, and were unable to find an increased incidence. This caused a lot of confusion since it suggested that mesothelioma was just related to an exposure to one certain type of crocidolite asbestos, from only one geographically specific area. Ian Webster, the brother-in-law of JC Wagner, still felt that there were unsolved problems in the relationship between asbestos and malignancy, in a paper he published in February 1973 in the *South African Medical Journal*. (Webster I. Asbestos and malignancy. *S Afr Med J* 1973;47(5):165–71.)

The relationship between peritoneal tumors and asbestosis was discussed in 1964 by Enticknap and Smither. (Enticknap JB, Smither WJ. Peritoneal tumours in asbestosis. *Br J Ind Med* 1964;21:20–31.) Later, Browne and Smither published a more complete analysis of the factors differentiating pleural and peritoneal mesotheliomas. (Browne K, Smither WJ. Asbestos-related mesothelioma: Factors discriminating between pleural and peritoneal sites. *Br J Ind Med* 1983;40:145–52.) The study included 143 cases of mesothelioma of which 22% were exposed for under 1 year, of whom 15% had no more than 6 months of exposure, and 6% no more than 3 months.

Irving Selikoff discussed the uncertainties about the pathology and epidemiology of mesothelioma in 1965. He stated,

In 1960 Wagner, Sleggs and Marchand had reported 33 cases of diffuse pleural mesothelioma from the North Western Cape Province of South Africa. The collection of such a large number of cases of a rare tumor within a short time (1956–1960) in one area was considered unusual enough. Even more striking was the fact that close questioning and investigation revealed that 32 patients had evidence, admittedly circumstantial in most cases, of some potential or actual contact with asbestos by virtue either of residence in mining areas or in industry twenty to forty years before.

This remarkable concentration of cases in one area of South Africa was explained by the hypothesis that mesothelioma was the result of exposure to one special type of asbestos (crocidolite), mined almost entirely in that region. The report of a mesothelioma associated with asbestosis in Western Australia, one of the few other regions of the world in which crocidolite is mined, was consistent with this hypothesis. Similarly, the occurrence of other cases of mesothelioma, including several of the peritoneum, in Great Britain was not disturbing since British asbestos companies have long been intimately related in ownership and management with the South African asbestos industry and the largest portion of crocidolite mined in South Africa had in previous years been imported into Great Britain.

Scattered reports of neoplasia of the pleural and peritoneal surfaces in association with asbestosis variously labeled 'undifferentiated carcinoma', 'endothelioma' and 'mesothelioma' have been available for thirty years. Although a special relation had been proposed such considerations faced the difficulty of the infrequency of reported cases and the absence of population and epidemiologic studies. Similar difficulties plagued the question of the relation between lung cancer and asbestos exposure until their resolution by adequate epidemiologic investigations, which confirmed the accurate but unverified pathological and clinical studies. It appears that a similar process is being completed regarding the complication of mesothelioma. Lung cancer has previously been demonstrated to be a frequent complication of asbestos exposure among insulation workers in the United States. The data in Table 3 may be considered an extension of previously reported observations, which were based upon age-specific death rates among 632 men with at least twenty years' elapsed time from onset of first exposure to asbestos and which were concerned with 255 consecutive deaths. There were 42 deaths due to lung cancer at that time (16.5 per cent). In the 52 additional deaths 11 have been due to lung cancer (21.2 per cent). [See Figure 15.1]

Originally, there were 4 mesotheliomas among the 255 deaths; there are now 10. Ten deaths from mesothelioma among 307 consecutive deaths is an extraordinarily high rate and permits the conclusion that this disease is an important complication of asbestos exposure. This conclusion, moreover, refers to such exposure

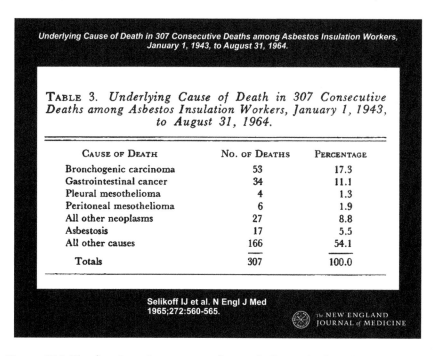

Underlying Cause of Death in 307 Consecutive Deaths among Asbestos Insulation Workers, January 1, 1943, to August 31, 1964.

TABLE 3. *Underlying Cause of Death in 307 Consecutive Deaths among Asbestos Insulation Workers, January 1, 1943, to August 31, 1964.*

CAUSE OF DEATH	NO. OF DEATHS	PERCENTAGE
Bronchogenic carcinoma	53	17.3
Gastrointestinal cancer	34	11.1
Pleural mesothelioma	4	1.3
Peritoneal mesothelioma	6	1.9
All other neoplasms	27	8.8
Asbestosis	17	5.5
All other causes	166	54.1
Totals	307	100.0

Selikoff IJ et al. N Engl J Med
1965;272:560-565.

The NEW ENGLAND
JOURNAL of MEDICINE

Figure 15.1 The first American report of mesotheliomas in American insulators.

in the United States, under working conditions of the recent past, with relatively light and intermittent asbestos exposure. It indicates, too, that mesothelioma may not necessarily be entirely a problem of only one kind of asbestos (crocidolite) and that it is surely not limited to South Africa. (Selikoff IJ, Churg J, Hammond EC. Relation between exposure to asbestos and mesothelioma. *N Engl J Med* 1965;272:560–5.)

In 1965, Dr. Sluis-Cremer of the Miner's Medical Bureau in Johannesburg, South Africa, gave a report to the New York Academy of Science that was published in 1965. Dr. Sluis-Cremer, in his discussion of mesotheliomas, pointed out that in his epidemiologic studies, he only found mesotheliomas in the Northwest Cape area of South Africa, and not in the Transvaal area, even though the two types of crocidolite were similar, and had no differences in surface area, solubility, or trace element content. The Northwest Cape fibers were thinner than the Transvaal fibers. The Transvaal amosite deposits had been actively developed for longer than this period, and he mentioned that in the 1940s, amosite was in fact at three times the level of production of the Northwest crocidolite, yet no mesotheliomas were seen in the area related to amosite exposure. Inhalation studies of both Transvaal and Northwest Cape crocidolite, performed on guinea pigs and rats in 1972, were unable to produce mesotheliomas, but the Northwest Cape fibers were more irritating and inflammatory than the Transvaal fibers for unknown reasons. (Botham SK, Holt PF. The effects of inhaled crocidolites from Transvaal and North-West Cape mines on the lungs of rats and guinea pigs. *Br J Exp Pathol* 1972;53:612–20.)

This was followed by an editorial in the *New England Journal of Medicine* on March 18, 1965, after the report of Drs. Selikoff, Churg, and Hammond of the increased incidence of mesotheliomas in their asbestos insulators. The editorial mentions "amosite, the third commercially used form of asbestos, has yet to be incriminated, but there are no definitive studies to date to confirm or deny such a connection." This statement is opposed by a statement in the same issue by Dr. Selikoff, who stated, "It indicates too that mesothelioma may not necessarily be entirely a problem of one kind of asbestos crocidolite, and that it is surely not limited to South Africa."

Dr. JS Harington wrote a chapter on mesothelioma in *The Prevention of Cancer* (Raven and Rowe, Eds. 1967). He stated, "The results of animal experimentation so far available suggests that crocidolite and chrysotile may be more active in inducing mesotheliomas than amosite" (Harington and Rowe 1965). "If the present trend is confirmed, substitution in mining and industry of amosite (e.g. for the more dangerous types of asbestos where they cannot be safely used) may be a practical and important preventative measure."

In an unsigned editorial in the *Journal of the Lancet* (March 5, 1966), the author stated,

A possible important clue to prevention was just uncovered by Wagner in South Africa, where after showing association between mesothelial tumors and exposure to crocidolite form of asbestos, he and his colleagues were unable to find any tumors in those exposed only to the amosite or chrysotile-types of fiber. The position in South Africa remains the same, despite continuing intensive search in the amosite and chrysotile mining areas.

The author goes on to say,

Mesothelioma tumors have been seen in a few individuals apparently exposed only to chrysotile in the United States and Canada, and other populations either industrial or residential exposed only to one type of fiber must now be investigated. This can be achieved only by international cooperation, because such exposures are almost entirely limited to those engaged in mining and milling of the fiber, which is done in the countries where the different types of asbestos are found.

Garrett Schepers, then working as an American pathologist for the Bureau of Health in Washington DC, and who was originally from South Africa, related his own experience, at the New York Academy of Sciences meeting (Schepers G. Comments. *Ann NY Acad Sci* 1965:595–602), in which he stated,

My first impression is that there is now less certainty that asbestos inhalation is associated with pulmonary neoplasia than there was 10 or 20 years ago. Perhaps this is due to greatly reduced dust exposures. Asbestos may after all prove to be carcinogenic only in overwhelming dosage. Thus, the high prevalence of neoplasia which was reported several decades ago may be a function of the severity of exposure rather than an indication of high carcinogenic potency. I suspect that the final analysis that the carcinogenicity of asbestos will be rated as of low order. Perhaps carcinogenicity will prove to be a correlate of asbestosis rather than a specific biological function of the mineral asbestos. This may be the crux of the matter. In all cases of asbestos-associated lung cancer, which I have personally studied (the number now exceeds two dozen), there invariably was well-established asbestosis. Not only was the asbestosis of marked degree in the areas where the cancer arose, but there generally was evidence from serial chest X-rays that asbestosis had been present in the lungs for a protracted period.

Dr. Wagner quickly discovered more cases, and developed an animal model for the production of mesotheliomas. In 1965, when he reported his updated series of cases at the New York Academy of Sciences, there was the general consensus that this indeed was a unique observation that there was an association between Cape Blue amphibole asbestos and mesothelioma. Some doubts about the association between asbestos exposure and mesothelioma continued after

1965, and eight case–control studies were conducted between 1965 and 1975, which confirmed the association between asbestos exposure and mesothelioma. (McDonald JC. Epidemiology of malignant mesothelioma—An outline. *Ann Occup Hyg* 2010;54:851–7.) Wagner's paper impacted the international scientific community significantly after 1965, when it began to evaluate regional experiences with mesothelioma and crocidolite exposure. (Riva MA, Carnevale F, Sironi VA et al. Mesothelioma and asbestos, fifty years of evidence: Chris Wagner and the contribution of the Italian occupational medicine community. *Med Lav* 2010;101(6):409–15.)

In hindsight in 1988, Dr. Selikoff mentioned that he reviewed the older literature on mesothelioma and states,

> During the 1950s there were several reports of deaths in asbestos workers caused by these diffuse tumors of the mesothelial surfaces. These isolated cases would have received little notice had it not been for the fact that the tumor has always been considered extraordinarily rare. It is no longer rare amongst asbestos workers. Indeed, it is so common a cause of death amongst them now. While still rare amongst individuals not known to be exposed to asbestos—it almost constituted tumor specific to asbestos exposure.

Furthermore, in 1988, Dr. Selikoff and coworkers state, "Nevertheless only in the past 25 years has malignant mesothelioma been widely accepted as an independent diagnostic entity." This means that, in his opinion, mesothelioma was not accepted as a diagnostic entity until 1963. Selikoff's review of the deaths of asbestos insulators in 1988, found that 175 deaths from mesothelioma occurred among 2221 men who died between 1967 and 1976, as well as 181 more deaths in the next 8 years, for a total of 356 deaths from mesothelioma, out a total of 3500 deaths from all causes by 1984. A total of 134 of these were pleural and 222 were peritoneal mesotheliomas. (Ribak J, Lilis R, Suzuki Y, Penner L, Selikoff IJ. Malignant mesothelioma in asbestos insulation workers: Clinical presentation, diagnosis, and causes of death. *Br J Ind Med* 1988;45:182–7.)

Selikoff, Hammond, and Churg reviewed the results of a study of an asbestos insulation manufacturing plant in Paterson, New Jersey, and published their results in the *Archives of Environmental Health* in September 1972. They pointed out, "Few data exist concerning the comparative neoplastic potential in man of the several kinds of asbestos, and particularly there has been no evidence concerning whether amosite variety is carcinogenic." They went on to say

> Whether or not amosite is carcinogenic is of some practical importance. Because this variety of asbestos has not been reported to cause cancer, there has been a tendency in Great Britain for example to substitute it for other types of asbestos, especially crocidolite.

Dr. Selikoff and coworkers emphasized the increased incidence of lung cancer and mesothelioma in this asbestos insulation plant because it was thought to be an example of pure exposure to amosite asbestos. (Selikoff IJ, Hammond EC, Churg J. Carcinogenicity of amosite asbestos. *Arch Environ Health* 1972;25:183–6.)

While it was generally accepted in the United States that pure amosite caused a high incidence of mesotheliomas and lung cancers, the paper by Selikoff and coworkers was not well accepted abroad. McCullagh published a paper in the *Journal of Society of Occupational Medicine* in 1980 (McCullagh SF. Amosite as a cause of lung cancer and mesothelioma in humans. *J Soc Occup Med* 1980;30:153–6) and pointed out that many of the Paterson, New Jersey cohorts studied by Selikoff, had previous exposure to asbestos from other manufacturing plants in the area. He felt that rather than 1/50th of the group, it seemed more likely that one-third of the group, or 300 members of the Paterson cohort, had been occupationally exposed to asbestos before entering the cohort. JC Wagner stated in 1979 (speaking for Europe) that "We feel very strongly that the material, which was milled in New Jersey for the Berkeley shipyards, was in fact, a mixture of crocidolite and amosite." (Wagner JC. The complexities in the evaluation of epidemiologic data of fiber-exposed populations. In: R Lemen, J Dement (Eds.), *Dust and Diseases*. Pathotox, 1979, pp. 37–9.) This is of import since crocidolite was being used in large quantities in asbestos factories in the same area. Dr. Selikoff felt that very little crocidolite had been used in the shipyards and in the United States, and therefore if a mesothelioma developed, it was most likely related to amosite, since there was very little crocidolite exposure. In fact, the monthly trade journal *Asbestos* mentions the early use of crocidolite and amosite asbestos in July 1919.

Drs. John Harington and Neil McGlashan reviewed the destination of South African exports of crocidolite and amosite asbestos, as well as chrysotile, from 1959 until 1993, and their studies indicated that the United States received considerable amounts of crocidolite asbestos right up until 1992. (Harington JS, McGlashan ND. South African asbestos: Production, exports, and destinations, 1959–1993. *Am J Ind Med* 1998;33:321–6.) Their study, and others, have suggested that there was actually more crocidolite asbestos used in the United States than had been previously recognized, and that the use of crocidolite asbestos is a major reason as to why there was an increased risk of mesothelioma. The issue of any fiber other than crocidolite being causative of mesothelioma remained controversial, and in February 1973, Ian Webster published an article in the *South African Medical Journal* entitled "Asbestos and malignancy." He looked at exposure to asbestos, and the association with 232 cases of pleural mesothelioma. Almost all of the individuals had been exposed to Cape Blue asbestos and only two miners had been exposed to amosite, as far as could be discerned. Thirty-two cases occurred in which there was no evidence of any asbestos exposure, presumably having only environmental exposure. Therefore, there were only two cases related to exposure to amosite, out of 232 confirmed cases of mesotheliomas. Dr. Webster remained skeptical as to why this previously rare tumor only seemed to be found in direct relationship to crocidolite exposure. He stated, "Furthermore it is difficult to conceive of amosite in the intermediate group of asbestos fibers causing malignancy, as suggested by Wagner et al. when there are so few cases in the employees of the amosite mines." He went on to say

> The production of amosite far exceeded that of Cape Blue asbestos. It is suggested that more attention should be paid to the determination of the nature of the substance of the Cape Blue areas and not in the Transvaal Blue, and apparently limited to the areas where amosite is mined. (Webster I. Asbestos and malignancy. *S Afr Med J* 1973:47(5):165–71.)

Selikoff, Peto, and coworkers further studied this population of asbestos workers, and they looked at the relationship between initial exposure and eventual development of a mesothelioma. (Peto J, Seidman H, Selikoff IJ. Mesothelioma mortality in asbestos workers: Implications for models of carcinogenesis and risk assessment. *Br J Cancer* 1982;45:124–34.) A "multi-stage" model of carcinogenesis was used to explain the long lag period between the initial exposure to asbestos and the subsequent development of a mesothelioma. They discovered that there was an association between the time of first exposure and the annual incidence of mesothelioma. They determined that mesothelium death rates appeared to rise proportionately to the time since first exposure to an exponent of 3.2 irrespective of age, fiber type, or dust level. They pointed out that this does not mean, of course, that risk is unrelated to fiber type and intensity of exposure, but that these factors influence only b, which is the constant factor in the incidence formula (annual incidence = $b.t^k$). The incidence of mesothelioma is, therefore, summarized by the constant b multiplied by time t to a given power k, usually between 3 and 4. Using this formula, they were able to reproduce the expected incidence of mesotheliomas.

Langer and Nolan wrote an article relating to the crocidolite exposure issue in the United States in 1998. In their appendix on crocidolite consumption in the United States, they pointed out that blue asbestos for boiler and steam coverings for locomotives was advertised in trade journals, such as *The Engine*, as early as 1897. The data from the U.S. Department of Commerce reveal significant crocidolite importation in the 1920s and 1930s, and this included the spraying of crocidolite in the form of Limpet up until 1966. The paper goes on to mention that all three major fiber types were permanently used on ships, and crocidolite was extensively applied in warships in the United Kingdom. Some international investigators outside the United States have interpreted this to mean that crocidolite was also used aboard American ships, and if mesotheliomas occurred among American insulation workers who worked in military shipyards, this was indirect evidence of crocidolite exposure. The authors went on to state,

> Still other investigators suggested that British ships were reoutfitted in U.S.A. ports during the war, and they have been the source of crocidolite exposure to American shipyard workers. This most certainly occurred and citations in the literature support this.

(Langer AM, Nolan RP. Asbestos in the lungs of persons exposed in the US. *Monaldi Arch Chest Dis* 1998;53(2):168–80.)

JC Wagner, by then the world's leading expert on mesothelioma, representing the British Medical Research Council, the International Agency of Cancer Research in Lyon, and the Environmental Health Commission of the European Economic Community, wrote in 1979, "Speaking on behalf of Europe, I would like to make it categorically clear that we believe that, in man, up until today, all mesotheliomas caused by commercial asbestos have been due to crocidolite. This is an emphatic statement." (Wagner JC. The complexities in the evaluation of epidemiologic data on fiber-exposed populations. In: *Dusts and Diseases*. Society of Occupational and Environmental Health, 1979, pp. 37–9.)

Wagner recapitulated his overview of the association between blue asbestos and mesotheliomas in 1991. (Wagner JC. The discovery of the association between blue asbestos and mesotheliomas and the aftermath. *Br J Ind Med* 1991;48:399–403.) He reviewed his story of the discovery of the association between asbestos and mesothelioma, and concluded that there was now evidence that all types of commercial asbestos, except anthophyllite, may be responsible for a mesothelioma. He stated, "The risk is greatest with crocidolite, less with amosite, and apparently less with chrysotile. With amosite and chrysotile, there appears to be a higher risk in manufacturing than in mining and milling." He went on to say "There is overwhelming evidence that crocidolite is a main fiber associated with mesotheliomas." This has primarily been the British view and Raymond Parkes in his classic book *Occupational Lung Disorders* (second edition, 1982) states, "Crocidolite is apparently the type of asbestos, which is overwhelmingly if not exclusively causally related to mesotheliomas in man." Meanwhile, American investigators began to examine the asbestos fiber content in workers with predominately chrysotile asbestos exposure, and noted an inverse relationship between the amount of tremolite asbestos contamination of chrysotile products, and the risk of mesothelioma. (Churg A, Wiggs B, Depaoli L, Kampe B, Stevens B. Lung asbestos content in chrysotile workers with mesothelioma. *Am Rev Respir Dis* 1984;130:1042–5; McDonald AD, Fry JS. Mesothelioma and fiber type in three American factories—Preliminary report. *Scand J Work Environ Heath* 1982;8(Suppl. 1):53–8; McDonald AD, McDonald JC, Pooley FD. Mineral fiber content of lung in mesothelial tumors in North America. *Ann Occup Hyg* 1982;26:417–22.)

More recent studies concerning the relationship between amphibole fibers and mesothelioma have been epidemiologic studies. Researchers in Germany, carefully analyzed fiber burdens in 66 cases of mesothelioma, and 66 controls, from hospitals in five German towns. (Rodelsperger K, Woitowitz HJ, Buckel B, Arheiger R, Pohlabein H, Jockel KH. Dose–response relationship between amphibole fiber lung burden and mesothelioma. *Cancer Diet Prev* 1999;23:183–93.) Lung tissue fiber analysis, by transmission electron microscopy, revealed a clearer dose–response relationship between the concentrations of amphibole fibers longer than 5 μm, and the relationship with mesothelioma causation. The relationship between amphibole asbestos was primarily related to the concentration of crocidolite fibers in the lung, but also amosite. The authors concluded that "amphibole fiber concentration in the lung tissue appears to be a good predictor of risk [of mesothelioma] and this risk was based almost entirely on amosite/crocidolite." The highest concentrations of chrysotile fibers were not observed in the mesotheliomas, but in the controls from Hamburg, Germany. There was no relationship between chrysotile concentration and mesothelioma. Woitowitz stated that Germany used 1.5 times more crocidolite than amosite, and also used sprayed asbestos after World War II. (Woitowitz HJ. Asbestos-related occupational diseases—The current situation. *Asbestos European Conference*, 2003.) Similarly, Ilg and colleagues suggested that the higher mesothelioma rate in France could be explained by different professional uses of asbestos, or a different proportion of amphibole fibers used in commercial asbestos. (Ilg A, Bignon J, Valleron A. Estimation of the past and future fiber burden of mortality from mesothelioma in France. *Occup Environ Med* 1998;55:760–5.)

The German authors published another article on the relationship between asbestos and man-made vitreous fibers, and the risk of malignant mesothelioma. (Rodelsperger K, Jockel KH, Pohlabeln H, Römer W, Woitowitz HJ. Asbestos and man-made vitreous fibers as risk factors for diffuse malignant mesothelioma: Results from a German hospital-based case–control study. *Am J Ind Med* 2001;39:262–75.) This was a German hospital-based case–control study. They concluded that for all measures of asbestos exposure, the odds ratio increased significantly up to 45 at the uppermost intervals. Even at low levels between 0 and 0.15 fiber-years, the odds ratio still was increased. This relationship could have been influenced by information bias, exposure assessment bias, and random error. Their conclusions were "these results confirmed the distinct dose-response relationship of the interview study even at a cumulative exposure below one-fiber year." Again, it needs to be pointed out that in this case–control study in Germany, we are dealing mostly with amphibole asbestos exposure, largely crocidolite, and actual fiber exposure levels were not measured but estimated. The conclusions about exposure levels are biased and based on speculation, because no actual measurements of exposure were available. Their dose estimates are not consistent with other case–control or cohort studies in asbestos product manufacturing, mining, or end-user exposures, in which actual exposures have been measured.

Mesotheliomas have not been found in South African chrysotile miners and millers, despite decades of producing over 100,000 tons of mineral per year. Low amounts of chrysotile and tremolite fibers were found in lung fiber analysis. Margaret Becklake summarized the work of Churg and others, on Canadian miners and millers, who had a geometric mean fiber concentration of nine tremolite fibers for every two chrysotile fibers. Mesothelioma cases in Canada have much higher concentrations of tremolite. (Becklake MR. Fiber burden and asbestos-related lung disease: Determinants of dose–response relationships. *Am J Respir Crit Care Med* 1994;150:1488–92.) The low concentration of tremolite contamination of South African chrysotile asbestos associated with the absence of mesothelioma generation demonstrates that chrysotile exposures, without significant amphibole tremolite contamination at an average exposure of about 1 fiber/cc, are not mesotheliogenic. (Rees D, Phillips JI, Garton E, Pooley FD. Asbestos lung fibre concentrations in South African chrysotile mine workers. *Ann Occup Hyg* 2001;45(6):473–7.)

Sluis-Cremer and coworkers from the Medical Bureau for Occupational Diseases in South Africa, noted that crocidolite asbestos had higher toxicity than amosite, for lung cancer and mesothelioma. Crocidolite-induced mesothelioma appeared only in men who had been exposed for long periods of at least 12 months, but on average 15 years. (Sluis-Cremer GK, Liddell FDK, Logan WPD, Bezuidenhout BN. The mortality of amphibole miners in South Africa, 1946–1980. *Br J Ind Hyg* 1992;49:566–75.) Rees et al. published another study of South African mesothelioma cases in 1999. A convincing history of asbestos exposure was obtained in the overwhelming majority of cases (only five cases had unlikely asbestos exposure). Twenty-three subjects had worked in Cape crocidolite mines (location of earlier case reports by Wagner), three at Penge (an amosite mine), three in mines producing amosite and Transvaal crocidolite and one in a Transvaal crocidolite mine. Exclusively environmental exposure accounted for at least 18% of cases; 91% of these cases (20/22 subjects) had had contact with Cape crocidolite. There was a relative paucity of cases linked to amosite, and no convincing chrysotile cases. Nonasbestos causes occurred rarely, if at all, in South Africa. This report and others demonstrate the importance of fiber size as well as fiber type. The crocidolite mined from the Transvaal area has a larger fiber than from the Cape area, and presumably this plays an important part in the significant difference in mesotheliogenic potential of these different types of crocidolite. (Rees D, Goodman K, Fourie E et al. Asbestos exposure and mesothelioma in South Africa. *S Afr Med J* 1999;89(6):627–34.)

This later data confirmed the earlier report of McCullagh that the majority of mesotheliomas were from crocidolite exposure, as compared to amosite asbestos. (McCullagh SF. Amosite as a cause of lung cancer and mesothelioma in humans. *J Occup Med* 1980;30:153–6.)

16

Chrysotile and mesothelioma

The issue of whether chrysotile asbestos causes mesothelioma has largely been related to the studies of Wagner (1982), Pooley and Mitha (1984), Churg (1984, 1988), Mossman (1990), and McDonald (1989, 1997), and others. (Churg A. Chrysotile, tremolite, and malignant mesothelioma in man. *Chest* 1988;93:621–8; McDonald JC, Armstrong B, Case B et al. Mesothelioma and fiber type. *Cancer* 1989;63:1544–7; Mossman BT, Bigon J, Corn A, Seaton A, Gee JBL. Asbestos: Scientific developments and implications for public policy. *Science* 1990;247:294–301.) McDonald and colleagues further supported what is called the "amphibole hypothesis." (McDonald AD, Case BW, Churg A et al. Mesothelioma in Quebec chrysotile miners and millers: Epidemiology and aetiology. *Ann Occup Hyg* 1997;41:707–19.)

The "amphibole hypothesis" is based on scientific and epidemiologic evidence that pure chrysotile without amphibole contamination (tremolite) does not cause mesothelioma. The McDonald article summarizes the study of a cohort of miners that included 11,000 men, born between 1891 and 1920, who were employed in the Quebec chrysotile production industry. The results of the long-term follow-up of these miners reveals that of 9780 men who survived until 1936, 8009 were known to have died before 1993, and 38 probably died from mesothelioma. Thirty-three of these 38 workers were miners and five were factory workers. The factory workers apparently had exposure to amphibole asbestos in the form of crocidolite and/or amosite. This leaves a total of 33 cases of mesothelioma out of 11,000 initial workers that were studied and about 10,000 that were followed. There appeared to be more mesotheliomas from the Thetford area of Quebec, than from other areas of Quebec where there was less contamination by tremolite in the rock where, asbestos was mined. The results of these careful studies of chrysotile-associated mesothelioma indicate that high concentrations of tremolite asbestos, a known contaminate of these ores, are associated with these mesotheliomas. There have been two careful mineralogical analyses of the Cary Canadian mine, which is unique, in that the studies have not yielded evidence of significant tremolite contamination, or epidemiologic evidence of mesothelioma.

Earlier studies had suggested that chrysotile might cause mesothelioma, and there was caution during the 1960s about chrysotile as an adequate replacement for crocidolite asbestos. With time and the careful studies of McDonald and coworkers in Canada, the evidence has come forth that there does not appear to be any risk of mesothelioma associated with pure chrysotile. Many of the Quebec cohort with mesothelioma were exposed to crocidolite and amosite. McDonald has suggested that these amphibole exposures were due to work in a plant that made military gas mask filters. (McDonald AD, Case BW, Churg A et al. Mesothelioma in Quebec chrysotile miners and millers: Epidemiology and aetiology. *Ann Occup Hyg* 1997;41:707–19.)

More recently, an analysis of lung fiber type and concentration in 123 Quebec asbestos workers, found that 85% had chrysotile fibers in their lungs, 76% had tremolite fibers, 64% had amosite fibers, and 43% had crocidolite fibers in their lungs. Half of the total fibers were short fibers, 30% were thin fibers and 20% were World Health Organization (WHO) fibers of length >5 μm and width between 0.2 and 3 μm. The worker population studied included 38 with asbestosis, 30 with pleural mesothelioma, and 70 with lung cancer. Of those with mesothelioma, 70% had amosite, 70% had chrysotile, 50% had crocidolite, and 70% had tremolite fibers in their lungs, with an average asbestos body count of 4271. (Adib G, Labreche F, De Guire L, Dion C, Dufrene A. Short, fine, and WHO asbestos fibers in the lungs of Quebec workers with an asbestos related disease. *Am J Ind Med* 2013;56:1–14.)

Many research studies have been performed since the 1960s, comparing tremolite-free asbestos to tremolite-contaminated asbestos, as a cause of mesothelioma. The problem with many of the epidemiologic studies of chrysotile asbestos workers, has been the contamination of the cohort by other amphibole exposures, as summarized by Dunnigan in 1988 and Pierce in 2008. (Dunnigan J. Linking chrysotile asbestos with mesothelioma. *Am J Ind Med* 1988;14:205–9; Pierce JS, McKinley MA, Paustenbach DJ, Finley BL. An evaluation of reported no-effect chrysotile asbestos exposures for lung cancer and mesothelioma. *Crit Rev Toxicol* 2008;38:191–214.)

The best recent study that confirmed that tremolite-free asbestos does not cause mesothelioma, was done by Bernstein and coworkers, comparing tremolite-free, Calidria chrysotile asbestos, with tremolite asbestos in rats. Their findings provide an important basis for substantiating both, kinetically and pathologically, the differences between chrysotile and the amphibole tremolite. As Calidria chrysotile has been certified to have no tremolite fibers, the results of this study, together with the results from toxicological and epidemiological studies, indicate that tremolite-free chrysotile asbestos fibers are not associated with mesothelioma, and short asbestos fibers do not induce fibrosis or lung disease in humans or animals. (Bernstein DM, Chevalier J, Smith P. Comparison of Calidria chrysotile asbestos to pure tremolite: Final results of the inhalation biopersistence and histopathology examination following short-term exposure. *Inhal Toxicol* 2005;17:427–49; Bernstein D, Dunnigan J, Hesterberg T et al. Health risk of chrysotile revisited. *Crit Rev Toxicol* 2013;43:154–83.)

The overall exposures to Canadian mixed chrysotile asbestos, contaminated with tremolite asbestos, in those who develop mesotheliomas, have been very high (i.e., more than twice the fiber concentration of comparable workers with asbestosis). (Liddell FD, McDonald AD, McDonald JC. The 1891–1920 birth cohort of Quebec chrysotile miners and millers: development from 1904 and mortality to 1992. *Ann Occup Hyg* 1997;41(1):13–36.) A recent review of fiber analysis performed on the lungs of Canadian Quebec chrysotile asbestos workers referred for compensation purposes, revealed that 85% of workers had chrysotile asbestos in their lungs, 74% had tremolite fibers, 64% had amosite fibers, and 43% had tremolite, amosite, and crocidolite fibers in their lungs. The fiber analysis of their 30 mesothelioma cases revealed that 50% had significant amounts of crocidolite, 70% had elevated amounts of amosite and/or tremolite asbestos, and 86.8% had elevated levels of chrysotile asbestos in their lungs. This lung fiber analysis study indicates that Quebec asbestos workers often have significant exposures to many different types of amphibole fibers. (Adib G, Labrèche F, De Guire L, Dion C, Dufresne A. Short, fine and WHO asbestos fibers in the lungs of Quebec workers with an asbestos-related disease. *Am J Ind Med* 2013;56:1001–14.)

Studies in Greece have also confirmed that chrysotile exposures high enough to produce lung cancer have not produced any mesotheliomas. (Sichletdi L, Chloros D, Spyratos D et al. Mortality from occupational exposure to relatively pure chrysotile: A 39-year study. *Respiration* 2009;78(1):63–8.) Others have claimed that pure chrysotile can cause a mesothelioma, such as the studies of asbestos miners in Balangero, Italy, where an excess number of mesotheliomas have occurred. (Miabelli D, Calisti R, Barone-Adesi F, Fornero E, Merletti F, Magnani C. Excess of mesotheliomas after exposure to chrysotile in Balangero, Italy. *Occup Environ Med* 2007;65:815–9.) Originally, this was thought to be an example of pure chrysotile asbestos-caused mesothelioma. However, a unique new fiber was found contaminating the asbestos ore called balangeroite. This fiber is similar to tremolite but mineralogically distinct. The balangeroite fiber contamination is thought to be the source of the mesotheliomas in this group of miners. (Turci F, Tomatis M, Compagnoni R, Fubini B. Role of associated mineral fibres in chrysotile asbestos health effects: The case of balangeroite. *Ann Occup Hyg* 2009;53(5):491–70.)

Studies in China have claimed mesotheliomas in amphibole-free chrysotile asbestos. (Yano E, Wang ZM, Wang XR, Wang MZ, Lan YJ. Cancer mortality among workers exposed to amphibole-free chrysotile asbestos. *Am J Epidemiol* 2001;154(6):538–43.) This article was refuted by Tossavianen and colleagues, who found amphibole contamination in Chinese chrysotile asbestos. (Tossavainen A, Kotilainen M, Takahashi K, Pan G, Vanhala E. Amphibole fibres in Chinese chrysotile asbestos. *Ann Occup Hyg* 2001; 45(2):145–52.)

Wang and others studied 1539 Chinese chrysotile asbestos miners and found an increased risk of lung cancer with increasing asbestos exposure, but no mesotheliomas were found in this heavily chrysotile-exposed cohort. Exposures were estimated and the high numbers of lung cancers and asbestosis suggests that exposures were underestimated. No increased risk of lung cancer was seen in smokers with <20 fiber-years of exposure and nonsmokers with <100 fiber-years of exposure. Furthermore, the Chinese data indicate a good correlation between no remarkable respiratory disease (NMRD) or asbestosis, and the risk of lung cancer. (Wang X, Yano E, Lin S et al. Cancer mortality in Chinese chrysotile asbestos miners: Exposure–response relationships. *PLoS One* 2013;8(8):e71899.)

In 1976, Fred Pooley performed quantitative electron microscopic counting of fibers recovered from lung tissue in Quebec chrysotile miners and millers. He found more tremolite asbestos in the lungs than chrysotile. This raises the question as to whether it was tremolite or chrysotile that caused the mesotheliomas. Later, Drs. Churg and Wiggs actually found levels of tremolite in the lung samples from five Quebec chrysotile workers with mesothelioma that were an order of magnitude higher than those for chrysotile fibers. It was these studies that gave birth to what was called the amphibole hypothesis. This hypothesis was that it is the needle-like long amphibole fibers that are predominantly, if not exclusively, associated with mesothelioma.

Dr. Churg further clarified his position in a letter to the editor of the *American Journal of Industrial Medicine* in 1988, in which he stated that his data indicated that chrysotile contaminated with tremolite could cause mesotheliomas in humans. (Churg A. Chrysotile, tremolite, and malignant mesothelioma in man. *Chest* 1988;93(3):621–8.) His studies were based on workers who had been exposed to chrysotile with tremolite contamination mined in Quebec. Churg has not studied workers with chrysotile exposure without tremolite contamination and none of these workers have developed mesothelioma. Dr. Churg also pointed out that the amphibole content of the chrysotile of exposed workers was more than two orders of magnitude greater than the amphibole content found in the lungs of shipyard workers, implying that the induction of mesothelioma from tremolite-contaminated chrysotile ore requires an extremely high exposure. He also referred to his 1984 article (Churg A, Wiggs B, Depaoli L, Kampe B, Stevens B. Lung asbestos content in chrysotile workers with mesothelioma. *Am Rev Respir Dis* 1984;130:1042–5) showing that the tremolite content in the lungs of chrysotile miners exposed to chrysotile equals or exceeds the chrysotile content of the lung tissue. This establishes that chrysotile does not seem to as readily accumulate in the lung as does amphibole tremolite fibers. He also pointed out that his later data indicated that lower ratios of chrysotile tremolite were found in the lungs of workers exposed to various types of processed chrysotile products.

Dr. Churg agreed that tremolite fibers could cause mesothelioma, and it is most likely the amphibole tremolite contamination of mined chrysotile asbestos fibers that is the cause a mesothelioma, but he was unable to rule out at that time whether extremely high doses of pure chrysotile could cause a mesothelioma.

Further studies were done so that by 1989, Sir Richard Doll, a medical giant in the field of epidemiology, concluded that

> While hesitating to give chrysotile a completely clean bill of health ... the difference between the effects of chrysotile and amphiboles ... is so great in relation to mesothelioma that it is not possible to argue that a man's occupational exposure to chrysotile, with the presence of unattended contamination with many minute amounts of tremolite, is the cause of mesothelioma. (Doll R. Mineral fibres in the non-occupational environment: Concluding remarks. *Non Occupational Exposure to Mineral Fibers IARC* 1989;90:511–8.)

One of the big issues that epidemiologists struggle with, is whether there is a threshold dose for a given toxin, below which, exposures to that toxin will not cause a measurable increase in disease. This was studied by Liddell and McDonald in 1997, who examined the mortality experience of 11,000 male Québec chrysotile miners and millers. They concluded that those exposed to less than 300 million particles per cubic foot years, which is equivalent to roughly 1000 fiber years, did not have a significant increase in death. (Liddell FD, McDonald AD, McDonald JC. The 1891–1920 birth cohort of Quebec chrysotile miners and millers: development from 1904 and mortality to 1992. *Ann Occup Hyg* 1997;41(1):13–36.)

McDonald, Case, and Churg summarized the findings establishing that the risk of developing a mesothelioma from exposure to chrysotile, was proportional to the contamination of the chrysotile ore with tremolite, in the central areas of Québec, particularly in the Thetford mine as compared to other mines. In a separate paper, they examined the cause a mesothelioma in the 33 of 11,000 workers who developed a mesothelioma. 22 of these cases were from Thetford, where there is significant tremolite contamination of the asbestos ore, and 5 were from Asbestos, Québec, where the tremolite contamination is lower. The risk of developing mesothelioma was proportional to the concentration of exposure to tremolite, and the risk was greater in the area of Thetford because of a higher concentration of tremolite fibers. (McDonald AD, Case BW, Churg A et al. Mesothelioma in Quebec chrysotile miners and millers: Epidemiology and aetiology. *Ann Occup Hyg* 1997;41:707–19.)

The issue of tremolite contamination of asbestos became very important. The Carey Canadian mine is located in a different geological setting from the major asbestos mining area in Quebec. Many years ago, in 1980, this area in Eastern Quebec was evaluated by a postgraduate student of Dr. Pooley, MA Butler, for his PhD thesis. Dr. Butler found no evidence of significant tremolite contamination. The chrysotile in the Carey deposit was found to be mainly of the slip fiber geological type with only small quantities of cross vein geological fiber present. This was unlike the chrysotile from other Quebec mines, which is mainly of the cross vein fiber type. The cross vein chrysotile fiber is of a higher quality than slip fiber chrysotile because it has longer fibers, which makes it more useful for textile applications. It is also more likely to be contaminated with amphibole tremolite asbestos. This data analysis was published in the PhD thesis of Dr. Butler in 1980.

The Carey chrysotile mine area was reevaluated by Dr. Mickey Gunter and others in 2007 and a careful analysis of ore samples, using polarized light microscopy and x-ray diffraction methods, found only extremely small trace amounts of amphibole, in the range of 50–120 parts per million. This level was thought to be an overestimate. The amount of tremolite amphibole in the Thetford, Quebec area is close to 1%, or 10,000 parts per million. This indicates that the Carey Canadian asbestos has extremely low, trace concentrations of amphibole contamination, and therefore Carey asbestos is unlikely to produce a mesothelioma. Furthermore, Carey chrysotile has never been reported to cause a mesothelioma in the medical literature. (Gunter M. *Can Mineral* 2007;45:263–80.)

Victor Roggli and others did a clinical pathological correlation study of 1445 cases of malignant mesothelioma; 268 of these cases underwent fiber burden analysis, and while chrysotile fibers were detectable in 36 cases, all but two of these cases had above background levels of commercial amphiboles. The presumption is that cases that do not have elevated levels of amphibole asbestos are most likely idiopathic or spontaneous mesotheliomas unrelated to an occupational exposure. (Roggli VL, Sharma A, Butnor KJ, Sporn T, Vollmer RT. Malignant mesothelioma and occupational exposure to asbestos: A clinicopathological correlation of 1445 cases. *Ultrastruct Pathol* 2002;26:55–65.) In a later paper published in 2006, Dr. Roggli used a larger case series of 396 mesothelioma cases and he concluded by fiber analysis that mesotheliomas in women had elevated tissue asbestos content in about 60% of cases, and that the main fiber identified was predominantly commercial amosite asbestos. Dr. Roggli stated that "chrysotile is a much less potent inducer of mesotheliomas in humans and there is no convincing evidence that chrysotile causes or contributes to development of a peritoneal mesothelioma." (Roggli VL. The role of analytical SEM in the determination of causation in malignant mesothelioma. *Ultrastruct Pathol* 2006;30:31–5.) In a 2007 paper, Dr. Roggli concluded that asbestos bodies were identified by light microscopy in 92% of his group 1 and 89% of his group 2 patients with mesothelioma. He also concluded that amosite was the most frequently detected fiber type, but that crocidolite asbestos showed an increased detection frequency with time (*Hum Pathol* 2007;20:1–9).

Other investigators have evaluated the relationship between asbestos fiber concentration and relative risk for mesothelioma and have found a dose–response relationship. (Rogers AJ, Leigh J, Berry G et al. Relationship between lung asbestos fiber type and concentration and relative risk of mesothelioma. A case–control study. *Cancer* 1991;67(7):1912–20; Tuomi T, Huuskonen MS, Virtamo M et al. Relative risk of mesothelioma associated with different levels of exposure to asbestos. *Scand J Work Environ Health* 1991;17(6):404–8.)

In 2007, a panel of international experts was invited to Montreal, Quebec, to evaluate the health hazards from exposure to chrysotile asbestos. The panel reviewed the literature, and noted that previous studies by Liddell and others in 1997, found that the dose of Quebec chrysotile asbestos required to produce a mesothelioma was more than twice the level necessary to produce asbestosis. Men exposed to high levels of asbestos at the level of 900 fiber-years showed no increased risk for developing a mesothelioma. (Liddell FD, McDonald AD, McDonald JC. The 1891–1920 birth cohort of Quebec chrysotile miners and millers: Development from 1904 and mortality to 1992. *Ann Occup Hyg* 1997;41:13–36.)

This confirms the work of Andrew Churg who also demonstrated by fiber analysis that extremely high levels of chrysotile and tremolite fibers are required to produce a mesothelioma. (Churg A. Analysis of lung asbestos content. *Br J Ind Med* 1991;48(10):649–52; McDonald AD, Case BW, Churg A et al. Mesothelioma in Quebec chrysotile miners and millers: Epidemiology and aetiology. *Ann Occup Hyg* 1997;41(6):707–19.) Studies on housewives living in Thetford, Quebec, and others never exposed to asbestos, who had environmental exposure to chrysotile, demonstrated that the ambient environmental level of asbestos fibers in the air was 100 times greater in the mining community, than in the general Canadian air, with an estimated exposure of 25 fiber-years. There was a small increased risk of mesothelioma in those women that were exposed to high levels of asbestos fibers, six of whom developed mesothelioma and lived in Thetford, of which five worked in the asbestos industry, but no cases of mesothelioma occurred in Asbestos, Quebec, where there was lower exposure to tremolite. The residential, domestic, and occupational exposures were huge and estimated at 226.1 fibers/mL-year. (Camus M, Richardson L, Parent MÉ, Desy M, Siemiatycki J. Preliminary findings for pleural mesothelioma among women in the Québec chrysotile mining regions. *Ann Occup Hyg* 2002;46(Suppl. 1):128–31; Camus M, Siemiatycki J, Case BW, Desy M, Richardson L, Campbell S. Risk of mesothelioma among women living near chrysotile mines versus US EPA asbestos risk model: Preliminary findings. *Ann Occup Hyg* 2002;46(Suppl. 1):95–8.) Bourgault and Belleville measured the ambient chrysotile fiber level in a mining town in Quebec at around 4 fibers/L of air, and chrysotile asbestos mining levels in the 1990s were estimated to be around 1000 fibers/L of air. (Bourgault MH, Belleville D. Presence of asbestos fibers in indoor and outdoor air in the city of Thetford mines: Estimation of lung cancer and mesothelioma risks. Montreal, Canada, 2010; Lajoie P, Dion C, Drouin L et al. Asbestos fibers in indoor and outdoor air—The situation in Quebec, Montreal, Canada, 2005.) The overall risk estimate for lung cancer and mesothelioma has been estimated by Bourgault et al. in the Thetford mining area of Quebec. These unit risks were then combined with recent environmental measurements made in the mining town, to calculate the estimated lifetime risk of asbestos-induced lung cancer and mesothelioma. Depending on the chosen potency factors, the lifetime mortality risks varied between 0.7 and 2.6 per 100,000 for lung cancer, and between 0.7 and 2.3 per 100,000 for mesothelioma. In conclusion, the estimated lifetime cancer risk for both cancers combined, is close to Health Canada's threshold for "negligible" lifetime cancer risks. However, the risks estimated are subject to several uncertainties and should be confirmed by future mortality rates attributed to present-day asbestos exposure (see Figures 16.1 and 16.2). (Bourgault MH, Gagné M, Valcke M. Lung cancer and mesothelioma risk assessment for a population environmentally exposed to asbestos. *Int J Hyg Environ Health* 2014;217(2–3):340–6.)

- Lifetime exposures in Eastern Quebec are several hundred times greater than those of typical urban dwellers without noting an increased incidence of mesothelioma in nonoccupationally exposed individuals.

- Several occupationally exposed populations with significant exposures have been studied but no excess risk of lung cancer or mesothelioma has been found.

Figure 16.1 Threshold data from asbestos mines in Quebec. (From Tubianam. The carcinogenic effects of low-dose asbestos. *Br J Ind Med* 1992;49:601.)

- Average exposure of the women with mesothelioma estimated at 226 fibers/cc-year
- Average exposure of control cases 84 fibers/cc-year
- All lived close to central mines (high tremolite mines)

Figure 16.2 Mesothelioma in women living in the Quebec mining townships showing high average exposures of women without mesothelioma. (From Camus et al. *Ann Occup Hyg* 2002;46:95–98; Case et al. *Ann Occup Hyg* 2002;46:128–131.)

A retrospective Cohort study in a chrysotile asbestos factory in Tianjin, China, revealed a high incidence of lung cancer associated with heavy exposure and asbestosis. No mesotheliomas were identified in this heavily exposed population. (Cheng WN, Kong J. A retrospective mortality cohort study of chrysotile asbestos workers in Tianjin 1972–1987. *Environ Res* 1992;59:271–8.)

These scientific data indicate a very low risk from the exposure to amphibole-contaminated chrysotile asbestos, and no risk from non- or minimally amphibole contaminated chrysotile, such as Carey Canadian chrysotile and certain chrysotile mines in China. (Wang X, Yano E, Lin S et al. Cancer mortality in Chinese chrysotile asbestos miners: Exposure–response relationships. *PLoS One* 2013;8(8):e71899.)

David Bernstein and John Hoskins evaluated the health effects of chrysotile based on recent data in 2006. They pointed out that one of the great difficulties in evaluating past exposure estimates in epidemiologic data is that many of the studies did not differentiate between chrysotile and amphibole exposure. Most of the epidemiologic studies had mixed exposure to commercial amphiboles as well as chrysotile asbestos. They concluded that chrysotile asbestos in heavy exposures causes lung cancer, but that there was no evidence that low exposures to pure chrysotile presented any detectable risk to health or caused mesothelioma. (Bernstein DM, Hoskins JA. The health effects of chrysotile: Current perspective based upon recent data. *Regul Toxicol Pharmacol* 2006;45:252–64.)

David Bernstein more recently reviewed the toxicological information on chrysotile asbestos, and concluded that bio-persistence and subchronic inhalation toxicology studies, have shown that exposure to chrysotile at up to 5000 times the current threshold limit value (0.1 fibers/cm) produces no pathological response. These studies demonstrate as well that following short-term exposure, the longer chrysotile fibers rapidly clear from the lung and are not observed in the pleural cavity. In contrast, short-term exposure to amphibole asbestos quickly results in the initiation of a pathological response in the lung and the pleural cavity. (Bernstein DM. The health risk of chrysotile asbestos. *Curr Opin Pulm Med* 2014;20(4):366–70.)

In 2007, Charles Yarborough evaluated the risk of mesothelioma from exposure to chrysotile asbestos. He reviewed the data from 71 occupational cohorts in the scientific literature in which there was asbestos exposure, and the number of mesotheliomas produced from those exposures. Of the 71 cohorts reported in the literature, 14 had exposure to chrysotile asbestos without any exposure to amphibole asbestos. Seven mesotheliomas reported in this series—but no pleural mesothelioma—could be confirmed and the diagnosis of these cases was questionable. Of 32,853 individuals exposed to amphibole asbestos, there were 404 cases of mesothelioma reported, or an incidence of 1.23%. In mixed chrysotile and amphibole exposures, the percentage of mesotheliomas was 0.67% or 994 out of 147,384. In contrast, only seven possible cases of mesothelioma were observed in 32,039 individuals, giving a percentage of 0.04% of those exposed only to chrysotile. Yarborough concluded that (1) pure amphiboles are the major causes of mesothelioma; (2) mixtures of chrysotile and amphibole develop fewer mesotheliomas than amphibole exposure alone; and (3) careful analysis of cohorts with chrysotile exposure alone, uncontaminated by amphibole, demonstrates no evidence of a risk for mesothelioma. (Yarborough CM. The risk of mesothelioma from exposure to chrysotile asbestos. *Curr Opin Pulm Med* 2007;13(4):334–8.)

One of the big problems in looking at epidemiologic studies is that many of the workers have died, and in retrospective analysis, no information is available as to whether workers had worked elsewhere in the asbestos industry and were exposed to amphibole asbestos in another factory or location prior to coming to work for the employer where the study was performed. Yarborough also pointed out that in another case–control study of 123 mesotheliomas in South Africa, no case with a history of chrysotile exposure alone had been identified. He further noted that the combined relative risk for chrysotile was not significantly elevated for neighborhood or household exposures. His final statement was that "the contention that airborne exposure to only chrysotile fibers is a risk factor for pleural mesothelioma is disputable. The basis for determining whether chrysotile asbestos causes mesothelioma should rest primarily upon the results of analytic epidemiological studies."

Drs. Graham Gibbs and Geoffrey Berry reviewed the epidemiologic data on mesothelioma and asbestos in 2008, and concluded that exposure to chrysotile in a pure form is likely to present a very low risk, if any, of mesothelioma. The majority of mesothelioma tumors result from exposure to asbestos minerals of the amphibole type. They concluded that it seems probable that chrysotile in a pure form may not cause mesothelioma in humans. Because experimental evidence suggests that different fiber lengths produce different mesothelioma risks, comparison should be done on a size basis based in such comparisons. (Gibbs GW, Berry G. Mesothelioma and asbestos. *Regul Toxicol Pharmacol* 2008;52(1 Suppl.):S223–31.)

Epidemiologists have reviewed the relationship between amphibole exposure at the Charleston, South Carolina, navy yard to workers in surrounding chrysotile-based industries. Workers with presumably pure chrysotile asbestos exposure often have unknown concurrent amphibole asbestos exposure. (Bernstein D, Dunnigan J, Hesterberg T et al. Health risk of chrysotile revisited. *Crit Rev Toxicol* 2013;43(2):154–83.)

Drs. Berman and Crump had previously prepared a report for the Environmental Protection Agency (EPA) on the potency factors and risk of asbestos-related lung cancer and mesothelioma. The EPA model for mesothelioma predicts that the mortality rate for mesothelioma increases linearly with the intensity of exposure, and for a given intensity, increases indefinitely after exposure ceases, approximately as a square of time since first exposure, lagged 10 years. The hypothesis that chrysotile asbestos and amphibole asbestos are equally potent was strongly rejected by every metric, and the notion that pure chrysotile is nonpotent for mesothelioma was not rejected by any metric. The best estimates of the relative potency for chrysotile range from zero to about a 200th of that of amphibole asbestos. The hypothesis that chrysotile and amphibole asbestos were equally potent for lung cancer was again rejected. The EPA work group concluded that amphiboles are four times as potent as chrysotile asbestos in inducing lung cancer and 800 times as potent in producing mesothelioma. (Berman DW, Crump KS. A meta-analysis of asbestos-related cancer risk that addresses fiber size and mineral type. *Crit Rev Toxicol* 2008;38(Suppl. 1):49–73; Berman DW, Crump KS. Update of potency factors for asbestos-related lung cancer and mesothelioma. *Crit Rev Toxicol* 2008;38(Suppl. 1):1–47.) Previous studies by Drs. Hodgson and Darnton, estimated the risk of mesothelioma for chrysotile versus amosite and crocidolite asbestos as 1:100:500, respectively. (Hodgson JT, Darnton A. The quantitative risks of mesothelioma and lung cancer in relation to asbestos exposure. *Ann Occup Hyg* 2000;44(8):565–601; Darnton A, Hodgson J, Benson P, Coggon D. Mortality from asbestosis and mesothelioma in Britain by birth cohort. *Occup Med (Lond)* 2012;62(7):549–52; Hodgson JT, Darnton A. Mesothelioma risk from chrysotile. *Occup Environ Med* 2010;67(6):432; Rake C, Gilham C, Hatch J, Darnton A, Hodgson J, Peto J. Occupational, domestic and environmental mesothelioma risks in the British population: A case–control study. *Occup Med (Lond)* 2012;62(7):549–52.)

Dr. Jennifer Pierce and others, in 2000, reported no affect from chrysotile asbestos for exposures relating to lung cancer and mesothelioma. The preponderance of cumulative no-effect exposure levels for lung cancer and mesothelioma fell into a range of 25–2000 fibers per cc/year for lung cancer and 15–500 fibers per cc/year for mesothelioma. The majority of studies did not report an increased risk of cancer at the highest estimated exposure. Pierce et al. felt that these data showed that there were no observed adverse effects from exposures to 2 fibers per cc/year of exposure. Occupational exposures, such as to friction products, have not produced any evidence of an increased risk of asbestos-related diseases or mesothelioma. They concluded that there should be further research into a nonlinear threshold cancer risk model for chrysotile-related respiratory diseases. (Pierce JS, McKinley MA, Paustenbach DJ, Finley BL. An evaluation of reported no-effect chrysotile asbestos exposures for lung cancer and mesothelioma. *Crit Rev Toxicol* 2008;38:191–214.) These results are extremely liberal estimates of risk, because they use a linear model for risk, rather than a more conservative model, which would use a minimal threshold model to determine risk.

THE FIBER TOXICOLOGY OF CHRYSOTILE ASBESTOS

Chrysotile asbestos is rapidly cleared from human and animal lungs, with a clearance half-time, of fibers longer than 20 μm, ranging from 0.3 to 11.4 days, depending on chrysotile fiber type. This means that chrysotile fibers do not stay in the lung for long periods compared to the sharp, needle-like fibers of amphibole asbestos, which have a clearance half-time of more than 20 years. Those chrysotile fibers that have been ingested by lung macrophages, may remain in the lung for longer periods because they are protected from further degradation. (Bernstein DM, Donaldson K, Decker U et al. A biopersistence study following exposure to chrysotile asbestos alone or in combination with fine particles. *Inhal Toxicol* 2008;20:1009–28.) Perhaps the best recent review on fiber toxicology is by Morton Lippmann from New York University in Tuxedo, New York. This paper is highly recommended to those desiring a much deeper review of fiber toxicology. (Lippmann M. Toxicological and epidemiological studies on the effects of airborne fibers: Coherence and public health implications. *Crit Rev Toxicol* 2014;44(8):643–95.) Lippmann's main conclusion is that mesothelioma, lung cancer, and asbestosis are caused by thin bio-persistent fibers longer than 20 µm. Furthermore, he points out the limitations of asbestos exposure analysis by the standard National Institute for Occupational Safety and Health (NIOSH) membrane filter phase-contrast microscopy technique, which does not count the small, thin, pathogenic fibers that can only be seen by electron microscopy.

Ken Donaldson and others have performed elegant experiments that demonstrate that the pleura stomata are the key sites of retention of long versus short fibers. Short fibers easily pass through these stomata and are removed by the pleural lymphatics. The inability of long, thin asbestos fibers to pass through these stomata leads to inflammatory changes at the edge of the visceral pleura that are thought to be the precursors of mesothelioma. Asbestos-related lung cancers have a different pathogenesis that seems to be related to the enhanced deposition of fibers at airway bifurcations rather than pleural stoma (see Figure 16.3).

The iron content of amphibole asbestos fibers is very important since iron catalyzes the Fenton reaction to convert nitric oxide to nitrite, which is toxic to living cells. It produces reactive oxygen species, which cause gene mutations and cell damage. Chrysotile is a magnesium silicate in contrast to the iron-rich

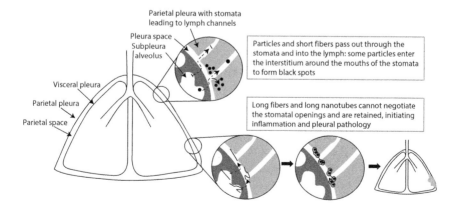

Figure 16.3 Demonstration of why only long, thin fibers are pathogenic for mesothelioma. (From Donaldson K, Murphy FA, Duffin R, Poland CA. *Part Fibre Toxicol* 2010;7(5):1–17. With permission.)

amphiboles. The lack of iron in chrysotile greatly reduces its ability to cause the release of free radicals and cellular and genetic damage. (Mossman BT, Churg A. Mechanisms in the pathogenesis of asbestosis and silicosis. *Am J Respir Crit Care Med* 1998;157:1666–80.) Japanese investigators have correlated body iron content with the risk for mesothelioma. (Toyokuni S. Iron overload as a major targetable pathogenesis of asbestos-induced mesothelial carcinogenesis. *Redox Rep* 2014;19(1):1–7.)

Recently, Italian investigators have investigated the surface reactivity of asbestos fibers:

The zeta (ξ) potential of pathogenic mineral fibres (chrysotiles, amphiboles and erionite) was systematically investigated to shed light on the relationship between surface reactivity and fibre pathogenicity. A general model explaining the zeta potential of chrysotile, amphiboles and erionite has been postulated. In double distilled water, chrysotiles showed positive values while crocidolite and erionite showed negative values. In contact with organic solutions, all fibres exhibited negative values of zeta potential. The decrease of the surface potential is deemed to be a defensive chemical response of the macrophage cells to minimize hemolytic damage. Negatively charged surfaces favor the binding of collagen and redox activated Fe-rich proteins, to form the so-called asbestos bodies and prompt the formation of HO via the reaction with peroxide ($H_2O_2 + e^- \rightarrow HO + HO^-$). An additional mechanism accounting for higher carcinogenicity is possibly related to the Ca^{2+} sequestration by the fibres with surface negative potential, impairing the mitochondrial apoptotic pathway. It was also found that with a negative zeta potential, the attractive forces prevailed over repulsions and favoured processes such as agglomeration responsible of a tumorigenic chronic inflammation. (Pollastri S, Gualtieri AF, Gualtieri ML et al. The zeta potential of mineral fibres. *J Hazard Mater* 2014;276C:469–79.)

One of the other issues related to the carcinogenicity of chrysotile asbestos is due to fiber dimensions, particularly fiber diameter and fiber length. Studies in animals have shown that long, thin fibers are carcinogenic, while short fibers do not pose a risk of causing either lung cancer or mesothelioma. One of the mysteries in science over the years, has been the question as to why there has been such a significantly increased risk of lung cancer related to exposures to chrysotile asbestos in the asbestos textile plants from North and South Carolina, as compared to the miners and millers of the asbestos in Quebec. Various experts had speculated over the years that the occurrence of lung cancer in the textile industry was related to fiber size, since long, thin fibers are present in great numbers in the production of asbestos-containing textiles. During the 1960s, the measurements taken in the plants used phase-contrast light microscopy that counted fibers but could not measure long, thin fibers.

Fortunately, slides of fiber counts from different areas of the plants were saved and reevaluated more recently using electron microscopy. John Dement's group at Duke University, was able to compare the number of long, thin fibers present in prior exposure specimens, to the incidence of lung cancer. They found that the correlation between the incidence of lung cancer and asbestos exposure was good when related to fiber dimensions, particularly long, thin fibers. (Loomis D, Dement J, Richardson D, Wolf S. Asbestos fiber dimensions and lung cancer mortality amounts workers exposed to chrysotile. *Occup Environ Med* 2010;67(9):580–4; Hein MJ, Stayner LT, Lehman E, Dement JM. Follow-up study of chrysotile textile workers: Cohort mortality in exposure–response. *Occup Environ Med* 2007;64:616–25.) There were only three mesothelioma deaths that occurred in this group of 3072 workers in South Carolina. These workers may have been exposed to crocidolite asbestos that was also used for a short time from the 1950s until 1975. Drs. Dement, Green, Case, Stayner, and others, do not feel that the small number of mesotheliomas was related to chrysotile exposure, but rather to amphibole exposure (see Figure 16.4).

Another important factor in the history of understanding asbestos fiber carcinogenesis, has been the fact that the incidence of mesothelioma in heavily exposed amphibole asbestos groups has ranged from 5% to 10%. Even though some individuals have been very heavily exposed to asbestos and have asbestosis, they never developed mesotheliomas. This suggests that there is a genetic factor that may increase susceptibility to the cancer-causing effects of the asbestos exposure, since one would expect that the incidence of mesothelioma would increase linearly with increasing asbestos exposure, but it does not. In fact, most of the mesotheliomas occur at low-to-moderate exposure levels,

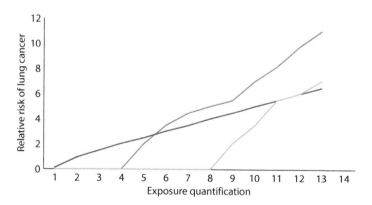

Figure 16.4 The red line is the Occupational Safety and Health Administration (OSHA)/National Institute for Occupational Safety and Health (NIOSH) calculation of risk based on interpolation rather than data. The red line assumes a linear risk model for low-dose exposure in spite of no data. The blue line is the epidemiologic data on risk from textile chrysotile exposure. The green line is the epidemiologic data from chrysotile miners/millers.

and continuous high-level exposures do not proportionately increase the risk of developing a mesothelioma. Michele Carbone and others had speculated that coinfection with the simian virus-40 may be an important factor in the causation of mesotheliomas. This monkey kidney virus contaminated the Salk poliovirus vaccine between 1955 and 1963. The authors have suggested that this virus increases the susceptibility to mesothelioma in individuals exposed to asbestos. (Qi F, Carbone M, Yang H, Gaudino G. Simian virus 40 transformation, malignant mesothelioma and brain tumors. *Expert Rev Respir Med* 2011;5(5):683–97.)

In the early 1980s, three brothers named Kinsman, died of mesothelioma after employment as insulators at the Puget Sound shipyard in Bremerton, Washington. Samuel Hammer and colleagues reported these cases in 1989, raising questions about the importance of familial genetic changes as significant causes of mesothelioma. (Hammar SP, Bockus D, Remington F, Freidman S, LaZerte G. Familial mesothelioma: A report of two families. *Hum Pathol* 1989;20(2):107–12.)

Other genetic data have been elucidated in the studies of groups of individuals in Turkey, and in other areas where there has been good evidence to demonstrate that some families carry an increased genetic susceptibility to mesothelioma. (Weiner SJ, Neragi-Miandoab S. Pathogenesis of malignant pleural mesothelioma and the role of environmental and genetic factors. *J Carcinog* 2008;7:3; Yang H, Testa JR, Carbone M. Mesothelioma epidemiology, carcinogenesis and pathogenesis. *Curr Treat Options Oncol* 2008;9(2–3):147–57; Bianchi C, Bianchi T. Susceptibility and resistance in the genesis of asbestos-related mesothelioma. *Indian J Occup Environ Med* 2008;12:57–60; Neri M, Ugolini D, Dianzani I et al. Genetic susceptibility to malignant pleural mesothelioma and other asbestos-associated disease. *Mutat Res* 2008;659:126–36.)

Interest in Mendelian genetic transmission has largely been supplanted by interest in epigenetics, since only a small percentage of mesotheliomas are familial in the United States, as compared with some areas of Turkey. I have been often asked about the role of asbestos exposure in familial mesothelioma cases. Certainly, in some cases the genetic defect seems to knock out certain regulatory genes that protect against cancer while leaving P53 intact. Additional damage from asbestos exposure provides the necessary genetic and epigenetic changes to produce mesothelial cell immortality. A recent Italian study detected 13 clusters and 34 familial cases, accounting for 3.4% of all mesotheliomas after analyzing a large data set from 10% of the Italian population:

> The most common clusters where those with affected siblings and unaffected parents. Asbestos exposure was occupational (n = 7 clusters), household (n = 2), environmental (n = 1), or not attributable for insufficient information (n = 3). There were 25 additional cancers in nine families. Some were cancer sites for which there is sufficient evidence (lung and larynx) or limited evidence (stomach and colon) of causal association with asbestos. The results suggest potential genetic recessive effects in mesothelioma that interact with asbestos exposure, but it is not possible to estimate

the specific proportion attributable to each of these components. (Ascoli V, Romeo E, Carnovale Scalzo C et al. Familial malignant mesothelioma: A population-based study in Central Italy (1980–2012). *Cancer Epidemiol* 2014;38(3):273–8; Hammar SP, Bockus D, Remington F, Freidman S, LaZerte G. Familial mesothelioma: A report of two families. *Hum Pathol* 1989;20(2):107–12.)

More recently, scientists have recognized epigenetic factors that are major players in cancer causation. William Nelson, a Johns Hopkins oncologist, was puzzled by why Asian men have only a 10% incidence of prostate cancer as opposed to Western men, in whom the majority have prostate cancer. Studies have revealed that as Asian men move to the United States, their risk of prostate cancer rises close to that of American men, suggesting that environmental factors, diet, drugs, and pollutants may play major roles in the incidence of prostate cancer, and other cancers as well, like mesothelioma. These increasing risks are thought to be mediated by epigenetic factors. Epigenetics does not involve the genes that encode proteins, but molecules that attach to DNA and determine how often gene instructions get read and acted upon (genetic metadata). These molecules affect what structures a cell builds and, among other things, whether a cell becomes cancerous. Increasing numbers of epigenetic molecules are being discovered that silence genes designed to protect cells from malignant transformation. The complexity of cancer formation is becoming increasingly obvious. Questions as to why some people with equal asbestos exposure develop cancer and others do not, are yet to be answered, but the evidence suggests that epigenetic factors will be increasingly important. Increasing evidence indicates that unresponsiveness to chemotherapy of mesotheliomas is due to epigenetic errors leading to inadequate gene expression in tumor cells. The availability of compounds that modulate epigenetic modifications, such as histone acetylation or DNA methylation, offers new prospects for the treatment of malignant pleural mesothelioma. (Valdés-Mora F, Clark SJ. Prostate cancer epigenetic biomarkers: Next-generation technologies. *Oncogene* 2015;34(13):1609–18; Mummaneni P, Shord SS. Epigenetics and oncology. *Pharmacotherapy* 2014;34(5):495–505; Huang B, Jiang C, Zhang R. Epigenetics: The language of the cell? *Epigenomics* 2014;6(1):73–88; Vandermeers F, Neelature Sriramareddy S, Costa C et al. The role of epigenetics in malignant pleural mesothelioma. *Lung Cancer* 2013;81(3):311–8.)

17

The tremolite hypothesis

The tremolite hypothesis states that it is amphibole asbestos of any sort that causes mesothelioma, and that chrysotile will not cause mesotheliomas without some amphibole contamination. Theoretically, this is related to the fact that amphibole asbestos is much more durable and therefore bio-persistent, and therefore its residence time in the lung is much longer than that of chrysotile asbestos. Chrysotile asbestos, as used in commercial joint compounds, has a very short half-life, and does not even reach the pleura in animal models of joint compound exposure, when compared to amosite asbestos. (Bernstein DM, Rogers RA, Sepulveda R et al. Quantification of the pathological response and fate in the lung and pleura of chrysotile in combination with fine particle compared to amosite asbestos following short term inhalation exposure. *Inhal Toxicol* 2011;23:372–91.) Therefore, pure chrysotile carries very little risk, if any, for mesothelioma. The current data from exposure to shorter-fiber, amphibole-free chrysotile asbestos from the Calidria asbestos mine, located in New Idria, California, have failed to demonstrate an increased risk of mesothelioma related to this particular fiber type. Only rarely have some "nonfriable" amphibole cleavage fragments been found in this mine. This fiber was used extensively by Georgia Pacific Co. in wallboard joint compounds. (Bernstein DM, Chevalier J, Smith P. Comparison of Calidria chrysotile asbestos to pure tremolite: Final results of the inhalation biopersistence and histopathology examination following short-term exposure. *Inhal Toxicol* 2005;17:427–49.) The Consumer Product Safety Commission banned the use of asbestos in joint compounds in 1978.

John T Hodgson and Andrew Darnton at the Epidemiology and Statistics Unit of the British Government, recently reviewed the quantitative risk for mesothelioma and lung cancer in relation to asbestos exposure. They embarked on a very ambitious plan to review the risk of lung cancer and mesothelioma associated with specific fiber types, based on an overall review of the medical literature. They reviewed a series of studies, and concluded that the exposure risk for mesothelioma from the three principle commercial asbestos types is broadly in the ratio of 1 for chrysotile, 100 for amosite, and 500 for crocidolite. For lung cancer, the conclusions were less clear-cut. It was felt that the risk differences between chrysotile and the two amphibole fibers for lung cancer were somewhere between 1–10 and 1–50. Furthermore, they felt that the risks for peritoneal mesothelioma were proportional to the square of cumulative exposure to asbestos. The lung cancer risk lay between a linear and square relationship, and pleural mesothelioma seemed to rise less than linearly with cumulative dose. Further analysis of their data in comparison to the more recent Environmental Protection Agency (EPA) data of Berman and Crump were published in a Chrysotile Asbestos Expert Panel report entitled *Chrysotile Asbestos Consensus Statement and Summary*, which appeared in Montreal, Canada, on November 13–14, 2007, but was not published until 2009.

In their discussion, the authors mention the controversy about whether chrysotile is a significant cause of mesothelioma based on the papers of Cullen, Stayner et al., Landergren and Nicholson, and Smith and Wright. (Stayner L, Smith R, Bailer J et al. Exposure–response analysis of risk of respiratory disease associated with occupational exposure to chrysotile asbestos. *Occup Environ Med* 1997;54:646–52; Cullen MR. Chrysotile asbestos: Enough is enough. *Lancet* 1998;351(9113):1377–8; Smith AH, Wright CC. Chrysotile asbestos is the main cause of pleural mesothelioma. *Am J Ind Med* 1996;30(3):252–66; Landrigan PJ, Nicholson WJ, Suzuki Y, Ladou J. The hazards of chrysotile asbestos: A critical review. *Ind Health* 1999;37(3):271–80.)

Frank, Dodson, and Williams reported cases of mesothelioma with only chrysotile fibers found in the lung by electron microscopy without any tremolite. No other scientists have reported similar findings. (Frank AL, Dodson RF, Williams MG. Carcinogenic implications of the lack of tremolite in UICC reference chrysotile. *Am J Ind Med* 1998;34(4):314–7.) These authors have argued that there is virtually no difference between the risks from different fiber types. This has been opposed by Doll and Peto in 1985, Hughes and Weil in 1986, the Health Effects Institute in 1991, and others. The authors point out the problem of bias associated with the articles chosen by Smith and Wright and others, who had ranked 25 cohort studies for the risk of pleural mesothelioma. The bias in their study was that there was contamination of the environment with amphibole asbestos in their "chrysotile cohorts," and therefore of the cohorts studied, there was no cohort with pure chrysotile exposure. Therefore, any conclusions drawn on review of these cohorts would be unacceptable because of the inherent bias of the bulk contamination of the chrysotile products with amphibole. They also point out in their article that the U.S. trade journal *Asbestos*, published monthly from 1919, made it clear that both amosite and crocidolite were used in the United States through the 1920s, though probably in limited quantities. Stayner and others who believe in the mesotheliogenic properties of chrysotile have used the argument that all forms of chrysotile can cause mesothelioma in experimental animals. The issue, of course, is that in humans the chrysotile fibers are cleared within weeks, months, or maybe a few years depending on dose, but the resident time of asbestos in a rat is long enough to cause a mesothelioma; in contrast to rats, the residence time of chrysotile asbestos in humans does not appear to be long enough to be causative of a mesothelioma. Rat studies are further complicated by the requirement of huge doses of asbestos fibers by pleural implantation, peritoneal implantation, or inhalation to cause cancer. Similar high exposures have not occurred in industrial processes. Studies of chrysotile miners and millers in Quebec have not demonstrated a statistically significant excess of lung cancer from exposures of up to 300 million particles per cubic foot-year, which is roughly equivalent to more than 1000 fibers/cc-year. (Liddell FD, McDonald AD, McDonald JC. The 1891–1920 birth cohort of Quebec chrysotile miners and millers: Development from 1904 and mortality to 1992. *Ann Occup Hyg* 1997;41:13–36.)

The inclusion of data from long fiber exposure in chrysotile textile factories skews the data on the risk analysis of chrysotile. It is like comparing apples with oranges. The risk for lung cancer in chrysotile textile workers is similar to the risk in many amphibole studies because of the carcinogenic effect of long fibers, which is unique to that particular industry. (Stayner L, Kuempel E, Gilbert S, Hein M, Dement J. An epidemiological study of the role of chrysotile asbestos fibre dimensions in determining respiratory disease risk in exposed workers. *Occup Environ Med* 2008;65(9):613–9; Loomis D, Dement JM, Elliott L et al. An epidemiological study of the role of chrysotile asbestos fibre dimensions in determining respiratory disease risk in exposed workers. *Occup Environ Med* 2012;69(8):564–8.) In some studies of chrysotile asbestos textile mills, the risk for asbestosis and lung cancer has been said to be as low as 25–100 fiber-years (Anon. Asbestos, asbestosis, and cancer: The Helsinki criteria for diagnosis and attribution. *Scand J Work Environ Health* 1997;23(4):311–6). A reevaluation of the data among North Carolina asbestos textile workers indicates that at 100 fibers/cc-year, the lung cancer risk is only 1.1. (Loomis D, Dement JM, Wolf SH. Lung cancer mortality and fiber exposures among North Carolina asbestos textile workers. *Occup Environ Health* 2009;66(8):535–42; Elliott L, Loomis D, Dement J et al. Lung cancer mortality in North Carolina and South Carolina chrysotile asbestos textile workers. *Occup Environ Med* 2012;69(6):385–90.) Risk analysis for chrysotile asbestos exposure can only be accurately performed by segregating populations at risk by fiber length. (Berman DW, Crump KS. A meta-analysis of asbestos-related cancer risk that addresses fiber size and mineral type. *Crit Rev Toxicol* 2008;38(Suppl. 1):49–73; Crump KS, Berman DW. Counting rules for estimating concentrations of long asbestos fibers. *Ann Occup Hyg* 2011;55(7):723–35; Berman DW. Comparing milled fiber, Quebec ore, and textile factory dust: Has another piece of the asbestos puzzle fallen into place? *Crit Rev Toxicol* 2010;40(2):151–88.)

Geoffrey Berry has also discussed the issue of proper models for mesothelioma following exposure to fibers in terms of timing and duration of exposure and the bio-persistence of the fibers. (Berry G. Models for mesothelioma incidence following exposure to fibers in terms of timing and duration of exposure and the biopersistence of the fibers. *Inhal Toxicol* 1999;11:101–20; Lippmann M. *Environmental Toxicants*, 2nd Edition. John Wiley & Sons, 2000, pp. 65–120.)

United States governmental agencies such as the EPA, National Institute for Occupational Safety and Health (NIOSH) and Occupational Safety and Health Administration (OSHA) have decided not to regulate asbestos fibers based on fiber type and fiber length. Their argument has been that while various experts recognize the vast differences in carcinogenicity of different fiber types, widths, and lengths, lay people may become confused by different labels and precautions based on fiber type and fiber length. They have decided that the best governmental policy for public safety is to label all asbestos products as equally hazardous.

Confusion arises from many historical studies evaluating the health risk of chrysotile, because of the ignorance or underestimation of environmental exposures from amphibole asbestos being used by other workers in the same area. This is best exemplified by studies of chrysotile exposure in electricians. Goodman and coworkers concluded, "Both mechanistic and epidemiology studies indicate chrysotile asbestos has a threshold below which it does not cause mesothelioma or lung cancer. Overall, the evidence does not indicate that exposure to chrysotile in electrical products causes mesothelioma or lung cancer in electricians." (Goodman JE, Peterson MK, Bailey LA, Kerper LE, Dodge DG. Electricians' chrysotile asbestos exposure from electrical products and risks of mesothelioma and lung cancer. *Regul Toxicol Pharmacol* 2013;68(1):8–15.)

Lippmann reviewed the literature on animal experiments on fiber type and size relationships in the induction of mesothelioma, and summarized these data in a table on page 90 of his treatise on chronic rat inhalation studies. Based on his review he states,

> I concluded that, for mesothelioma, the relatively low tumor yields seemed to be highly dependent on fiber type. Combining the data from various studies by fiber type, the percentages of mesotheliomas were 0.6% for Zimbabwe (Rhodesian) chrysotile, 2.5% for various amphiboles as a group, and 4.7% for Quebec (Canadian) chrysotile. This difference, together with the fact that Zimbabwe chrysotile has two to three orders of magnitude less tremolite than Quebec chrysotile, provides support for the hypothesis that the mesotheliomas that have occurred among chrysotile miners and millers could be largely due to their exposures to tremolite fibers. The chrysotile may be insufficiently biopersistent because of the dissolution during translocation from the sites of deposition to sites where more durable fibers can influence the transformation or progression to mesothelioma. (Lippmann M. Asbestos and other mineral fibers. In: *Environmental Toxicants III: Human Exposures and Their Health Effects*, 3rd Edition. New York: John Wiley, 2009; Lippmann M. Toxicological and epidemiological studies on airborne fibers: Coherence and public health implications. *Crit Rev Toxicol* 2014;44(8):643–95.)

In summary, over the last 40 years there has been an increasing interest in fiber type and their ability to cause a mesothelioma. The initial studies by Wagner suggested that only crocidolite from a specific area of South Africa, called the Northwest Cape, was the cause of malignant mesothelioma. There was very little evidence of a risk from the area of the Transvaal, where there was also a form of crocidolite fiber present. The fibers found in Transvaal were thicker and therefore thought to be less likely to cause a mesothelioma. The amosite deposits were also contaminated with some of this crocidolite. There were no significant numbers of mesotheliomas found in this area of South Africa in the early 1960s, and it was not until the end of the 1960s that a few cases of amosite-induced mesothelioma were discovered. Up until that time, it was generally thought that amosite was perhaps the safest form of asbestos. A paper by Selikoff and coworkers published in September 1972 pointed out that up until that time, there had not been good evidence of any risk for mesothelioma related to amosite exposure.

An important issue has been the translocation of chrysotile asbestos fibers to the pleura. Suzuki et al. found large numbers of short chrysotile fibers in the pleural space, indicating that chrysotile fibers breach the pleura. There is no evidence that these short chrysotile fibers are causative of mesothelioma. (Suzuki Y, Yuen SR, Ashley R. Short, thin asbestos fibers contribute to the development of human malignant mesothelioma: Pathological evidence. *Int J Hyg Environ Health* 2005;208:201–10.) If we assume that these short fibers are instrumental in the production of mesothelioma, then the chrysotile asbestos mining industry would have the highest incidence of mesothelioma in the world, since these mining operations produce huge amounts of short chrysotile asbestos fibers.

In 2012, a distinguished expert group from the International Agency for Research on Cancer in Lyon, France, estimated asbestos-related lung cancer burden from mesothelioma mortality. This was a very thorough and critical study of different types of asbestos exposures and the risk of lung cancer and mesothelioma. The study group reviewed the 55 best epidemiologic studies published in the world's literature and performed 68 risk analyses. The authors concluded that, for chrysotile asbestos, asbestos-related lung cancers cannot be robustly estimated from the few mesothelioma deaths, and the latter cannot be used to infer there being no excess risk of lung or other cancers. They concluded that many of the mesothelioma deaths in primarily chrysotile-exposed cohorts are actually due to amphibole exposure. (McCormack V, Peto J, Byrnes G, Straif K, Boffetta P. Estimating the asbestos-related lung cancer burden from mesothelioma mortality. *Br J Cancer* 2012;106(3):575–84.) This study was criticized by a group of plaintiff asbestos experts. McCormack and others replied to Lemen's criticisms. (Lemen RA, Frank AL, Soskolne CL, Weiss SH, Castleman B. *Br J Cancer* 2013;109(3):823-5; McCormack V, Peto J, Byrnes G, Straif K, Boffetta P. Reply: Comment on 'estimating the asbestos-related lung cancer burden from mesothelioma mortality'. *Br J Cancer* 2013;109(3):825–6.)

The risk that is present in the miners and millers in Quebec for mesothelioma appears primarily to be related to the contaminated tremolite asbestos, unless there has been exposure to amosite or crocidolite. It is felt by many that the low concentration of tremolite asbestos contaminating the chrysotile asbestos ore, is the cause for the low numbers of mesotheliomas found in this group of heavily exposed miners and millers. More recently, the health risks of chrysotile asbestos were reassessed by a group of scientists from Europe, Canada, Mexico, and the United States. Their conclusion was that heavy and prolonged exposure to chrysotile causes lung cancer, and that studies reporting mesotheliomas from low-to-moderate exposures to chrysotile, uncontaminated with amphibole asbestos, do not have sufficient merit to prove causation from pure chrysotile exposure.

They stated that the studies they report "show that low exposures to chrysotile do not present a detectable risk to health." Furthermore, they suggested that "the risk of an adverse outcome may be low with even high exposure, experienced over short duration." (Bernstein D, Dunnigan J, Hesterberg T et al. Health risk of chrysotile revisited. *Crit Rev Toxicol* 2013;43:154–83.)

Up until recently, there has been a lot of discussion over the relative risks of different forms of asbestos in causing mesothelioma, but now, some of the shouting has stopped and the air is clearing. In 1997, Liddell and coworkers reported data from a cohort of Quebec asbestos miners and millers, of 51.30 thousand person-years at risk in men from the age of 55 years and older, with exposure to the age of less than 300 million particles per cubic foot-years of exposure (one million particles per cubic foot is approximately equivalent to 6 fibers/cc), which was estimated to be above 900 fiber-years (fibers/cc/year). (Liddell FD, McDonald AD, McDonald JC. The 1891–1920 birth cohort of Quebec chrysotile miners and millers: Development from 1904 and mortality to 1992. *Ann Occup Hyg* 1997;41:13–36.) These asbestos-exposed workers showed no increases in risk of lung cancer or mesothelioma at this level of exposure. There was an increased risk of lung cancer above this level, but these data indicate that the risk of lung cancer and/or mesothelioma only occurs at extremely high levels of exposure, which are generally several orders of magnitude higher than the exposures present when using chrysotile-containing products such as automobile brakes, gaskets, and wallboard paste.

Bourgalt and others, in another paper, recently estimated the risk of lung cancer and mesothelioma from environmental exposure in the chrysotile mining town of Thedford, Quebec. Asbestos-related cancer risk is usually a concern restricted to occupational settings. Recently published data on asbestos environmental concentrations in Thetford mines, provided the authors with an opportunity to undertake a prospective cancer risk assessment in the general population exposed to these concentrations. Using an updated Berman and Crump dose–response model for asbestos exposure, they selected population-specific potency factors for lung cancer and mesothelioma. These factors were evaluated on the basis of population-specific cancer data attributed to the studied area's past environmental levels of asbestos. They also used more recent population-specific mortality data, along with the validated potency factors, to generate corresponding inhalation unit risks. These unit risks were then combined with recent environmental measurements, made in the mining town, to calculate estimated lifetime risk of asbestos-induced lung cancer and mesothelioma. Depending on the chosen potency factors, the lifetime mortality risks varied between 0.7 and 2.6 per 100,000 for lung cancer, and between 0.7 and 2.3 per 100,000 for mesothelioma. In conclusion, the estimated lifetime cancer risk for both cancers combined is close to Health Canada's threshold for "negligible" lifetime cancer risks. However, the risks estimated are subject to several uncertainties and should be confirmed by future mortality rates attributed to present-day asbestos exposure. (Bourgault MH, Gagné M, Valcke M. Lung cancer and mesothelioma risk assessment for a population environmentally exposed to asbestos. *Int J Hyg Environ Health* 2014;217(2–3):340–6.)

It is becoming increasingly obvious that amphibole asbestos in the forms of crocidolite, amosite, and tremolite are the major sources of malignant mesothelioma. There are other forms of asbestos-like fibers that are present in the environment that also produce a high risk of mesothelioma, such as erionite in Turkey, but these exposures are only relevant to some focal areas in the United States and Turkey. I do not believe that pure chrysotile asbestos, uncontaminated by tremolite, may cause mesothelioma. However, very high concentrations of tremolite-contaminated chrysotile, sufficient to cause asbestosis and lung cancer, have caused mesothelioma in the past.

There remain a few stalwarts who have opined that chrysotile is the main case of mesothelioma. I hope my well-referenced, up-to-date discussion of the subject will have been an adequate rebuttal to those who continue to expound the view that chrysotile is the main cause of mesothelioma. (Smith AH, Wright CC. Chrysotile asbestos is the main cause of pleural mesothelioma. *Am J Ind Med* 1996;30:252–66.) Berman and others have reviewed the evidence and have found that the potency of commercial asbestos with varying tremolite contamination is one to two orders of magnitude lower than amphibole fiber exposure. They postulated a zero risk for pure chrysotile exposure, and a 700-fold difference in mesothelioma potency, between amphibole and commercial chrysotile. Crocidolite asbestos appears to be five times more potent than amosite asbestos. (Berman DW, Crump KS. A meta-analysis of asbestos-related cancer risk that addresses fiber size and mineral type. *Crit Rev Toxicol* 2008;38(Suppl. 1):49–73; Berman DW, Crump KS. Update of potency factors for asbestos-related lung cancer and mesothelioma. *Crit Rev Toxicol* 2008;38(Suppl. 1):1–47; Donaldson K, Oberdorster G. Continued controversy on chrysotile biopersistence. *Int J Occ Environ Health* 2011;17:98–9; Hodgson JT, Darnton A. Mesothelioma risk from chrysotile. *Occup Environ Med* 2010;67(6):432; Rake C, Gilham C, Hatch J, Darnton A, Hodgson J, Peto J. Occupational, domestic and environmental mesothelioma risks in the British population: A case–control study. *Occup Med (Lond)* 2012;62(7):549–52.)

Finally, the careful analysis of mesothelioma incidence trends in the United States has not demonstrated a significant change in the incidence of mesotheliomas in women from 1907 to 2005. The low incidence in women, in spite of universal low-level background exposure to asbestos fibers, indicates that there is a safe level of exposure and that a threshold level for exposure to asbestos exists. (Price B, Ware A. Mesothelioma trends in the United States: An update based on surveillance, epidemiology, and end results program data from 1973–2003. *Am J Epidemiol* 2004;159:107–12; CDC. Malignant Mesothelioma Mortality—United States, 1999–2005. *MMWR Morb Mortal Wkly Rep* 2009;58(15):393–6.) The safe level of asbestos exposure is based on fiber type, fiber diameter, fiber length, and intensity and duration of fiber exposure. In short, the scientific evidence as reported in the literature, has established amphibole asbestos fiber type, and not pure chrysotile asbestos, as the cause of mesothelioma. All types of asbestos cause asbestosis and lung cancer, but not mesothelioma.

18

Mesothelioma latency and risk

There is a mathematical equation that indicates that individuals who have early exposure to asbestos are going to be affected primarily by these earlier exposures rather than later exposures, since the primary factor on incidence of mesothelioma is latency. The time from the first significant exposure to amphibole asbestos, to the time of the beginning of enough genetic and epigenetic changes to produce cell immortality or cancer, is properly called the *induction period*. The time required for that cancer to develop from the first cell division until the time of diagnosis is called the *initiation period*. The time from the first exposure to asbestos to the time of the discovery of a cancer is called the *latency period* and is the sum of the *induction period* and the *initiation period*. Lanphear and Buncher reviewed the latency period, from first exposure to diagnosis, for malignant mesothelioma (MM) of occupational origin, in an article published in the *Journal of Occupational Medicine*. (Lanphear BP, Buncher CR. Latent period for malignant mesothelioma of occupational origin. 1992;34:718–21.) They discovered after reviewing a large number of studies that the latency period for MM is going to be greater than 20 years in 95% of the cases, and there is a greater than 99% probability of there being a latency of 15 years or longer. This 15–20-year *initiation period* is the time required for cell division, usually 40 doublings of tumor cells, before the tumor is identified. Thus, it is highly unlikely that any mesothelioma is going to be related to any exposure to any asbestos products less than 20 years prior to the discovery of that tumor because of its long initiation period. Again, this reinforces the data of Peto and Selikoff in 1982 that earlier exposures are most likely to be causative of a mesothelioma.

Mesotheliomas today have longer latency times because there is an inverse relationship between fiber burden and latency. (Roggli V, Vollmer R. Twenty five-years of fiber analysis: What have we learned? *Hum Pathol* 2008;39:307–15.) This means that lower exposures produce longer *induction periods*, but the *initiation period* will remain unaffected. French scientists also recently confirmed that the risk of asbestos-related neoplasm was related to exposure intensity, but that the risk does not increase with the duration of exposure. (Clin B, Morias F, Lannoy G et al. Cancer incidence within a cohort occupationally exposed to asbestos: A study of dose–response relationships. *Occup Environ Med* 2011;68:832–6.) Bianchi, Hilliard, and later Newman, agreed that high cumulative exposure to asbestos, such as in pipe insulators, results in shorter latency periods as compared with individuals with relatively low exposures. (Bianchi C, Giarelli L, Grandi G, Brollo A, Ramani L, Zuch C. Latency periods in asbestos-related mesothelioma of the pleura. *Eur J Cancer Prev* 1997;6:162–6; Newman V, Günthe S, Mülle KM, Fischer M. Malignant mesothelioma register 1987–1999. *Int Arch Occup Environ Health* 2001;74:383–95; Hilliard AK, Lovett JK, McGavin CR. The rise and fall in incidence of malignant mesothelioma from a British naval dockyard, 1979–1999. *Occup Med (Lond)* 2003;53:209–12.)

The Western Australia group in Perth, reviewed six large epidemiologic studies with a combined total of 22,048 people, and also concluded that the risk of MM increases proportionally to the cumulative exposure to asbestos, and to the third or fourth power of time since first exposed. However, little is known about the risk of MM after more than 40 years since first exposure, because most epidemiological studies do not have follow-up for sufficient periods of time. While the rate of increase appears to start to level out after 40–50 years, no one survives long enough for the excess risk to disappear. (Reid A, de Klerk NH, Magnani C et al. Mesothelioma risk after 40 years since first exposure to asbestos: A pooled analysis. *Thorax* 2014;69(9):843–50.)

Bruce Robinson, also of Perth, has noted that disease incidence varies markedly within and between countries. The highest annual rates of disease—approximately 30 cases per million—are reported in Australia and Great Britain. The risk of disease increases with age and is higher in men. Time from asbestos exposure to disease diagnosis is on average, greater than 40 years. (Robinson B. Malignant pleural mesothelioma: An epidemiological perspective. *Ann Cardiothorac Surg* 2012;1(4):491–6.) There are marked regional differences in the rates of mesothelioma in the United States. In 1998, the incidence ranged from 4.5 per million in Hawaii, to 23.3 per million in the Seattle–Puget Sound area. (Pinheiro GA, Antao VC, Bang KM et al. Malignant mesothelioma surveillance: A comparison of ICD 10 mortality data with SEER incidence data in nine areas of the United States. *Int J Occup Environ Health* 2004;10:251–5.) Generally, the incidence of mesothelioma, which is higher in Europe than the United States, is related to the greater use of crocidolite asbestos. In the United States, mesothelioma cases are predominately located along coastal areas where there has been ship construction. In a few scattered areas of the world, environmental exposures have produced a very high incidence of mesothelioma, particularly in Turkey due to erionite asbestos exposure, and in New Caledonia, with incidence rates above 1000 per million. (Metintas S, Metintas M, Ucgun I et al. Malignant mesothelioma due to environmental exposure to asbestos: Follow-up of a Turkish cohort living in a rural area. *Chest* 2002;122:2224–9; Baumann F, Maurizot P, Mangeas M et al. Pleural mesothelioma in New Caledonia: Associations with environmental risk factors. *Environ Health Perspect* 2011;119:695–700.)

Frost, who studied 614 workers who died from mesothelioma between 1978 and 2005, has disputed the issue of fiber dose and latency. Total follow-up time was 9280 person-years, with a median latency of 22.8 years (95% confidence interval [CI]: 16.0–27.2 years). In the fully adjusted model, latency was around 29% longer for females compared with males (time ratio [TR]: 1.29; 95%

CI: 1.18–1.42) and 5% shorter for those who died with asbestosis compared with those who did not (TR: 0.95; 95% CI: 0.91–0.99). There was no evidence of an association between latency and occupation. Frost did not find sufficient evidence that greater-intensity asbestos exposures would lead to a shorter latency time for mesothelioma, in contrast to other authors. However, the shorter latency of workers with asbestosis in his study, indicating heavy exposure, and the longer latency of females, which suggests lower exposure, produces the opposite conclusion. (Frost G. The latency period of mesothelioma among a cohort of British asbestos workers (1978–2005). *Br J Cancer* 2013;109(7):1965–73.) The methodology of Frost's calculations and assumptions has been challenged by Mirabelli and Zugna in a letter to the editor of the *British Journal of Cancer* (Mirabelli D, Zugna D. Comment on 'The latency period of mesothelioma among a cohort of British asbestos workers (1978–2005)'. 2014;111(8):1675; Consonni D, Barone-Adesi F, Mensi C. Comment on 'The latency period of mesothelioma among a cohort of British asbestos workers (1978–2005)': Methodological problems with case-only survival analysis. *Br J Cancer* 2014;111(8):1674; Farioli A, Mattioli S, Curti S, Violante FS. Comment on 'The latency period of mesothelioma among a cohort of British asbestos workers (1978–2005)': The effect of left censoring. *Br J Cancer* 2014;111(11):2197–8.)

The Frost data did not account for the importance of historical factors in calculating dose and latency. For instance, most of the asbestos insulators were included in the cohort that was first exposed before 1978, at which time 85% of the cohort members were alive. The asbestos-removers were a second, later cohort, with a much lower and distinct asbestos exposure. The fact that the exposure type, and level or intensity of exposure, changed radically over time, makes it difficult to come to a conclusion when there is such a mixture of exposure groups in the underlying cohort.

In summary, most experts agree that the latency period shortens linearly with dose (the greater the exposure, then the shorter the latency period) and latency rises exponentially with time, which is the same conclusion that Peto et al. made in 1982 (Table 18.1; Figures 18.1 and 18.2). (Peto J, Seidman H, Selikoff IJ. Mesothelioma mortality in asbestos workers: Implications for models of carcinogenesis and risk assessment. *Br J Cancer* 1982;45:124–35.)

Darnton, Hodgson, and others have confirmed that mortality from mesothelioma is highest among men born between 1939 and 1943, and asbestosis deaths are highest in men born between 1924 and 1938 in Great Britain. They concluded that mortality from mesothelioma is determined from exposures in early working life, when higher occupational exposures were present, due to inadequate environmental reductions in exposures, prior to 1970. The strong effect of early exposures can be explained by random DNA damage associated with increased cell turnover as a consequence of chronic inflammation related to retained asbestos fibers. The carcinogenic effect continues after removal from exposure, due to the long half-life of amphibole asbestos. This carcinogenic process takes many years because it requires many genetic and epigenetic events to occur before a mesothelioma cell becomes immortalized. The data indicate that exposures before 45 years of age are the most relevant to risk. The risk for mesothelioma

Table 18.1 Worldwide trends is epidemiologic features of malignant mesothelioma[a]

Country or region	Incidence (cases/ million population)	Predicted peak year	Predicted No. of deaths in next 40 Yr[b]	Predicted cost[c] (billions of U.S. dollars)
United States	15	2004	72,000	200
Europe	18[d]	2015–2020	250,000	80
Japan	7	2025	103,000	–
Australia	40	2015	30,000	5–10

Source: Robinson B.W.S. et al. N Engl J Med 2005; 353:1591–1603.

[a] The sources of the data on the incidence (most recent figures), predicted peak year, and predicted number of deaths in the next 40 years are as follows: United States, Roushdy-Hammady et al.; Europe, Pelin et al.; Japan, Sebastien et al.; and Australia, Wagner et al. The sources of the date on predicted cost are as follows: United States, Shah and Williams; Europe, Lee et al.; and Australia, Wagner et al. Costs for Japan are unknown.

[b] The predicted number of deaths is estimated from data on annual incidence and predicted peak year.

[c] The costs shown are for compensation only; health care costs are excluded.

[d] The incidence, in number of cases per million population, is 33 in Great Britain, 30 in the Netherlands, 15 in Germany, 16 in France, and 19 in Italy (range in Europe, 15 to 33).

continues to rise until at least 85 years of age. (Darnton A, Hodgson J, Benson P, Coggan D. Mortality from asbestosis and mesothelioma in Britain by birth cohort. *Occup Med* 2012;62:549–52.)

A report of the risk of mesothelioma and lung cancer in women assembling gas masks, containing 20% crocidolite asbestos, has demonstrated that the risk of mesothelioma begins after as little as 1 year of exposure, and is related to the duration of exposure. Goff and Gaensler reported a case of asbestosis in a man who worked as a cigarette filter manufacturer, who transferred raw crocidolite asbestos to a carding machine for 9 months, and 13 years later developed signs of asbestosis. Brief but heavy exposures can cause asbestosis and mesothelioma. (Goff AM, Gaensler EA. Asbestosis following brief exposure to cigarette filter manufacture. *Respiration* 1972;29:83–93.) No risk of mesothelioma was seen in women assembling gas masks prior to 1940, when using chrysotile

> For 2008, Price and Ware estimate 2400 new cases of mesothelioma with asbestos being the likely cause in 58% and by 2042 asbestos will no longer be a factor in mesothelioma cases. For 2008–2042, there will be 68,000 total cases of mesothelioma with asbestos the likely cause in 34% of cases.

Figure 18.1 Time trend of U.S. mesothelioma cases and projection of future cases: an update based on SEER data for 1973 through 2005. (From Price and Ware, *Crit Rev Toxicol* 2009;39:575–88.)

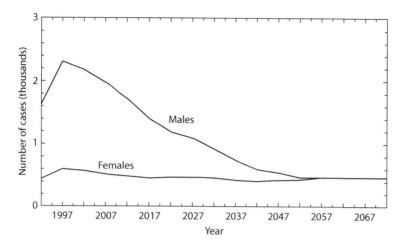

Figure 18.2 American projected incidence of mesothelioma 1997–2067. (From Price B, *Am J Epidemiol 1997.*)

asbestos in gas mask production. After an initial lag period of 22 years, the risk of mesothelioma rose progressively and then fell at 50–55 years after exposure to crocidolite asbestos when assembling gas masks. The authors thought that the risk fell 50 or more years after exposure due to gradual elimination of these crocidolite fibers with time. Because the average age of these women was >70 years, competing causes could also play major roles in risk reduction many years after exposure. (McDonald JC, Harris JM, Berry G. Sixty years on: The price of assembling military gas masks in 1940. *Occup Environ Med* 2006;63(12):852–5; Cherrie JW, Cowie HA, Jones AD. Modelling mesothelioma risk for workers assembling military gas masks. *Occup Environ Med* 2007;64(11):785–6.)

La Vecchia and Boffetta evaluated the model of asbestos-related mesothelioma and the time since first exposure (latency) as the key determinant of subsequent risk. They conducted a literature review to the end of 2010. In a cohort of 1966 Italian textile workers, the standardized mortality ratio, on the basis of 68 deaths from mesothelioma, was 6627 for workers employed only under the age of 30 years, 8019 for those employed both under the age of 30 years and at the age of 30–39 years, and 5891 for those employed both under the age of 30 years and at the age of 40 years or more. In a cohort of Italian asbestos cement workers, including 135 deaths from pleural cancer, compared with workers who had stopped being exposed for 3–15 years, the relative risk (RR) was similar for those still employed (RR = 0.67) and for those who had stopped for 30 years or more (RR = 0.65). In a British case–control study including 622 cases of mesothelioma and 1420 population controls, the RR substantially increased with increasing duration of exposure under the age of 30 years, but not with exposure at the age of more than 30 years. In the Great Britain Asbestos Workers Survey, including 649 deaths from mesothelioma compared with workers who were still employed and/or had stopped their exposure for less than 10 years, the multivariate RRs were 0.90 for 10–20 years after stopping their exposure and 0.99 for both 20–30 years and more than 30 years after stopping their exposure. The authors concluded that there is consistent evidence showing that, for workers exposed in the distant past, the risk of mesothelioma is not appreciably modified by subsequent exposures, and that stopping exposure does not materially modify the subsequent risk of mesothelioma. (La Vecchia C, Boffetta P. Role of stopping exposure and recent exposure to asbestos in the risk of mesothelioma. *Eur J Cancer Prev* 2012;21(3):227–30.)

RISK MODELING

The scientific basis for mesothelioma risk analysis began around 1958, when the medical community began to become aware that cancer is not due to a single change in a gene that transforms a cell from noncancerous to cancerous. Cancer is the result of multiple epigenetic and genetic events in which there is damage, change in function, inactivation, or deletion of chromosomes. Numerous events have to occur before there is cell transformation into the malignant stage. This process is called the induction phase for the initiation of the actual malignant tumor or cancer.

To recapitulate, a mesothelioma is a malignant tumor that has developed properties of unrestricted growth and spread to other organs. Several genes have to be altered in their function for the cancer cell to become immortalized. Several cellular mechanisms that regulate cell growth need to be effected before a specific cell can be immortalized into a cancer cell with unlimited growth (Schiller J. *N Engl J Med* 2008;359(4)):

- Evasion of apoptosis or programmed cell death
- Self-sufficiency in growth signaling
- Insensitivity to antigrowth signals
- Sustained angiogenesis
- Limitless replicative potential

The total number of genetic and epigenetic events that have to occur before induction of a mesothelioma develops, is unknown but most likely involves several genes, and probably more than a dozen genes. This process takes many years and the average mesothelioma I see today has had a latency period from first exposure to asbestos of >50 years. This means that if the average tumor growth time for a mesothelioma takes >15–20 years from the development of the first cancer cell until diagnosis, then it usually takes 15–30 years for several genetic and epigenetic events to occur before there is enough cell transformation for the malignancy to begin. It is very unusual for all of these genetic changes in cell regulation, and then unregulated cell growth, to occur in a period as short as 20 years.

Once there has been adequate duration for these genetic and epigenetic changes to occur, the tumor begins to double at a rate that will vary with the tumor type, but is generally considered to be at least 15 or more years, and usually 20 or more years, after initial exposure to asbestos in patients with a mesothelioma. It usually takes more than 40 years from first exposure until the development of a clinical mesothelioma. This number comes from the work of Bruce Lanphear at the University of Cincinnati. (Lanphear BP, Buncher CR. Latent period for malignant mesothelioma of occupational origin. *J Occup Med* 1992;34:718–21.) Drs. Lanphear and Buncher have shown that we have a 99%, or greater, degree of certainty that any mesothelioma that occurs in a worker must have a latency period of at least 15 years, before any occupational exposure can be associated with the subsequent development of this malignancy. There is a 95% probability that the last 20 years are not causative. Therefore, if there is continuous exposure, we traditionally subtract that last 20 years of exposure prior to the diagnosis of a mesothelioma, from the accounting of probability of causation, since our data indicate that this last 20 years would have a 95% probability of not being causative of the tumor. This leaves the earlier years—those exposures greater than 20 years prior to the year of diagnosis—as the most likely years for causing a mesothelioma. The Health Effects Institute presented formulas relating to mesothelioma occurrence with dose and time from exposure, according to duration of exposure (brief or extended) and constant or variable exposure. (Health Effects Institute—Asbestos Research. *Asbestos in Public and Commercial Buildings.* Cambridge: Health Effects Institute—Asbestos Research, 1991.) The study of a cohort of crocidolite miners in Western Australia, by Musk et al., presented results in respect to exposure intensity and duration separately; proportionality was observed for both exposure metrics. (Musk AW, deKlerk NH, Olsen N et al. Mortality in miners and millers of crocidolite in Western Australia: Follow-up to 1999. *Ann Occup Hyg* 2002;46(Suppl. 1):90–92; Musk A, deKlerk NH, Reid A et al. Mortality of former crocidolite (blue asbestos) miners and millers at Wittenoom. *Occup Environ Med* 2008;65:541–3.)

The earlier the exposure, the more likely that exposure is to be causative, since the original works of Pike (Pike MC. A method of analysis of a certain class of experiments in carcinogenesis. *Biometrics* 1966;22:142–61) and the subsequent studies of Cook, Doll, and Fellingham, as well as Berry and JC Wagner in 1969, indicated that the mathematical model best describing the times of occurrence of mesotheliomas in rats, and then in humans, seems to be related to the time of exposure to an exponential power, usually between 3 and 4. In 1982, a classic paper in the *British Journal of Cancer* by Peto and coworkers suggested the exponent would be 3.2, and in another paper, he used the exponent 3.5. (Peto J, Seidman H, Selikoff IJ. Mesothelioma mortality in asbestos workers: Implications for models of carcinogenesis and risk assessment. *Br J Cancer* 1982;45:124–35.) Most experts agree that the exponent is somewhere between 3 and 4, and for the purposes of our own analysis, we use an exponent of 3.2, since this is the most widely accepted exponent, and the most conservative way of estimating the impact of a given exposure. Morgan has developed a very useful and practical model for demonstrating the contribution of a given exposure in a given year to the overall risk of developing a mesothelioma. (Morgan RW, Whodunit? Liability for mesothelioma cases. *J Occup Med* 191;33:956–7.) By using a risk model from the work of Peto, Seidman, and Selikoff, the number of years of exposure from first exposure to diagnosis is used to estimate the probability of a given year of exposure as causative of a mesothelioma, which is listed as the number of years that the patient was exposed. The model used by Peto was $\wp = \theta t^{\hbar}$. The letter $\wp$ represents the incidence in any one year. The letter θ is a constant and the letter t is the time in years since the first exposure and where $\hbar$ is an exponent between 3 and 4. Once the probability is calculated for each year of exposure, then those probabilities can be totaled. Each year's portion of the total probability can then be calculated. Experts are often asked to opine about the contrition of a given exposure during a known timeframe to the causation of an asbestos-related mesothelioma. The advantage of this model is that it is empirical and practical.

If a person was exposed from 1960 to 1970, and then developed a mesothelioma in 1994, then only that 10-year period would be used in our calculation, since there would be no other years in which asbestos exposure occurred. Then, based on the Peto model, we would estimate which years would be most likely to be causative of that particular mesothelioma. The earlier exposures are more likely to cause a mesothelioma simply because of the long latency time of this tumor. Later exposures usually are not causative if earlier exposures are present.

In an example case, the subject was potentially exposed to asbestos between 2003 and 2006. His mesothelioma was diagnosed in 2008. The question now has been raised about even a very small contribution to the causation of his mesothelioma related to possible asbestos exposure in the 3 years prior to his diagnosis. Our understanding of mesothelioma cell growth is that this tumor has a similar cell doubling time to a primary lung adenocarcinoma. It takes about 40 cell doublings to get to a large stage 4 mesothelioma. This means that from the time the tumor begins to grow independently, it will take a minimum of 15 years (99% certainty) and more likely, more than 20 years (95% certainty) for this tumor to grow to a size that is diagnosable. This means that, in this case, the tumor induction and growth would have had to transpire extremely fast, so fast that it is no longer scientifically credible. It also means that more recent exposures, within 20 years prior to diagnosis, could not contribute to the causation of a mesothelioma statistically on a more-probable-than-not basis.

Table 18.2 demonstrates the actual contribution of a specific exposure at any given year. For instance, the individual in the table worked in shipyards from 1953 to 1960, and the contribution of the shipyard exposure would be 56.68%. If this individual was exposed to certain asbestos-containing products in 1965, then the contribution of that exposure in 1964 would be 4.25% of the total cause. If this same individual was exposed to an asbestos product for 1 week in 1964 with similar exposure to other asbestos products that year, then the contribution of that 1-week exposure would be 0.08%, or a very negligible contribution to the causation of the mesothelioma.

The data reveal that early exposures are the most important and that later exposures contribute very little to causation. The advantage of this type of statistical modeling is that it is unbiased and very fair to all parties. The intensity of exposure during these different years does not play a major role in the pathogenesis of mesothelioma, since changes in intensity are of importance, but the effects of intensity, above the threshold dose for developing mesothelioma,

Table 18.2 Sample risk analysis report

Date of mesothelioma diagnosis: 2008				
First exposure: 1953	Last exposure: 1972	Exponent 3.2	$p = \mathcal{B} \cdot t^x$	$p = t^x/\Sigma t^x \times 100$
Years exposed		Latency	Exponent	Probability
1953		55	370,817.83	8.68%
1954		54	349,671.33	8.19%
1955		53	329,369.05	7.71%
1956		52	309,892.24	7.26%
1957		51	291,222.26	6.82%
1958		50	273,340.52	6.40%
1959		49	256,228.51	6.00%
1960		48	239,867.80	5.62%
1961		47	224,240.03	5.25%
1962		46	209,326.91	4.90%
1963		45	195,110.23	4.57%
1964		44	181,571.87	4.25%
1965		43	168,693.78	3.95%
1966		42	156,457.98	3.66%
1967		41	144,846.61	3.39%
1968		40	133,841.86	3.13%
			Subtotal: 83.25%	

(Continued)

Table 18.2 (*Continued*) Sample risk analysis report

BJ, born September 25, 1935				
Date of mesothelioma diagnosis: 2008				
First exposure: 1953	**Last exposure: 1972**	**Exponent 3.2**	$p = \vartheta \cdot t^k$	$p = t^k/\Sigma t^k \times 100$
Years exposed		**Latency**	**Exponent**	**Probability**
1969		39	123,426.02	2.89%
1970		38	113,581.48	2.66%
1971		37	104,290.68	2.44%	Subtotal: 95.32%
1972		36	95,536.21	2.24%
			0.00	
			$\Sigma = 4{,}271{,}333.21$	100.00%

are probably linear rather than exponential. It is for this reason that the exponential effect of time plays a much larger role than the actual intensity of exposure. It is also for this reason that we do not make any allowances for differences in exposure during the years of the probability analysis. The data analysis that is displayed takes into account the year of diagnosis. What we traditionally do is subtract 20 years from the year of diagnosis and say any exposure during the 20 years prior to diagnosis would be noncausative and needs to be disregarded for consideration of causation. We then disregard any other exposures in which there is no asbestos present in the environment, as well as later years in which there has not been any further asbestos exposure.

Price and Ware calculated the number of mesotheliomas projected from current Surveillance, Epidemiology, and End Results (SEER) data to 2050. The commercial asbestos-related mesotheliomas will gradually decline due to lack of exposure. Between 2008 and 2054, the projected number of mesotheliomas in women, due to asbestos exposure, will be 0.2%–0.7%, and in men it will be 42.1%–42.4% of the total projected number of cases of mesothelioma. The number of women who worked in World War II industries and shipyards, or who were married to men exposed to amphibole asbestos in the workplace, has slowly declined with time, and by 2040, the incidence of mesothelioma will return to baseline for both sexes. In 2008, 58% of U.S. cases were due to asbestos exposure, and between 2008 and 2042, 34% of all U.S. cases will be due to asbestos exposure. (Price B, Ware A. Time trend of mesothelioma incidence in the United States and projection of future cases: An update based on SEER data for 1973 through 2005. *Crit Rev Toxicol* 2009;39(7):576–88.)

In summary:

1. Asbestos latency of less than 20 years after exposure is unlikely to be related to that exposure with a 95% degree of certainty.
2. The first year of exposure to amphibole asbestos is most likely to be the most important cause.
3. All mesotheliomas are not due to asbestos exposure, and the number of cases due to asbestos exposure is slowly declining.
4. Actual risk for a given exposure can be calculated.

19

Household and neighborhood exposure to asbestos

The next issue that I would like to address is whether neighborhood and household exposures to asbestos have resulted in risk of adverse health effects. The first possible para-occupational case of asbestos exposure was described by Dr. AC Haddow, of a man who was not employed in the asbestos industry, but who lived next door to an asbestos factory, and asbestos bodies were found in his lung. However, no one recognized this case report as a potential warning about para-occupational asbestos exposure. This was reported at a meeting of the British Medical Association under the title "Occupational diseases" in *The Lancet* in 1929.

Some experts have tried to establish a 1960 South African case of Wagner as the sentinel case that established the risk of mesothelioma from low-level household-type exposure. Wagner reported a case of a professional accountant who played on asbestos mine tailings as a child, and lived in the vicinity of a crocidolite asbestos mill until 7 years of age, before moving away from the Northwestern Cape Province. Unfortunately, a chest mass developed, and a surgical biopsy performed in June of 1957, at the accountant's age of 35, was consistent with a pleural mesothelioma. An autopsy was not performed. Most experts at that time would have felt that the diagnosis of a mesothelioma was inconclusive without a thorough postmortem examination. Wagner and coauthors on page 269 of their paper stated, "The pathological evidence associating these tumors with asbestos exposure is not conclusive." Attempts to produce mesotheliomas in animals had largely been unsuccessful, except for the production of a few sarcomas in rats. Some have questioned whether this was a case of a low-dose environmental or para-occupational type of exposure. (Wagner JC, Sleggs CA, Marchand P. Diffuse pleural mesothelioma and asbestos exposure in the North Western Cape Providence *Br J Ind Med* 1960;17:260–71.)

We know that histological evidence of asbestosis was found in eight out of ten cases reported by Wagner, in which some lung parenchyma was included in the pathological specimens. This case of a short-term exposure from the age of 1–7 cannot be considered a true low-level household type of exposure, because it is likely that the exposures were very high when he was playing on the crocidolite asbestos mine tailings. The short latency period is very suggestive of a heavy exposure. He developed an asbestos-related pleural effusion at 22 years of age with recurrent pleurisy beginning at 31 years of age, again suggesting high exposure. (Wagner JC, Sleggs CA, Marchand P. Diffuse pleural mesothelioma and asbestos exposure in the North Western Cape Province. *Br J Ind Med* 1960;17:260–71.) Later experts have not mentioned this case as an example of a mesothelioma related to low-level exposure for the reasons mentioned above. The importance of para-occupational or environmental exposure to asbestos was ignored, and not again emphasized until the papers of Newhouse and Thompson were published in 1965, 1976, and 1985. (Newhouse ML, Thompson H. Mesothelioma of pleura and peritoneum following exposure to asbestos in the London area. *Br J Ind Med* 1965;22:261–9; Newhouse ML, Berry G. Predictions of mortality from mesothelial tumours in asbestos factory workers *Br J Ind Med* 1976;33:147–15; Newhouse M, Berry G, Wagner JC. Mortality of factory workers in East London 1933–80. *Br J Ind Med* 1985;42:4–11.)

Generally, beginning in 1965 with Newhouse and Thompson (Newhouse ML, Thompson H. Mesothelioma of pleura and peritoneum following exposure to asbestos in the London area. *Br J Ind Med* 1965;22:261–69) and later with Harries (Harries PG. Asbestos hazards in naval dockyards. *Ann Occup Hyg* 1968;11:135–45), there were some scattered reports suggesting that workers living close to factories, or not working directly with asbestos, were at increased risk of health effects from exposure to asbestos in the workplace. Newhouse and Thompson found nine family member cases (seven female and two male) among 76 mesothelioma cases. A series of 42 mesotheliomas was reported to be related to exposure to an asbestos manufacturing plant in Southeast Pennsylvania (Lieben J, Oistawka H. Mesothelioma and asbestos exposure. *Arch Environ Health* 1967;14:559–63). Three female cases were classified as exposed to asbestos through family contacts. One other family contact case was reported by Milne in 1976. Two out of three subjects with peritoneal mesothelioma were women who were siblings and had no known exposure to asbestos. These women had a strong family history of cancer and this may have been the first reported cases of genetically induced peritoneal mesotheliomas. (Milne JE. Thirty-two case of mesothelioma in Victoria, Australia: A retrospective survey related to occupational exposure. *Br J Ind Med* 1976;33:115–22.) Selikoff measured the elevated concentration of asbestos in the home of a child with some type of tumor in 1973, but the data were never published. If a mesothelioma could develop from exposure to the clothing of a worker manufacturing asbestos products, then a similar condition could probably occur from exposure to the clothing of an asbestos insulator. His group of investigators began to research this issue further.

GF Rubino et al. presented 54 case reports of mesothelioma in 1972 in Turin, Italy, of which three men and one woman (16%) were associated with possible home contamination. This study was limited by the fact that only 22 of the suspected 54 cases of mesothelioma were confirmed pathologically. (Rubino GF, Scansetti G, Conna A et al. Epidemiology of pleural mesothelioma in northwestern Italy. *Br J Ind Med* 1972;29:436.) Their study was further limited by the fact that actual first-person interviews were not available in this retrospective study for determining exposure. The investigators relied on occupational and asbestos exposure histories from the mesothelioma cases by their nearest relatives, which is a poor substitute for first-person statements on probable exposure. This study was important in that it reviewed the recent published literature regarding environmental and take-home exposures and suggested the need for further studies.

Information on exposure to family members through the practice of bringing home work clothes, and then laundering these clothes that were contaminated with asbestos, was noted by lung fiber analysis by Ashcroft and Heppleston in 1973, Dalquen et al. in 1970, Edge and Choundry in 1978, Lander and Viskum in 1985, Gibbs et al. in 1989 and 1990, and Giarelli in 1992, who found asbestos fibers in household members' lungs. It was the first cohort of case–control studies performed by Anderson in 1976, 1979, and 1983 and Vienna and Polan in 1978, that grabbed the medical profession's attention as to the risk of take-home asbestos exposures. (Ashcroft T, Heppleston AG. The optical and electron microscopic determination of pulmonary asbestos fibre concentration and its relation to the human pathological reaction. *J Clin Pathol* 1973;26(3):224–34; Dalquen P, Hinz I, Dabbert AF. Pleural plaques, asbestosis and exposure to asbestos. An epidemiological study from the Hamburg area. *Pneumonologie* 1970;143(1):23–42; Edge JR, Choudhury SL. Malignant mesothelioma of the pleura in Barrow-in-Furness. *Thorax* 1978;33(1):26–30; Lander F, Viskum B. The occurrence of benign pulmonary changes in the spouses of previously employed asbestos workers. *Ugeskr Laeger* 1985;147(22):1805–6; Gibbs AR, Jones JS, Pooley FD et al. Non-occupational malignant mesotheliomas. *IARC Sci Publ* 1989;90:219–28; Gibbs AR, Griffiths DM, Pooley FD et al. Comparison of fibre types and size distributions in lung tissues of paraoccupational and occupational cases of malignant mesothelioma. *Br J Ind Med* 1990;47(9):621–6; Giarelli L, Bianchi C, Grandi G. Malignant mesothelioma of the pleura in Trieste, Italy. *Am J Ind Med* 1992;22(4):521–30.)

Sahmel and coworkers have made efforts to better characterize take-home asbestos exposures, by performing a study to measure the relationship between airborne chrysotile concentrations in the workplace, the contamination of work clothing, and take-home exposures and risks. The study included air sampling during two activities: (1) contamination of work clothing by airborne chrysotile (i.e., loading the clothing) and (2) handling and shaking out of the clothes. The measured airborne concentrations for the clothes handler were 0.2%–1.4% (8-hour time weighted average (TWA) or daily ratio) and 0.03%–0.27% (40-hour TWA or weekly ratio) of loading TWAs. Cumulative chrysotile doses for clothes handling at the airborne concentrations tested, were estimated to be consistent with lifetime cumulative chrysotile doses associated with ambient air exposure (range for take-home or ambient doses: 0.00044–0.105 fibers/cc-year). These values were surprisingly lower than expected. (Sahmel J, Barlow CA, Simmons B et al. Evaluation of take-home exposure and risk associated with the handling of clothing contaminated with chrysotile asbestos. *Risk Anal* 2014;34(8):1448–68.)

The 1970s and early 1980s have been characterized by a greater understanding of what are called "para-occupational exposures" from people working near an area in which asbestos is being used, but not using asbestos directly themselves. Case reports were published in "Insulation Hygiene Progress Reports" from the insulation industry hygiene research program in the fall of 1973 and later in the summer of 1975, before these studies reached the peer-reviewed medical literature in 1976. The relationship between distance from the primarily site of asbestos exposure and the number of fibers inhaled was made more recently by Donovan et al., who estimated that exposures 1–5 feet from source are 50%, 5–10 feet away 35% and greater than 10 feet away from the source are 10%. (Donovan E, Donovan B, Sahmel J, Scott PK, Paustenbach DJ. Evaluation of by stander exposure to asbestos in occupational settings: A review of the literature and application of a simple eddy diffusion model. *Crit Rev Toxicol* 2011;41:52–74; Donovan EP, Donovan BL, McKinley MA, Cowan DM, Paustenbach DJ. Evaluation of take home (para-occupational) exposure to asbestos and disease: A review of the literature. *Crit Rev Toxicol* 2012;42:703–31.)

Anderson and others from the Selikoff group reported mesothelioma cases among household contacts of asbestos manufacturing workers in 1976 and 1979. (Anderson HA, Lilis R, Daum B, Fischbein AS, Selikoff IJ. Household-contact asbestos neoplastic risk. *Ann NY Acad Sci* 1976;271:311–23; Anderson HA, Lilis R, Daum SM, Selikoff IJ. Asbestos among household contacts of asbestos factory workers. *Ann NY Acad Sci* 1979;330:387–99.)

The Mt. Sinai Selikoff group found a high incidence of asbestos-related pleural and parenchymal changes on x-rays of household contacts of asbestos manufacturing workers from an amosite asbestos insulation factory, which produced amosite asbestos insulation between 1941 and 1954 in Paterson, New Jersey. They reported four mesotheliomas out of 3100 family contacts of 1664 workers. They were able to investigate approximately a third of the available living household contacts (679/2200). Approximately 35% of these household contacts had radiographic abnormalities. Wives of asbestos workers had the highest prevalence of x-ray abnormalities at 48% (25% small opacities and 36% pleural abnormalities with a mean duration of employment of the spouse of 2.2 years). Some of those exposed had x-ray evidence of asbestosis (17%), of which 10% had rales. Although published measurement of asbestos fibers in households was not made until 1980–1983, the inference obviously must be made that there must be very high exposures in homes of asbestos workers, to the nonoccupationally exposed family members, if parenchymal x-ray changes of asbestosis were present after a mean exposure of only a little more than 2 years. Unfortunately, no actual measurements of asbestos fibers were made in the homes of these exposed household members during the time of exposure. (Anderson HA, Lilis R, Daum SM et al. Asbestosis among household contacts of asbestos factory workers. *Ann NY Acad Sci* 1979;330:387–99.)

In 1978, Vianna and Polan reported a case–control study from New York of 52 female mesotheliomas, again emphasizing potential exposure from washing the clothing of an asbestos-exposed spouse. (Vianna NJ, Polan AK. Nonoccupational exposure to asbestos and malignant mesothelioma in females. *Lancet* 1978;1:1061–3.) By 2012, a total of 60 articles had been published concerning take-home exposures and the development of asbestos-related disease.

In 1972, the U.S. Department of Health, Education, and Welfare (USDHEW), Public Health Service, and Centers for Disease Control and Prevention (CDC)/ National Institute for Occupational Safety and Health (NIOSH) published the *Criteria for a Recommended Standard of Occupational Exposure to Asbestos*, which reviewed the literature on the health hazards from asbestos exposure. Recommended standards for safe practices and exposure limits were made, but there was no mention about the risk of household exposure until the Asbestos Standard was revised in 1976. (*NIOSH Revised Asbestos Standard*, 1976.)

It was felt during the 1960s and 1970s that if the asbestos exposure could be capped within the suggested limits, future asbestos-related lung disease, including mesothelioma, would be prevented. Based on the literature available during the 1960s and early 1970s, one would not have anticipated that household exposure through the laundering of clothing would have resulted in any cumulative asbestos exposure above the permissible exposure limits recommended at that time.

Nicholson et al. in 1980 reported measurement of a specific contamination in workers' homes. He measured chrysotile asbestos in 13 air samples from the homes of miners and millers in California and Newfoundland, which averaged out to be about 0.01 fibers/cc. This fiber exposure is well below the Occupational Safety and Health Administration (OSHA) maximum permissible concentration of 0.1 fibers/cc. (Nicholson WJ. Tumor incidence after asbestos exposure in the USA: Cancer risk of the non-occupational population. In: D Reinishd, HW Schneider, KF Birkner (Eds.), *Fibrous Dusts—Measurement, Effects, Prevention*. Dusseldorf: DI-Verlag, pp. 161–77; Nicholson WJ, Rohl AN, Weisman I et al. Environmental asbestos concentrations in the United States. *IARC Sci Publ* 1980;30:823–7.)

Epidemiologic studies suggested that the respirable doses were much higher, since epidemiologic studies by many authors, such as Anderson, found substantial amounts of early asbestosis, as well as asbestos-related pleural disease in radiologic surveys of household-exposed members. Unfortunately, we do not have environmental exposure data from take-home clothing exposure to amphibole asbestos in shipyards. No measurements of clothing as a source of the contamination were made. There were no published studies evaluating the relationships between home contamination by asbestos, contamination of clothing brought home from work, and exposures during home laundering. There were no studies performed on exposures during home laundering. A maximum of 1.2 fibers/cc was found during the full laundry operation by Sawyer in 1977. (NIOSH Report to Congress on Worker's Home Contamination Study conducted under The Workers Family Protection Act [29 U.S.C, 671a, September 1995, DHHS (NIOSH) Publication No. 95–123].) The published data on fiber measurements show that these reports were snap-shot measurements of exposures to a process such as laundering clothes or to measurements of asbestos on clothing. Household members are exposed up to 24 hours a day to house contamination of asbestos fibers. These fibers may float around in the air for prolonged periods before they settle on surfaces. No exposure data are available of ambient levels during the work years of these asbestos insulation manufacturing workers reported by Anderson or others. Margaret Becklake stated in 1982, after reviewing the then-current literature, "What are described in the present review as "casual" exposures (i.e., usually domestic or neighborhood) are exposures that are intermittent but have turned out to be very heavy dust clouds of fine particles." (Becklake MR. Exposure to asbestos and human disease. *N Engl J Med* 1982;306:1480–2; Gloag D. Asbestos—Can it be used safely? *Br Med J* 1981;282:551–3.) I agree with Dr. Becklake that household exposures of asbestos workers were much higher than reported in recent retrospective studies.

In 1991, Roggli and Longo published asbestos lung content information on six female household contacts exposed to men with asbestosis. The lung fiber count of uncoated fibers ranged from 17,000 uncoated commercial fibers/gram (UG/gm) to 120,00 uncoated fibers/gram (UF/gm) with a median count of 24,300 UG/gm and a normal background level of 3100 UG/gm. The asbestos body count (AB) ranged from 2 to 8200 with a normal background level of <20 AB/g. Almost half of the fibers analyzed were commercial amphiboles, amosite, or crocidolite. These data confirm that these household contacts had very substantial exposure to commercial asbestos related to take-home exposure. (Roggli VL, Longo WE. Mineral fiber content of lung tissue in patients with environmental exposures: Household contacts vs. building occupants. *Ann NY Acad Sci* 1991;643:511–8.) A later update by Roggli et al. found that, in an analysis of 1445 cases of mesothelioma, 57% of household contacts had pleural plaques and 7.9% had asbestosis. Most of these household contacts had elevated concentrations of commercial amphiboles (amosite–crocidolite) or noncommercial amphiboles. (Roggli VL, Sharma A, Butnor KJ et al. Malignant mesothelioma and occupational exposure to asbestos: A clinicopathological correlation of 1445 cases. *Ultrastruct Pathol* 2002;26:55–65.) Gibbs et al. found similar elevations of lung tissue fiber counts in mesotheliomas from para-occupational exposures. (Gibbs AR, Griffiths DM, Pooley FD et al. Comparisons of fiber types and size distributions in lung tissues of paraoccupational and occupational cases of malignant mesothelioma. *Br J Ind Med* 1990;47:621–6; Dawson A, Gibbs AR, Pooley FD et al. Malignant mesothelioma in women. *Thorax* 1993;48:269–74.)

There has been confusion regarding the attribution of home renovation exposures in the United States, with the exception of vermiculite exposure in Libby, Montana, with home exposures in other countries, where home renovation products or insulation, contain hazardous amounts of amphiboles, like crocidolite in Australia. Crocidolite, a type of amphibole asbestos, does increase the risk of mesothelioma during home maintenance and renovation work in Western Australia, but this type of asbestos has never been used in home renovation products or home insulation in the United States. (Olsen NJ, Franklin PJ, Reid A et al. Increasing incidence of malignant mesothelioma after exposure to asbestos during home maintenance and renovation. *Med J Aust* 2011;195:271–4.)

This type of data indicates that a chronic low-level exposure of the right fiber type, diameter, and length in sufficient concentrations, can produce a mesothelioma. The question now being argued relates to what dose of asbestos is necessary to produce a mesothelioma in this type of para-occupational exposure. The Canadian report from the Royal Commission in Ontario suggested that doses of less than 5 fiber-years were unlikely to produce mesotheliomas.

More recently, there has been increased attention to the fact that many mesotheliomas produced, particularly in women, are spontaneous mesotheliomas, and some mesotheliomas may be caused by a variety of other causes, such as genetics, viruses such as simian virus-40, radiation, chronic inflammation of any cause such as tuberculosis or other chronic infections, radiation, familial Mediterranean fever, various drugs, environmental exposure to noncommercial fibrous minerals such as zeolites like erionite, tremolite, Libby asbestiform fiber, balangeroite, antigorite, fluoro-edenite, Luto, winchite, richterite, actinolite, carbon nanotubes, and other long, thin fibers, and many other factors, further complicating the issue of causation at low-level exposures. (Ontario Ministry of the Attorney General. *Report of The Royal Commission on Matters of Health and Safety Arising from the Use of Asbestos in Ontario.* Toronto: Queen's Printer for Ontario, 1984.)

Household exposures among Libby, Montana, household contacts of workers with direct exposure to amphiboles found in Libby vermiculite, revealed no increase in pleural or parenchymal radiographic abnormalities, even though the workers themselves had a 45% incidence of pleural abnormalities, and an 8% incidence of parenchymal abnormalities, at an estimated exposure of <2 fibers/cc/ year. The low incidence of household member abnormality was thought to be related to the work safety practices of showering before going home (63.9%) and the use of coveralls by 96.2% of the most heavily exposed workers. (Hilbert TJ, Franzblau A, Dunning KK et al. Asbestos-related radiographic findings among household contacts of workers exposed to Libby vermiculite: Impact of workers' personal hygiene practices. *J Occup Environ Med* 2013;55:1300–4.)

Younger people seem to be more resistant to asbestos-associated mesothelioma, suggesting that immunodeficiency may also play a role in susceptibility to mesothelioma with age. (Bianchi C, Bianchi T. Susceptibility and resistance in the genesis of asbestos-related mesothelioma. *Ind J Occup Environ Med* 2008;12:57–60; Comar M, Zanotta N, Pesel G et al. Asbestos and SV40 in malignant pleural mesothelioma from a hyperendemic area of north-eastern Italy. *Tumori* 2012;98(2):210–4.) The most difficult diagnostic consideration in all mesothelioma cases is differentiating a true mesothelioma from a metastatic or primary tumor of the pleura or abdomen.

The overall incidence of pleural mesothelioma in North America is low, or about 2 cases/million, in women, and around 10–15 cases/million, in men in the United States. Recently, the incidence in men has been falling to about 7.5 million cases permillion each year, while the incidence in women has remained stable. A recent survey in Denmark, of malignant mesothelioma cases, found that the incidence in women between 1943 and 2009 remained stable, while being elevated in men during that period. (Skammeritz E, Omland Ø, Hansen J, Johansen JP. Regional differences in incidence of malignant mesothelioma in Denmark. *Dan Med J* 2013;60/3:1–5.) Peritoneal mesotheliomas are usually related to high amphibole asbestos exposure in men, and usually develop spontaneously in women without any asbestos exposure. (Sebag G, Sugarbaker PH. Peritoneal mesothelioma proposal for staging system. *Eur J Surg Oncol* 2001;27:223–4.) The increased risk of peritoneal mesothelioma related to high exposure has been confirmed by others. (Mensi C, Bonzini M, Macchione M et al. Differences among peritoneal and pleural mesothelioma: Data from the Lombardy Region Mesothelioma Register (Italy). *Med Lav* 2011;102(5):409–16.)

"The overall stable low incidence of mesothelioma in women suggests that very few are related to asbestos exposure." (Spiritas R, Heineman EF, Bernstein L et al. Malignant mesothelioma: Attributable risk of asbestos exposure. *Occup Environ Med* 1994;51:804–11; Carbone M, Ly BH, Dodson RF et al. Malignant mesothelioma: Facts, myths, and hypotheses. *J Cell Physiol* 2011;227:44–58; Smith DD. Women and mesothelioma. *Chest* 2002;123:1885–6.)

Spanish investigators have evaluated the pleural cancer mortality rate and time trends through to 2020. Most of these workers (70%) were exposed in the fiber/cement industry. They found 6037 mesothelioma deaths from 1975 to 2010. The number of cases in men was 2.7 times higher than in women, and beginning in 1981–1985, the number of cases in women slowly began to level off with a gradual decline beginning in the 1980s from 2.5 cases per million to 1.5 cases per million. It is estimated that 63% of pleural cancers in women were mesotheliomas. The first preventive measures targeting asbestos use were implemented in 1984 and the ban on the production and marketing of asbestos products came into effect in December 2002. These investigators felt that most of the pleural cancers in women were occupationally related, rather than related to household exposure. (López-Abente G, Garcia-Gomez M, Menendez-Navarro et al. Pleural cancer mortality in Spain: Time-trends and updating of predictions up to 2020. *BMC Cancer* 2013;13:528.)

Most mesotheliomas in women are idiopathic. McDonald and McDonald reported that 98% of female cases in Canada, and 95% in North America, were idiopathic or had no known asbestos exposure. (McDonald AD, McDonald JC. Malignant mesothelioma in North America. *Cancer* 1980;46:1650–58.) Enterline and Henderson studied U.S. death rates from malignant tumors of the pleura between 1968 and 1981 and found an increase in death rates for men >65 years of age, but not for younger men or women. (Enterline PE, Henderson VI. Geographic patterns for pleural mesothelioma deaths in the United States, 1968–1981. *J Natl Cancer Inst* 1987;79:31–7.) Later, Roggli used lung fiber analysis to determine the causation of mesothelioma in women. He estimated that approximately 40% of mesotheliomas in women were idiopathic in this group of cases referred to him by attorneys, which leads to bias in attributing more cases of mesothelioma to asbestos exposure, as compared to the general population. (Roggli VL. The role of analytical SEM in the determination of causation of malignant mesothelioma. *Ultrastruct Pathol* 2006;30:31–5.) Dodson et al. performed a much smaller study to analyze asbestos fiber burden in 15 attorney-referred women, and found that nine women had significant asbestos fiber burdens (60%) and six (40%) had background or borderline elevated levels of asbestos bodies. (Dodson RF, O'Sullivan M, Brooks DR et al. Quantitative analysis of asbestos burden in women with mesothelioma. *Am J Med* 2003;43:188–95.)

A retrospective analysis of all cases of mesothelioma in women was performed of all the people registered during 1975–1980 in Los Angeles County, the New York State Cancer registry, and 39 Veterans Administration Hospitals, where the authors found 208 mesotheliomas. In men, 88% had significant asbestos exposure as compared with 23% of women. (Spiritas R, Heineman EF, Bernstein L et al. Malignant mesothelioma: Attributable risk of asbestos exposure. *Occup Environ Med* 1994;51:804–11.)

Hemminki and Li found that a large percentage of peritoneal mesotheliomas in Sweden were unrelated to asbestos exposure. Moreover, the increasing trends in incidence over the period of 1961–1998, were probably attributable to factors other than asbestos. (Hemminki K, Li X. Time trends and occupational risk factors for peritoneal mesothelioma in Sweden. *J Occup Environ Med* 2003;45:451–5.)

Pleural and peritoneal mesotheliomas in Surveillance, Epidemiology, and End Results (SEER) 1973–2005 data in terms of age-adjusted rates of pleural mesothelioma among women, have remained more or less constant at about 2.5 per million person-years. Age-adjusted rates for peritoneal mesothelioma in both men (1.2 per million person-years) and women (0.8 per million person-years) exhibit no temporal trends over the period of the study. We estimate that approximately 94,000 cases of pleural and 15,000 cases of peritoneal mesothelioma will occur in the United States over the period 2005–2050. (Moolgavkar SH, Meza R, Turim J. Pleural and peritoneal mesotheliomas in SEER: Age effects and temporal trends, 1973–2005. *Cancer Causes Control* 2009;20:935–44.)

Burdorf et al. examined the incidence of peritoneal mesothelioma in Sweden and The Netherlands over 1989–2003, and concluded that the incidence rate of peritoneal mesothelioma over the past 15 years may point to a limited role of occupational exposure to asbestos in the etiology of peritoneal mesothelioma, especially among women. (Burdorf A, Järvholm B, Siesling S. Asbestos exposure and differences in occurrence of peritoneal mesothelioma between men and women across countries. *Occup Environ Med* 2007;64:839–42.)

A similar study was performed in 2002 in Italy by Gennaroa et al., who found that 57.5% of mesotheliomas in women were idiopathic and had no known asbestos exposure, versus only 15% of males. (Gennaroa V, Ugolini D, Viarengo P et al. Incidence of pleural mesothelioma in Liguria region, Italy (1996–2002). *Eur J Cancer* 2005;41:2709–14.)

Later reports from the Italian National Register of Pleural Mesotheliomas collected cases into five groups: occupational, household, environmental, leisure, and unknown exposure. The authors found that men had an occupational cause in 81% of mesotheliomas and women in only 33% of cases. Only 14% of men and 37% of women had idiopathic (without any known cause) mesotheliomas. (Marinaccio A, Binazzi A, Di Marzio D et al. Pleural malignant mesothelioma epidemic: Incidence, modalities of asbestos exposure and occupations involved from the Italian National Register. *Int J Cancer* 2012;130:2146–54.)

Boffetta from the International Agency for Research on Cancer reported that there was a strong correlation between heavy asbestos exposure in occupational cohorts, and the incidence of pleural and peritoneal mesothelioma, but a low correlation between the incidence of pleural and peritoneal mesothelioma in population-based registries. This finding suggests that in the general population, a smaller fraction of peritoneal than pleural mesotheliomas is attributable to asbestos exposure. (Boffetta P. Epidemiology of peritoneal mesothelioma: A review. *Ann Oncol* 2007;18:985–90.) The dose–response relationship between occupational asbestos exposure and peritoneal mesothelioma risk has been investigated on the basis of the studies providing information on quantitative asbestos exposure. The risk of peritoneal mesothelioma for workers exposed to amphiboles was proportional to the square of cumulative exposure, while a similar estimate could not be obtained for chrysotile-exposed workers. (Boffetta P. Epidemiology of peritoneal mesothelioma: A review. *Ann Oncol* 2007;18:985–90.)

It is my opinion—based on my review of the literature, and consistent with Boffetta—that all asbestos-induced peritoneal mesotheliomas are due to amphibole exposure, and that chrysotile exposure does not cause peritoneal mesotheliomas. The dose of amphibole required to produce a peritoneal mesothelioma is equivalent to the dose of amphibole asbestos exposure required to produce asbestosis.

The incidence of mesothelioma has been 2% (356/17,800 workers) in American and Canadian insulation workers exposed to mixed varieties of asbestos fibers and reached a high of 4.7% (329/6908) in former Australian crocidolite miners and millers. This Australian study also confirmed the relationship between high exposures and the increased risk of peritoneal mesothelioma. (Berry G, Reid A, Aboagye-Sarfo P et al. Malignant mesotheliomas in former miners and millers of crocidolite at Wittenoom (Western Australia) after more than 50 years follow-up. *Br J Cancer* 2012;106(5):1016–20; Ribak J, Lilis R, Suzuki Y et al. Malignant mesothelioma in a cohort of asbestos insulation workers: Clinical presentation, diagnosis, and causes of death. *Br J Ind Med* 1988;45(3):182–7.)

A recent characterization of a French series of female cases of mesothelioma, revealed that more than 80% of mesothelioma cases in men are attributable to occupational asbestos exposure, compared to only 40% in women. The objective of the study was to characterize a series of female pleural mesotheliomas according to known and suspected risk factors. From the exhaustive recording of 318 female mesothelioma cases in the French National Mesothelioma Surveillance Program between 1998 and 2009, multiple correspondence analysis and hybrid clustering were performed to characterize these cases according to expert-assessed occupational and nonoccupational exposure to asbestos and man-made vitreous fibers, x-ray exposure, and history of cancer and nonmalignant respiratory diseases. Four clusters were identified: (1) occupational exposure to asbestos and man-made vitreous fibers (7.9% of subjects); (2) radiation exposure during radiotherapy (12.9%); (3) increased asbestos exposure (19.8%); and (4) "nonexposure" characteristics (59.4%). (Camiade E, Gramond C, Jutand MA et al. Characterization of a French series of female cases of mesothelioma. *Am J Ind Med* 2013;56(11):1307–16.) The low incidence of asbestos exposure in women of 19.8% is strikingly similar to the 23% incidence of asbestos exposure in women with mesothelioma reported by Spiritas et al. (Spiritas R, Heineman EF, Bernstein L et al. Malignant mesothelioma: Attributable risk of asbestos exposure. *Occup Environ Med* 1994;51:804–11.)

The risk of mesothelioma is very high if the exposed workers have asbestosis from amphibole asbestos exposure, indicating a very high fiber burden and high exposure. The risk was 13.7% or 17/124 workers with asbestosis in Hong Kong exposed to mixed chrysotile and amphibole asbestos. (Chen M, Tse L, Au R et al. Mesothelioma and lung cancer mortality: A historical cohort study among asbestosis workers in Hong Kong. *Lung Cancer* 2012;76(2):165–70.) However, the risk is much lower in workers who had much lower exposure. The risk of mesothelioma in 98,912 British workers with some asbestos exposure was 0.6% (649/98,912). This relatively low risk is related to the low incidence of asbestosis (477/98,912). Again, the risk was significantly related to asbestosis. (Harding AH, Darnton AJ. Asbestosis and mesothelioma among British asbestos workers (1971–2005). *Am J Ind Med* 2010;53:1070–80.)

We know that warnings about the health hazards of asbestos were placed on the boxes of Johns-Manville Thermobestos pipe insulation on September 10, 1964, and warnings were placed on Kaylo asbestos pipe insulation in 1966. The major manufacturers of asbestos-containing pipe insulation stopped manufacturing these products by 1971–1972. This seems reasonably prudent based on the information available at that time. In the mid-1960s, papers were published from Great Britain and the United States on the health hazards of individuals living near asbestos manufacturing plants. Most of the physicians at the time paid little attention to this information and it was not until the mid-to-late 1970s and early 1980s that workers' clothing became a concern of the general medical community. NIOSH reported in 1995 that

> Several studies of asbestos worker's families inferred that asbestos-related diseases were due to home contamination emanating from clothes contaminated at work, especially due to laundering the clothes (Anderson et al. 1979a,b; Bianchi et al. 1987; Giarelli et al. 1992; Gibbs et al. 1990; Huncharek et al. 1989, Nicholson et al. 1980). However, no studies evaluated the relationships between home contamination by asbestos of clothing brought home from work, and exposures during home laundering. The few studies reported and reviewed in this section indicate that clothing probably was a source of home contamination by asbestos and support the hypothesis that home laundering of asbestos contaminated clothing could be especially hazardous. One study reported measurements of asbestos contamination in workers' homes; however no measurements of clothing as a source of the contamination were made. (Report to Congress on Worker's Home Contamination Study, Conducted under the Worker's Family Protection Act (29 U.S.C. 671a) September 1995, DHHS (NIOSH) Publication No. 95–123.)

> Two studies of workplace clothing contamination by asbestos have been reported [Seixas and Ordin 1986; Driscoll and Elliott 1990]. Chrysotile asbestos was found in all clothing vacuumed as employees left work at a brake shoe manufacturing facility, neither report provided quantitative data on asbestos recovered from the worker's clothing.

No studies of exposure during home laundering were found by NIOSH in their review published in 1995.

> However, a study on laundering clothing contaminated by an asbestos removal operation produced an average of 0.4 fibers/ mL while picking up clothing and loading the washer. A maximum of 1.2 fibers/mL was found during the total laundry operation [Sawyer 1977]. Although the study was not conducted in a home laundry and measurements of the level of clothing contamination that generated these concentrations were not made, the study is consistent with the hypothesis that home laundering of asbestos-contaminated clothing is hazardous. Another important aspect of laundering asbestos contaminated clothing is that the fibers can transfer to uncontaminated clothing washed with the contaminated clothing, as was found by NIOSH (1971) in a study of dry cleaning a coat made with 8% asbestos fiber. (Report to Congress on Worker's Home Contamination Study, Conducted under the Worker's Family Protection Act (29 U.S.C. 671a) September 1995,DHHS (NIOSH) Publication No. 95–123.)

It is important to note that the reports and literature issued were all directed to the medical community. Due to the technical nature of these reports, a layperson would likely have had a difficult time grasping the scientific significance of the find-ings. The initial reports of domestic exposure were all in asbestos manufacturing facilities and not in end users. No information of exposure in housewives of end users was available until the mid-1970s and early 1980s. The production of meso-thelioma in nonmanufacturing facilities located near shipyards and nonasbestos end users was not really reported until the studies of Bianchi and others in 1982 and 1987 in the shipbuilding area of Trieste, Italy. (Bianchi C, Brollo A et al. *Adv Pathol* 1982;2:545–48; Bianchi C, Brollo A, Bittesini L, Ramani L. Hyaline plaques of the pleura and domestic exposure to asbestos. *Med Lav* 1987;78:44–9; Bianchi C, Bianchi T. Mesothelioma among shipyard workers in Monfalcone, Italy. *Indian J Occ Environ Med* 2012;3:119–23.) Bianchi noted a familial aggregation in these Italian mesothelioma cases and others have confirmed this fact. (de Klerk N, Alfonso H, Olsen N et al. Familial aggregation of malignant mesothelioma in former workers and residents of Wittenoom, Western Australia. *Ind J Cancer* 2013;132:1423–8.)

Bianchi, Brollo, and others reported in 2001 on asbestos exposure and malig-nant mesothelioma in a major shipbuilding area of Italy, where a substantial amount of crocidolite asbestos was used rather than amosite asbestos. The major-ity of the 557 cases of mesothelioma worked in shipyards. The duration of expo-sure to asbestos of 348 cases of mesothelioma was reported to be from less than 1 year to more than 50 years. Only 0.6% of cases of mesothelioma had an exposure duration of less than 1 year and only 6.8% had an exposure duration of 1–4 years. The latency time or the time between the first exposure to asbestos to the time of diagnosis of a mesothelioma was a mean of 48.8 years and a median of 51.0 years. The authors reported on 21 (3.8% of the total) cases in women with domestic exposure attributed to cleaning work clothes at home. In this series of women, 51% had pleural plaques and 57.1% had an asbestos body count of <1 asbestos body per 1000 g of dried lung tissue, which is equivalent to background exposure to asbestos and suggests that more than half of these women had idiopathic mesotheliomas. (Bianchi C, Brollo A, Ramani L et al. Asbestos exposure in malignant mesothelioma of the pleura: A survey of 557 cases. *Ind Health* 2001;39:161–7.)

It was the Anderson study of workers employed in the amosite manufacturing plant in Paterson, New Jersey, that provided enough epidemiologic information to confirm the earlier case reports. Mesotheliomas associated with household exposure are generally pleural rather than peritoneal (259 versus 19). Peritoneal mesotheliomas in women are almost always idiopathic unless there is a history of very heavy exposure to amphibole asbestos that is usually sufficient to cause asbestosis (Walker et al. 1983, Albin et al. 1990, Goldblum and Hart 1995, Spiritas et al. 1994, McDonald 1985, McDonald and McDonald 1994, Huncharek 2002, Price and Ware 2004, Moolgavkar 2009).

In summary, mesotheliomas in women usually do not meet the dose requirements for causation of pleural mesothelioma, and very rarely is the dose of sufficient fiber type, diameter, fiber length, concentration, and duration of exposure to be considered a probable cause of a peritoneal mesothelioma (see Figure 19.1).

The issue of the need for warnings about wearing clothing contaminated with asbestos home from the job site are certainly pertinent in many cases. Recommendations to never wear asbestos-contaminated clothing home were only made for those individuals who directly worked with asbestos, such as insulators in 1972. The new NIOSH standard for clothing was provided in Section I-8 of the *Criteria for a Recommended Standard... Occupational Exposure to Asbestos 1972, US Public Health Service, CDC, National Institute of Occupational Health and Safety 1972 HSM 72–10267* and applied only to workers exposed to an average exposure of >1 fiber/cc of asbestos over an 8-hour day or peak exposures of >5 fibers/cc (Page I-3).

This warning was not given to workers with incidental or para-occupational asbestos exposure who would not have been expected to meet the exposure criteria, since they never worked directly with asbestos-containing products. It was also in 1972 that Owings Corning stopped manufacturing asbestos products,

---

What do the data show?

- All individuals have significant enviromental asbestos burden.

- Individuals with background levels 100 times those of the normal urban workers who live near the asbestos mines in Quebec, but who are not asbestos workers, have no elevated risk for lung cancer or mesothelioma.

- Only those workers with significant asbestos exposure are at risk for asbestos-related disease and malignancy.

Figure 19.1 Risk of mesothelioma is based on dose, fiber type, and fiber size. (From Camus *NEJM* 1998;338:565.)

including Kaylo asbestos pipe insulation. The recommended standard in 1972 was lowered to 5 fibers/cc of asbestos from 5 million particles/cubic foot of asbestos dust (approximately 30 fibers/cc) and then lowered further to 2 fibers/cc of asbestos in 1976.

It is always difficult to review science by hindsight, and estimate when enough information was available to determine with a reasonable degree of medical certainty, when a warning should have been issued related to domestic exposure to asbestos products. The NIOSH and its panel of experts did not feel that there was sufficient scientific data to warn of bystander or household exposures in 1972. The suggested clothing and laundry standard only applied to workers with an average exposure higher than 1 fiber/cc over an 8-hour day or <1 fiber/year if an individual was continuously exposed to asbestos for 50 years, as this would be an accumulative exposure of nearly 50 fiber-years. Today's standard is 0.1 fibers/cc of asbestos for a total of 5 fiber-years. An exposure of 50 fiber-years would be considered excessive today, but based on the knowledge and safety standards in 1972, this was thought to be an acceptable level of exposure.

I believe that the papers by Anderson and others published in 1976 and later republished in 1979 and 1982 (Anderson HA, Lilis R, Daum SM et al. Asbestosis among household contacts of asbestos factory workers. *Ann NY Acad Sci* 1979;330:387–99), followed by Vianna and Polan in 1978 and Nicholson in 1980 and 1983, were the most important published scientific papers signaling a very significant asbestos exposure to household contacts of asbestos workers. This is because they proved by their x-ray survey of household contacts that high asbestos exposures could be produced in a domestic environment, simply by bringing asbestos-contaminated clothing into a domestic environment. These studies were landmark studies because they represent the first cohort studies of take-home exposure to amphibole asbestos from a manufacturing plant of amosite asbestos insulation in Paterson, New Jersey. Previous case reports did not give enough information to estimate exposures in a domestic environment. However, it was not until September 1995 that the NIOSH published a study on home contamination by take-home exposures of potentially toxic materials, as authorized by the Workers Family Protection Act (29 U.S.C. 671a, NIOSH 1995).

Once high exposures were proven in a household setting, then warnings should have been issued. There was not adequate information available to warn of the hazard of nonoccupational exposure to asbestos of family members, as well as para-occupational bystander exposure, in the 1940s, 1950s, 1960s, and early 1970s.

A review article was published in 2012 (Donovan EP, Donovan BL, McKinley MA, Cowan DM, Paustenbach DJ. Evaluation of take home exposures (para-occupational) exposure to asbestos and disease: A review of the literature. *Crit Rev Toxicol* 2012;42:703–31). The authors reviewed nearly 60 articles that described cases of asbestos-related disease thought to be caused by para-occupational exposure. Over 65% of these cases were in persons who lived with workers classified as miners, shipyard workers, insulators, or others involved in the manufacturing of asbestos-containing products, with nearly all remaining workers identified as craftsmen. A total of 98% of the available lung samples of the persons with diseases indicated the presence of amphibole asbestos. Eight studies provided airborne asbestos concentrations during (i) handling of clothing contaminated with asbestos during insulation work or simulated use of friction products; (ii) ambient conditions in the homes of asbestos miners; and (iii) wearing previously contaminated clothing. Their review indicated that the literature was dominated by case reports, the majority of which involved household contacts of workers in industries characterized, generally, by high exposures to amphiboles or mixed mineral types. The available data did not implicate chrysotile as a significant cause of disease for household contacts. Also, the analysis indicated that there was insufficient information in the published literature that would allow one to relate airborne asbestos concentrations in a workplace to those that would be generated from subsequent handling or contact with clothing that had been contaminated in that environment. Ideally, a simulation study should be conducted in the future to better understand the relationships between the airborne concentrations in the workplace and the fiber characteristics that influence retention on fabric, as well as the concentrations that can be generated by handling the contaminated clothing by the persons in the home. The authors discovered that 98% of available lung fiber analysis studies indicated the presence of amphibole asbestos. Furthermore, the authors concluded that chrysotile asbestos exposure could not be implicated as a cause of mesothelioma in these take-home exposure cases. A detailed bibliography is included with this article with reference to all reports in the literature on this subject (Donovan EP, Donovan BL, McKinley MA et al. 2012).

Goswami et al. provided a comprehensive review of epidemiologic (cohort, case–control, and case reports and series) and exposure data regarding domestic exposure and its relationship to mesothelioma, lung cancer, pleural disease, and asbestosis. By the fall of 2013, there were 143 published articles with some reference to household and bystander asbestos exposure by searching for key words such as domestic, household, laundry, para-occupational, take-home, asbestos, asbestosis, lung cancer, mesothelioma, and/or pleural changes in a MEDLINE search. Only 108 studies had enough information to be relevant to this study. Only 32 case reports were specific for mesothelioma and are listed in Table 1 of their paper. (Goswami E, Craven V, Dahlstrom DL et al. Domestic asbestos exposure: A review of epidemiologic and exposure data. *Int J Environ Res Public Health* 2013;10(11):5629–70.) This report is the most comprehensive review of the literature to date. The authors concluded that domestically exposed individuals via workers involved in occupations with a traditionally high risk of disease from exposure to asbestos (i.e., asbestos product manufacturing workers, insulators, shipyard workers, and asbestos miners) had an increased risk of an asbestos-related disorder and mesothelioma. The epidemiologic studies also showed an elevated risk of interstitial, but more likely pleural abnormalities (n = 6), though only half accounted for confounding exposures. The studies are limited with regards to lung cancer (n = 2). Several exposure-related studies describe results from airborne samples collected within the home (n = 3), during laundering of contaminated clothing (n = 1), or in controlled exposure simulations (n = 5) of domestic exposures, the latter of which were generally associated with low-level chrysotile-exposed workers. Lung burden studies (n = 6) were also evaluated as a surrogate of exposure. Lung fiber burden studies have indicated elevated tissue levels of amphibole asbestos. In general, the available results for domestic exposures are lower than the workers' exposures. While domestic exposure has been associated with pleural plaques and mesothelioma, the data on domestic exposure as a cause of lung cancer have not been supportive. Recent simulations of low-level chrysotile-exposed workers indicate asbestos levels commensurate with background concentrations in those exposed domestically.

Lacourt and others from the French Mesothelioma Study Group found 437 cases of mesothelioma with 874 controls between 1998 and 2002. Asbestos exposure by job title was estimated by two expert industrial hygienists. The problem with this paper is in the estimates of these hygienists regarding exposures. Their estimates of exposure are much higher than others have published in the literature for similar occupations. They also are publishing from a French database in which there is more exposure to crocidolite asbestos then there would be in a U.S. population. They have assessed that 80% of male cases of mesothelioma are related to occupational asbestos exposure, whereas only 40% of women with mesothelioma have an occupational asbestos exposure. They defined nonoccupational asbestos exposure as a group that had domestic, environmental, or para-occupational exposures to asbestos. I have reviewed other papers published by the same French group of investigators, elsewhere in my book, and again the major problem with their published data has been their high estimates of exposures, which result in very low estimates of the minimal asbestos exposure responsible for a mesothelioma. They do not distinguish the exposure by fiber types or give information on exposures (see Figures 19.2 through 19.4). (Lacourt A, Gramond

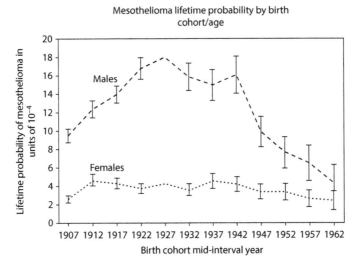

Mesothelioma lifetime probability by birth cohort/age

Figure 19.2 Risk for females has been very low and stable in spite of the great increase in industrial and consequently household exposures to asbestos from 1930 to 1970. (From Price B, Ware A, Mesothelioma trends in the United States: An update based on Surveillance, Epidemiology, and End Results Program data for 1973 through 2003. *Am J Epidemiol* 2004;159:107–12. With permission.)

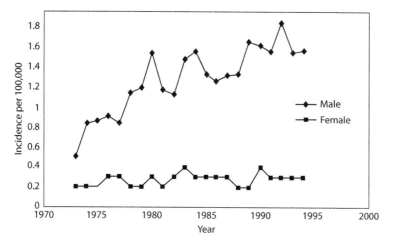

Figure 19.3 The age-adjusted risk has remained stable for women. (From Price B, Ware A, Mesothelioma trends in the United States: An update based on Surveillance, Epidemiology, and End Results Program data for 1973 through 2003. *Am J Epidemiol* 2004;159:107–12. With permission.)

- Age-adjusted rates of pleural mesothelioma among women have remained more or less constant at about 2.5 per million person-years over the period 1973–2005.

- Age-adjusted rates for peritoneal mesothelioma in both men (1.2 per million person-years) and women (0.8 per million person-years) exhibit no temporal trends over the period of the study.

- We estimate that approximately 94,000 cases of pleural and 15,000 cases of peritoneal mesothelioma will occur in the United States over the period 2005–2050.

- Mesotheliomas in women rarely meet the dose requirments for causation and rarely is the dose of sufficient fiber type, diameter, fiber length, concentration, and duration of exposure to be considered a probable cause of a peritoneal mesothelioma.

Figure 19.4 The lifetime risk for mesothelioma remains near baseline in women, suggesting that the contribution of household exposures to the production of mesothelioma is small. (From Moolgavkar SH, Meza R, Turim J. Pleural and peritoneal mesotheliomas in SEER: Age effects and temporal trends, 1973–2005. *Cancer Causes Control* 2009;20:935–944.)

C, Rolland P et al. Occupational and non-occupational attributable risk of asbestos exposure for malignant pleural mesothelioma. *Thorax* 2014;69(6):532–9.)

In summary, case reports of mesotheliomas associated with asbestos exposure are potentially useful in suggesting a possible relationship between an exposure and subsequent disease. Case reports do not prove an association between a given exposure and disease. Large epidemiologic studies with measurement of the amount of a potential toxic substance in the place of exposure (dose response) are necessary to strongly suggest a possible causation in an exposed population. While there were a few scattered case reports of household environmental and take-home exposures to amphibole asbestos in the 1960s, scientific evidence was not forthcoming of a proof of mesothelioma causation from asbestos in para-occupational exposures until the mid-1970s in asbestos manufacturing facilities, and later in take-home exposures by "end users" of asbestos materials in the 1980s. Case reports of domestic exposure to chrysotile and mesothelioma are rare and most mesotheliomas that occur in women are spontaneous and idiopathic.

20

What did asbestos pipe insulation manufacturers and the U.S. Navy understand about the risk to manufacturing employees and end users?

It is my opinion that the information on the health hazards of asbestos exposure and mesothelioma was generally accepted by the scientific community in the mid-1960s, largely due to the work of Dr. JC Wagner, beginning in 1960, related to exposure to a particular type of blue crocidolite asbestos in a particular location in South Africa. Since it was thought that little crocidolite asbestos was used in the United States, experts were wary of accepting the risk of mesothelioma in U.S. asbestos workers until 1964 and 1965, when articles began to be published regarding insulation workers in this country. The information was summarized on December 31, 1965, with the release of the *Annals of the New York Academy of Sciences*, International Meeting on Asbestos in 1964.

It would be my opinion that as of 1966, various manufacturers of asbestos insulation had been notified of the health hazards of their products, based on the international consensus suggested by the publication of the New York Academy Symposium in January 1966, and would need to have appropriately placed warning labels on any insulation products produced that contained asbestos. Manufacturers of asbestos insulation products began to place warning labels on their products in the 1966–1967 era. No specific epidemiological studies of these U.S. asbestos pipe insulation manufacturing facilities were performed until 1971, beginning in an amosite pipe insulation company in Paterson, New Jersey. In the 20-year period between 1974 and 1994, approximately 35 cohort studies were performed and published concerning the health effects from asbestos exposure during the application or manufacturing of these products.

Initially, it was thought in the 1960s that crocidolite and chrysotile asbestos were the major culprits in the causation of mesothelioma. It was felt, at that time, that it was most likely that amosite asbestos was the safest form of asbestos insulation, since relatively few cases had been reported in amosite miners and millers in South Africa. In 1972, Dr. Selikoff and coworkers published an article based on a study of amosite insulation workers in Paterson, New Jersey, with a high incidence of mesothelioma. Subsequent studies have confirmed that insulation products containing amosite asbestos are associated with a high incidence of mesothelioma. Subsequently, manufacturers of amosite-containing insulation removed amosite asbestos from their products.

The information on the health hazards of asbestos was carefully followed by the International Asbestos Workers Union, and was published in its journal, *The Asbestos Worker*, during the 1960s. During the 1960s, the permissible exposure limit for asbestos-containing products was 5 million particles/ft^3, as suggested by the U.S. Public Health Service and the American Conference of Governmental Industrial Hygienists (ACGIH), which is roughly equivalent to 30 fibers/cc. In 1968, the British government recommended that the exposure to asbestos products for insulators be reduced to 5 fibers/cc. The ACGIH recommended that the standard in the United States be lowered to 2 million particles of asbestos/cc (12 fibers/cc) in response to the new British standard. They later recommended that the level of exposure be lowered further, in 1971, to 5 fibers/cc. This recommendation was promulgated in the United States by a ruling by the newly formed Occupational Safety and Health Administration (OSHA) in 1972. The exposure level was further reduced, in 1976, to 2 fibers/cc. The OSHA standard assumes a continuous exposure to asbestos over an 8-hour day and 40-hour week, or roughly 2000 hours per year. It was felt at that time that if the asbestos exposure could be capped at a level sufficient to prevent asbestosis, then future asbestos-related lung disease, including mesothelioma, would be prevented.

We know that warnings about the health hazards of asbestos were placed on the boxes of Johns-Manville Thermobestos pipe insulation on September 10, 1964. Mundet Corporation stopped production of asbestos insulation products before November 6, 1963, because of poor sales, with less than a 2% market share and low profits. Later, in 1966, after publication of the reports in the *Annals of the New York Academy of Sciences* of the meeting on December 31, 1965, warnings were place on Kalo pipe insulation and Pittsburgh Corning Unibestos. This seems reasonably prudent based on the information available at that time. In the mid-1960s, papers were reported from Great Britain and the United States on the health hazards for individuals living near asbestos manufacturing plants. Most of the physicians at the time paid little attention to this information and it was not until the mid-to-late 1970s and early 1980s that workers' clothing became a concern of the general medical community.

The initial asbestos health hazard epidemiologic studies were performed on asbestos insulators, asbestos textile workers, and asbestos product manufactures. It took about 10 years for the scientific community to begin studying the risk from asbestos exposure in refineries, chemical plants, electric power plants, and other large end users of asbestos insulation. The only report of an asbestos-related health hazard in electricity-generating power plants, was an early nonpublished report of medical officers in a power plant in London in 1965, which was mentioned in a paper by Bonnel and others at the 13th International Congress on Occupational Health in Brighton, England, in 1975. In October 1971, RC Browne warned about the potential of exposure in power plants, but did not present any data from any epidemiological studies. (Browne RC. Health in power stations. *Proc R Soc Med* 1971;64:1075–7.) In 1975, Fontaine and Trayer published a report entitled "Asbestos control in steam-electric generating plants" (Fontaine JH, Trayer DM. *Am Ind Hyg Assoc J* 1975;36:126–30). This was followed by a paper by Hirsh et al. in the *Annals of New York Academy of Science* in 1979. (Hirsch A, Di Menza L, Carre A et al. Asbestos risk among full-time workers in an electricity-generating power station. 1979;330:137–45; Bonnel JA et al. A review of the control of asbestos processes in the Central Electricity Board. Presented at: *XVIII International Congress in Occupational Health*, Brighton, England. This paper was not published and is unavailable for review, but is quoted in the paper by Hirsh et al.)

My conclusion is that the risk of asbestos-related mesothelioma and other health effects, was not recognized in America until 1966 in asbestos insulators, and not until 1975 in U.S. power plants and many other large end users of asbestos insulation. The "middleman," or wholesaler of asbestos-containing insulation products, would not be responsible for the health effects related to the end use of a properly labeled product with appropriate warnings. This situation is no different than holding Walmart or any sporting goods store responsible for selling ammunition to someone who shoots and kills someone.

Finally, the issue of the need for warnings about wearing asbestos-contaminated clothing home from the job site, is certainly pertinent in many cases. In 1972, recommendations to never wear asbestos-contaminated clothing home were made, but only for those individuals who directly worked with asbestos, such as insulators. The new National Institute for Occupational Safety and Health (NIOSH) standard for clothing was provided in Section I-8 of the *Criteria for a Recommended Standard. Occupational Exposure to Asbestos 1972, US Public Health Service, CDC, National Institute of Occupational Health and Safety 1972 HSM 72–10267.* The new standard applied only to workers exposed to an average of >1 fiber/cc over an 8-hour day or with peak exposures of >5 fibers/cc (Page I-3). They suggested regulations for protective clothing.

NAVAL AND SHIPYARD EXPOSURE

Commercial ships, passenger vessels, and warships are all very vulnerable to fires on board as exemplified by the ship *General Slocum*, which caught fire in 1904 and resulted in the death of 137 individuals. This incident is similar to what happened on the ship *Moro Castle* in September 1934, again with the loss of 137 lives. Many other ship fires occurred with significant loss of life in the early 20th century. This made government and naval safety staff aware of the need to provide better fire protection on any type of naval vessel. Ship under-writers refused to insure ships without adequate fire protection around 1935, and their requirements increased in 1939, at the onset of World War II. By 1940, the U.S. Navy, Coast Guard, and Maritime Commission, demanded asbestos insulation in critical parts of ships under construction, including high-temperature applications, packings, boiler casings, piping, gaskets, tape, and electrical insulation. Amosite felt insulation began to be used in 1934 by the Navy, originally only on turbine insulation. Amosite pipe covering was developed in late 1935 and early 1936. It was first used on naval vessels in 1937. Water-repellent amosite felt was developed in the early part of 1942, as a replacement for hair felt in the insulation of cold water lines, to prevent sweating. (Fleisher WE et al. A health survey of pipe covering operations in constructing naval vessels. *J Ind Hyg Toxicol* 1946;28:9–16.)

Ernest Brown conducted a survey of the New York Navy Yard for asbestosis and found no cases of asbestosis. (Brown EW. Industrial hygiene and the navy in national defense. *War Med* 1941;1:3–14.) Minimum requirements for safety and industrial health in shipyards were published by the Navy and Maritime Commission in 1942. Asbestos, as used in covering pipes, was an exposure requiring respiratory equipment such as respirators. (*J Ind Hyg Toxicol* 1943;4:259–63.)

During World War II, employment in U.S. shipyards rose from 168,000 in 1940 to 1,772,000 in November 1943. There was a high rate of worker turnover resulting in high numbers of American workers being exposed to asbestos.

When information about the health hazards of asbestos from ship construction appeared in 1964–1965, the Navy was resistant to using nonasbestos substitutes, which were thought to provide inferior fire protection. Asbestos substitutes were slowly developed so that asbestos insulation requirements could be slowly phased out over the next 10 years. After the Fleisher–Drinker report, Navy officials focused on maintaining safety standards. The *General Safety Rules Manual, Puget Sound Naval Shipyard of 1950* stated on page 8 that "Wherever there are fumes, irritating vapors, or heavy dusts present in the atmosphere, respiratory equipment is necessary for your protection."

Meanwhile, Navy physicians and epidemiologists carefully followed the scientific literature in order to establish appropriate safety standards for naval personnel. The Navy had precise military specifications for the construction of Navy vessels in private shipyards, including specifications and requirements for the use of asbestos-containing materials. The Navy recognized that excessive exposure to asbestos dust could cause asbestosis, and in 1950, recommended respiratory protection when exposed to dusty conditions, and that manufacturers provide materials to the Navy, where required, so as to provide warnings associated with their products.

All construction was also required to meet Navy safety requirements. During this period, the Navy continued to require amosite insulation, but in 1964, recommended wetting down the insulation and wearing respirators. In 1964, the ACGIH recommended the same 5 million particles per cubic foot (mppcf) of asbestos dust standard, which was reviewed and lowered to 2 mppcf or 12 fibers/cc in 1968 and 5 fibers/cc in 1970. Proof that the general work environment aboard ships and engine rooms was unsafe occurred in the mid-1960s. In 1964,

William T Marr, who was an industrial hygienist at the Long Beach Naval Shipyard in California, noted five employees, averaging 15 years exposure to asbestos, to be receiving disability, and one pipe coverer/insulator had died in 1962. Marr noted that many employees were involved in asbestos removal after the war, and many of those with more than 20 years of exposure had disease, but the average exposure was roughly within the 5 mppcf standard. Subsequently, many more reports of asbestos-related disease in shipyards were published. (Marr W. Asbestos exposure during naval vessel overhaul. *Am Ind Hyg Assoc J* 1964;25:264–8; Selikoff I, Churg J, Hammond E. Relation between exposure to asbestos and mesothelioma. *N Engl J Med* 1965;272:560–5; Harries PG. Asbestos hazards in naval dockyards. *Ann Occup Hyg* 1968;11:135–45; Balzar JL, Cooper WC. The work environment of insulating workers. *Am Ind Hyg Assoc J* 1968;29(3):222–7; Sheers G, Templeton AR. Effects of asbestos in dockyard workers. *Br Med J* 1968;3:574–9; Stumphius J. Epidemiology of mesothelioma on Walcheren Island. *Br J Ind Med* 1971;28:59–66; Harries PG. Asbestos dust concentrations in ship repairing: A practical approach to improving asbestos hygiene in naval dockyards. *Ann Occup Hyg* 1971;14:241–54; Murphy RL, Ferris BG, Burgess WA et al. Effects of low concentrations of asbestos—Clinical, radiologic, and epidemiologic observations in shipyard pipe covers and controls. *N Engl J Med* 1971;285:1271–8; Selikoff IJ, Lilis R, Nicholson WJ. Asbestos disease in United States shipyards. *Ann NY Acad Sci* 1979;330:295–311; Sheers G. Mesothelioma risks in a naval dockyard. *Arch Environ Health* 1980;35:276–82; Franke KD, Paustenbach D. Government and Navy knowledge regarding health hazards of asbestos: A state of the science evaluation (1900 to 1970). *Inhal Toxicol* 2011;23(Suppl. 3):1–20.)

Amphibole asbestos products were used intermittently as needed, and there was thought to be no significant exposure to crocidolite in the United States compared to British and European shipyards, since U.S. naval specifications required 85% mag pipe insulation. This required the use of amosite, which in the 1960s was thought to be the safest form of asbestos. The Navy was one of the biggest consumers of asbestos and monitored the workers and workplace carefully. Little was known about the risk to end users until 1964. (Franke K, Paustenbach D. Government and Navy knowledge regarding health hazards of asbestos: A state of the science evaluation (1900–1970). *Inhal Toxicol* 2011;23(Suppl. 3):1–20; Hollins D, Paustenbach DJ, Clark K et al. A visual historical review of exposure to asbestos at Puget Sound naval shipyard (1962–1972). *J Toxicol Environ Health B* 2009;12:124–56.)

I am frequently asked about the minimum duration of exposure to amphibole asbestos required to produce a mesothelioma in a shipyard. Little was known about the difference in risk to insulators working in ships compared to insulators working elsewhere, until the 1970s. Selikoff et al. reported in 1979 that a comparison of insulation worker deaths between 1967 and 1976 revealed that the incidence of asbestosis was 17.8% in shipyard insulators versus 7.8% in insulators employed elsewhere. (Selikoff IJ, Lilis R, Nicholson WJ. Asbestos disease in United States shipyards. *Ann NY Acad Sci* 1979;330:295–311.) No specific information about the minimum dose of asbestos required to produce a mesothelioma, from only American shipyard exposures, is available to answer that question. Employment in shipyards in the Tidewater of Virginia, using asbestos insulation prior to 1968, was associated with a tenfold increased risk of mesothelioma to shipyard employees who had no known direct contact with asbestos, and an 18-fold increased risk in career shipyard workers who handled asbestos directly, according to Tagnon, Blot, and coworkers. Unfortunately, only limited data are available as to the minimum duration of employment in American naval shipyards capable of increasing the risk of mesothelioma. (Tagnon I, Blot WJ, Stroube RB et al. Mesothelioma associated with the shipbuilding industry in coastal Virginia. *Cancer Res* 1980;40:3875–9.)

Bianchi, Brollo, and others reported on asbestos exposure and malignant mesothelioma in a major shipbuilding area of Italy, where a substantial amount of crocidolite asbestos was used rather than amosite asbestos. The majority of the 557 cases of mesothelioma worked in shipyards. The duration of exposure to asbestos of 348 cases of mesothelioma was reported to be from less than 1 year to more than 50 years. Only 0.6% of cases of mesothelioma had an exposure duration of less than 1 year, and only 6.8% had an exposure duration of 1–4 years. The latency time, or the time between the first exposure to asbestos and the time of diagnosis of a mesothelioma, was a mean of 48.8 years and a median of 51.0 years. (Bianchi C, Brollo A, Ramani L, Bianchi T, Giarelli L. Asbestos exposure in malignant mesothelioma of the pleura: A survey of 557 cases. *Ind Health* 2001;39:161–7.)

Indirect information is available from British asbestos manufacturing facilities, but not shipyards, where there was heavy exposure to crocidolite asbestos, unlike the predominately amosite and mixed asbestos exposure in American shipyards. Browne and Smither studied 144 cases of mesothelioma and related their duration of exposure to the incidence of mesothelioma. These confirmed British cases of mesothelioma were identified among employees of an organization using asbestos in the manufacturing of insulation (crocidolite exposure in factories A and B as compared with factories C, D, and E, where there was no crocidolite exposure, but exposure to amosite and chrysotile asbestos). Some outside laggers worked at various outside jobs not mentioned by the authors, and shipyard exposures were not mentioned. The primary sites of mesothelioma were peritoneal in 74 cases, pleural in 66 cases, and undetermined in four cases. All employees had been exposed to amphibole asbestos, and evidence from different factories confirmed the predominant role of crocidolite in the production of mesothelioma; there were 133 cases of mesothelioma in crocidolite asbestos-using factories operating between 1913 and 1967 with approximately 10,000 employees in factory A, and factory B operating between 1939 and 1968 with 2000 employees. Only four mesotheliomas occurred in factories C, D, and E, with 7500 employees operating between 1948 and 1980 using mixed amosite and chrysotile asbestos. No cases of mesothelioma occurred from a plant manufacturing textiles and friction materials from 1902 to 1980 with 15,000 employees exposed only to chrysotile asbestos. Approximately 22% of the mesothelioma cases of those workers exposed to amphibole asbestos were exposed for less than 1 year, 15% under 6 months and 6% no more than 3 months in this very heavily exposed cohort to predominately crocidolite asbestos. The higher exposures were responsible for the increased risk of peritoneal versus pleural mesothelioma. No direct comparison is available, however, comparing the asbestos exposure in these British insulation manufacturing plants to shipyard exposures. (Browne K, Smither WJ. Asbestos related mesothelioma: Factors discriminating between pleural and peritoneal sites. *Br J Ind Med* 1983;40:145–52.) This finding is similar to the finding of Victor Roggli, who found that only 6% of his mesothelioma study populations were exposed for less than 6 months. (Roggli V. Malignant mesothelioma and duration of asbestos exposure: Correlation with tissue mineral fibre content. *Ann Occup Hyg* 1995;39:363–74.)

21

The intervention of government to provide safety standards

The first U.S. standard for controlling exposure to asbestos dust was recommended by Dreesen, of the U.S. Public Health Service, in 1938, following a study of 541 employees of four asbestos textile plants in which massive exposures had occurred. A tentative limit of asbestos dust recommended for the textile industry was 5 million particles per cubic foot (mppcf) of asbestos dust as determined by the midget impinger technique and area samplers. The limitation of the midget impinger is that it can produce errors if the sampling rate is not set properly, and according to Drinker and Hatch, "midget impinger efficiency varied directly with sampling rate and inversely with particle size of the collected dust." (Drinker P, Hatch T. *Industrial Dust*. New York: McGraw-Hill, 1954, p. 151.) The authors found numerous cases of asbestosis at an exposure level above 5 mppcf. The four textile mills evaluated had been in operation for only 6–16 years. Those 75% of workers employed for more than 15 years had at least early stages of asbestosis. Those workers with disabling asbestosis had left the workplace and could not be evaluated. Only three doubtful cases were seen at a concentrations below 5 mppcf. The limitations of the study were that only 66 persons had been exposed as long as 10 years and only two for more than 20 years. None of the 39 persons exposed to less than 2.5 mppcf showed evidence of asbestosis, but only six of these had been employed for more than 5 years. The authors recognized the many limitations of the study and stated that "5 mppcf may be regarded tentatively as the threshold value for asbestos dust exposure until better data are available." It is important to point out that during the 1940s, Vigliani did a similar epidemiologic study to Dr. Dreesen on asbestos textile workers in northern Italy and he came to the same conclusions about a safe level of asbestos dust as did Dr. Dreesen in 1938. One of the problems with early dust measurement was that the measurement tools were inaccurate. Merewether-Price used an Owens Jet Counter that only took "snap-shot" samples and Dreesen used this same technique. The Owens Jet sampler was used to determine particle size and length and count fibers in a sample by oil immersion microscopy. It could not distinguish thin cotton fibers from asbestos fibers, but was able to estimate the percentage of fibers versus nuisance dust in a sample. The median length of fibers ranged from 7 to 16.3 μm, but very long fibers of 400 μm in length were noted in the study of weavers. Asbestos textile mills studied by Dreesen were extremely dusty with concentrations of total dust of more than 200 mppcf. Once an estimate of the percentage of fibers in an area sample was performed, then the actual "asbestos dust" concentration could be estimated from the total measurements in mppcf.

The thermal precipitator was a much better tool for determining the percentage of fibers versus nuisance dust in a sample, but was not used in asbestos factories in Britain until 1951. The membrane filter method was not used in Britain until the late 1960s. (Dreesen WC, Dallavalle JM, Edwards TL et al. *A Study of Asbestosis in the Asbestos Textile Industry*. US Treasury Department, Public Health Service Bulletin No. 241. Washington DC: U.S. Government Printing Office, 1938, p. 117; Sayers RR, Dreessen WC. Asbestosis. *Am J Pub Health* 1939;29:205–14; Wikeley NJ. Measurement of asbestos dust levels in British factories in the 1930s. *Am J Ind Med* 1993;24:509–20.) Selikoff, speaking in 1982 in a report to the U.S. Department of Labor, stated that the lack of reliable exposure data necessarily limits the accuracy of estimates of dose–response relationships.

The U.S. Navy was about to embark on a massive shipbuilding program in 1941. Ernest Brown, a Captain in the Navy Medical Corps, investigated the New York Navy Yard, and was concerned about the potential hazard from inhalation of asbestos, so he x-rayed workers exposed to asbestos for up to 17 years and found no cases of asbestosis. The safety practice was to moisten the material, use localized exhaust ventilation and respirators in the dustiest areas, and continue x-ray surveillance. In July 1942, the Navy Department, in cooperation with the Maritime Commission, agreed to sponsor a joint project. The study was supervised by Philip Drinker, who was the inventor of the iron lung and a world authority on industrial hygiene and dust control. The first author was Walter Fleischer, a Navy Commander, and the report is commonly called the Fleischer–Drinker report. The authors concluded that asbestos pipe covering was a safe occupation and that while these workers intermittently were exposed to asbestos levels far above the 5 mppcf standard, overall, the 5 mppcf standard seemed adequate to protect workers. The authors studied four Navy shipyards in which standard procedure was to wet down asbestos material before installation. The incidence of asbestosis was 0.29%, or three cases out of 1074 pipe coverers. The exposures to asbestos were high, at up to 142 mppcf. The apparent discrepancy between such high exposures and safety was thought to be due to the fact that pipe coverers did multiple tasks, some with low asbestos exposure and some with high asbestos exposure. It was felt that the constantly changing work environment resulted in a low overall exposure within the 5 mppcf standard. The integrity of the dust measurement data obtained by Fleisher and co-workers was supported more than 20 years later by Murphy and coworkers from Boston in 1965–1966. Murphy and colleagues found the estimates of exposure of Fleisher and Drinker to be accurate by using the same Konimeter method as Kotze and the same midget impinger technique. Total dust counts were made and then separate fiber counts were also made. (Murphy R, Ferris B, Burgess W, Worcester J, Gaensler E. Effects of low concentrations of asbestos. *N Engl J Med* 1971;285:1271–8.) Asbestosis became evident after 13 years of exposure or a total exposure of 60 mppcf/year, which is equivalent to 90 fibers/cc/year.

Fleischer and Drinker assumed that asbestosis results from breathing asbestos fibers of long length, based on Lanza's 1935 publication. (Lanza AJ. *Effects of the Inhalation of Asbestos Dust in the Lungs of Asbestos Workers. Public Health Report* (vol. 50). Washington, DC: U.S. Treasury, 1935.) Fleisher and Drinker assumed that "chopped-up" asbestos, or short fibers of 1–2 μm, were inert. They concerned themselves with long fibers having a width-to-length ratio of 3 or greater, which could be seen microscopically. It was assumed that medium-length fibers would be deposited in the upper airways. According to Nowinski, a concentration of 6 mppcf of total dust would be equivalent to 0.2 mppcf of asbestos dust with a fiber length >15 μm. The authors mentioned that "petrographic analysis of asbestos cement indicate that the amount of diatomaceous earth may be as high as 87%." The published text states 5 mppcf of "total dust" as being safe, which remains controversial in that many claim that Fleischer and Drinker meant to say "asbestos dust," as did Dreesen. For example, Kenneth Smith, Medical Director of Johns-Manville Corp., wrote to Detroit-Edison Company in February 1959 about the health hazards of Thermobestos asbestos insulation. Smith assumed that since the product contained approximately 10% asbestos, using the American Conference of Governmental Hygienists (ACGIH) standard of 5 mppcf of asbestos dust would permit exposures to 50 mppcf of total dust. (Nowinski P. Chronology of asbestos regulation in United States workplaces. In: K Antman, J Aisner (Eds.), *Asbestos-Related Malignancy.* New York: Grune & Stratton, 1986, pp. 99–134.)

The Navy regulations required amosite insulation chemical composition to be 47.5% silica, 45% iron oxide, and 6% magnesium oxide. This was called "85% mag" insulation. The only type of insulation to meet Navy standards was a mixture of chrysotile (high magnesia content) and amosite (high silica content). (Fleischer WE et al. A health survey of pipe covering operations in constructing naval vessels. *J Ind Hyg Toxicol* 1946;28:9–16.)

The ACGIH recommended a standard of 5 mppcf of asbestos dust, and not total dust, between 1946 and 1968. The federal government in 1951 adopted the 5 mppcf standard under the Walsh–Healy Act to protect all government workers.

This preliminary standard remained the Navy, state regulatory agencies, and industry standard until 1972. It was in the 1960s that there was an increased incidence of asbestosis and asbestos-associated neoplasms found in workers whose workplaces were in compliance with these regulations, at which point it became very clear that the regulations were not stringent enough, and that the exposures obviously had been excessive. Much of these data were reviewed in the *Annals of Occupational Hygiene* in 1968, when the Committee on Hygiene Standards of the British Occupational Hygiene Society, revisited the issue of a safe level of asbestos dust exposure, and felt that a safe level of asbestos dust exposure would be a level at which less than 1% of the exposed workers developed asbestosis. The development of basilar rales (an early sign of asbestosis) was thought to be more sensitive than chest x-ray abnormalities from exposure to asbestos. The results of this study were that exposures below 100 fiber/year, with a lower confidence limit of 51 fiber-years and an average of 112 fiber-years, were thought to be protective from asbestosis. This level was an average level of 2 fibers/cc of asbestos dust over an 8-hour day for 50 years. The authors concluded their paper by stating,

> The quantitative relationship between asbestos and cancer risk is not known, nor is it known exactly why these two are related, nor even whether all kinds of asbestos present a risk. Consequently, it is not possible at this time to specify an air concentration, which is known will be free of risk in this respect.

NIOSH/ACGIH STANDARDS

Prior to 1971, the responsibility for regulating exposure to asbestos was primarily left with the states, who followed the AGGIH-suggested standards. Each state promulgated permissible exposure limits for asbestos exposure. Different states had different regulations as to what was a safe exposure. Because of the increasing problems with asbestos, as well as for other reasons, the federal government decided to step in and form the Occupational Safety and Health Administration (OSHA) as the regulatory/enforcement division, and the National Institute of Occupational Safety and Health (NIOSH) as the research arm of the U.S. Department of Labor. This was done in 1971, and OSHA began regulating asbestos in 1972, according to NIOSH-recommended standards. On June 7, 1972, OSHA enacted a permissible exposure limit of 5 fibers/cc, later to be reduced to 2 fibers/cc in 1976. The chronology of these regulations is nicely summarized by Brownson (Table 21.1; Figures 21.1 and 21.2). (Brownson. *Monaldi Arch Chest Dis* 1998;53(2):181–5; Homa DM, Garabrant DH, Gillespie BW. A meta-analysis of colorectal cancer and asbestos exposure. *Am J Epidemiol* 1994;139:1210–22.)

Table 21.1 Exposure levels: Ambient and regulatory

USPHS	1938	30 fibers/cc
ACGIH-proposed standard	1968	12 fibers/cc
ACGIH-proposed standard	1970	5 fibers/cc
ACGIH-proposed standard	1972	2 fibers/cc
ACGIH-proposed standard	1983	0.5 fibers/cc
ACGIH-proposed standard	1986	0.2 fibers/cc
ACGIH-proposed standard	1990	0.1 fibers/cc
Urban ambient air		0.0001 fibers/cc
Building with/ACM		0.0002 fibers/cc
Quebec mining towns		0.1 fibers/cc
Historic epi studies		1–5 fibers/cc

Source: Homa DM et al. *J Epidemiol* 1994;1939:1210.
Note: American Conference of Governmental Hygienists (ACGIH)-proposed asbestos standards.

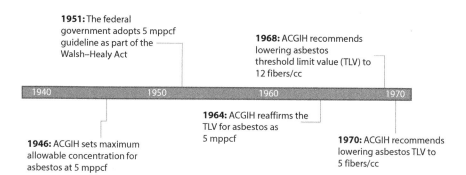

Figure 21.1 Timeline of asbestos exposure limits and recommendations, 1946–1970.

The bases of these regulations have been published since 1972 in what are called NIOSH Asbestos Criteria Documents. These documents are based on reviews of the world's literature and what was known about the health effects of asbestos, and it is on the basis of these documents that further regulations on establishing a safe level of asbestos are then made. When one reviews these documents, it is clear that for regulatory purposes, the U.S. Department of Labor has chosen to use a linear model to extrapolate risk. A linear model is a model based on calculating the risk of adverse health effects from historical cohorts in which the dose was high enough to produce a significant amount of disease. These historical cohorts that were chosen for risk assessment were always the cohorts that had the highest risk, such as the risk of lung cancer in asbestos

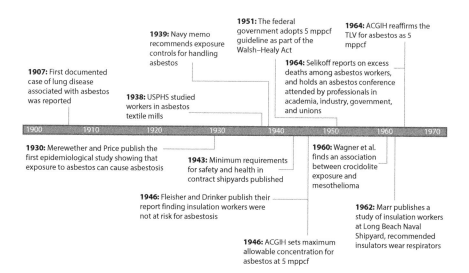

Figure 21.2 Regulatory time line for asbestos. (From Franke K, Paustenbach D. *Inhal Toxicol* 2011;23(Suppl. 3):1–20.)

textile workers, and workers that were primarily exposed to amphibole asbestos. This method has been chosen because it would seem to best protect the safety of the average American.

Another problem with NIOSH risk assessment has been the failure to account for the effects of fiber length and diameter, and type of work exposure when evaluating risk for lung cancer. Repeated studies have demonstrated increased risk of lung cancer in asbestos textile workers as opposed to asbestos miners and millers. The inclusion of asbestos textile workers in the mix with other asbestos exposures overestimates the risk for nontextile asbestos exposures. (Wang X, Lin S, Yano E et al. Exposure-specific lung cancer risks in Chinese chrysotile textile workers and mining workers. *Lung Cancer* 2014;85(2):119–24.)

In summary, the main problems with NIOSH risk analysis are that they do not take into account the fact that different processes and different fiber types have different risks, which may be much lower (by one or two magnitudes) than the risks of some of these historical cohorts. Secondly, using the linear model extrapolates back to a level of zero, whereas zero risk only occurs when there is zero exposure. In all biological models, there is a threshold dose below which no risk exists. Every adult human has been exposed to some environmental asbestos and therefore the zero risk concept used in back extrapolation is an oxymoron. There are few good exposure data on risk at low levels of exposure. Government agencies ignore the threshold dose and assume that it is zero. Thirdly, all biological models of the relationship between a given toxic exposure and its health effects are exponential and nonlinear. Therefore, one would have to conclude that the only safe dose of asbestos on the basis of this regulatory model would be no exposure whatsoever. This is unscientific, and in reality, government agencies like the Environmental Protection Agency (EPA) and NIOSH define risk as any exposure at which the risk of an adverse health effect, including death, is less the 1 in 100,000. OSHA stated in its promulgation of the proposed 1986 standard of 0.1 fibers/cc that the expectation was that 3.4 deaths from cancer would occur per 1000 individuals exposed to asbestos. (Federal Register Vol. 51,119: Table 6, p. 22644.) Government agencies can be accused of double-speak because, on the one hand, they claim that a variety of potentially toxic substances are unsafe, such as arsenic in drinking water, while on the other hand stating that some exposure to arsenic in drinking water is at a "safe level." The word "safe" as used by government agencies really means "relatively safe or safe enough," but not absolutely safe at any level of exposure.

There are two problems with this type of safety analysis. First of all, it is widely recognized by all experts that there is no such thing as no or zero exposure to asbestos since it is present in the ambient air. There is environmental exposure to asbestos in all individuals due to airborne asbestos, predominantly from the constant erosion of asbestos-bearing rocky surfaces. The average person in North America has an asbestos concentration of 1 million fibers per gram of dry lung in their lung at the age of 50 years or older. Also, historical studies of the risk in residents of the town of Thetford, Quebec, have demonstrated that ambient environmental levels in asbestos-producing areas are usually 100 times the average environmental exposures of those in nonasbestos-producing areas. This means that the average concentration of asbestos in the air is in the order of two magnitudes higher (100 times) than what we would find in the average city in the United States or in nonexposed Canadian residents. The residents of this city do not have an increased risk of mesothelioma, lung cancer, or asbestosis based on the exposure to this increased amount of asbestos in their environment. (Case BW, Sebastien P. Environmental and occupational exposures to chrysotile asbestos: A comparative microanalytic study. *Arch Environ Health* 1987;42:185–91; Sebastien P, Begin R, Case BW, McDonald JC. Inhalation of chrysotile asbestos dust. *Accomplish Oncol* 1986;1:19–29.) The Quebec information indicates that even at much higher exposure levels to chrysotile asbestos, there is no risk of adverse health effects.

Health risks have to be balanced with public safety. AE Martin wrote in February 1970:

Mesotheliomas may be caused by the inhalation of very small numbers of fibers, and it therefore becomes a question of how far it is reasonable to attempt to limit exposure to the general public. The use of asbestos is essential for protection of the public against fire and other risks, and its value must therefore be weighed against the degrees of risk, which arise from its use and the practical difficulties of control. (Martin AE. Asbestos in the environment, possible hazards to the general population. In: *Health Trends*. London: Her Majesty's Stationary Office, 1970, reprinted in *Med Bull* 1971;31:164–73.)

There are other examples in the United States in which the ambient concentrations of environmental asbestos are really quite high, but there is no evidence of significant disease in these areas. This type of evidence as well as animal studies has suggested that there is a threshold dose for the adverse health effects of asbestos. A threshold dose for asbestosis has been nicely shown in animals by Illgren and Wagner in a publication in *Regulatory Toxicology and Pharmacology* in 1991. Similar studies by JMG Davis and others have shown a threshold dose for not only mesothelioma, but also lung cancer. We do not find lung cancer in animals unless the dose of asbestos has been sufficient to produce asbestosis. Davis and Cowie reviewed some of these relationships in 1990. (Davis JMG, Cowie HA. The relationship between fibrosis and cancer in experimental animals exposed to asbestos and other fibers. *Environ Health Perspect* 1990;88:305–9; Ilgren EB, Browne K. Asbestos-related mesothelioma: Evidence for a threshold in animals and humans. *Regul Toxicol Pharmacol* 1991;13:116–32; Davis JMG. Experimental studies on mineral fiber carcinogenesis: An overview. In: *Mechanisms in Fiber Carcinogenesis*. NY: Plenum Press, 1991, pp. 51–8; Davis JMG. Mineral fibre carcinogenesis: Experimental data relating to the importance of fibre type, size, deposition, dissolution, and migration. In: J Bignon, J Peto, R Saracci (Eds.), *Non-Occupational Exposure to Mineral Fibers*. Lyon, France: International Agency for Research on Cancer, 1989, pp. 33–45; Davis JMG, Bolton RE, Miller BG, Niven K.

Mesothelioma dose response following intraperitoneal injection of mineral fibres. *Int J Exp Pathol* 1991;72:263–74.)

Why is this information important? This information is important because the evidence from biological models in animals and other studies of human workers, who have been exposed to significant amounts of asbestos in various industries shows that, while there has been significant exposure, there has been no significant disease. All of this suggests that there is a threshold dose below which adverse health effects from asbestos exposure do not occur. This means that there is a safe level of asbestos exposure below which adverse health effects will not occur. Furthermore, no more than 8% in the largest series, to 20% in one small series, of workers heavily exposed to amphibole asbestos develop mesothelioma. Once a threshold dose of amphibole asbestos has been reached, further exposures do not increase the risk. (La Vecchia C, Boffetta P. Role of stopping exposure and recent exposure to asbestos in the risk of mesothelioma. *Eur J Cancer Prev* 2012;21:227–30.) This suggests that there are significant genetic and other cofactors that increase mesothelioma risk. (Jasani B, Gibbs A. Mesothelioma not associated with asbestos exposure. *Arch Pathol Lab Med* 2012;136(3):262–7; Carbone M, Ly B, Dodson R et al. Malignant mesothelioma: Facts, myths, and hypotheses. *J Cell Physiol* 2012;227(1):44–58; Kalogeraki AM, Tamiolakis DJ, Lagoudaki ED et al. Familial mesothelioma in first degree relatives. *Diagn Cytopathol* 2013;41(7):654–7; Clin B, Morlais F, Launoy G et al. Cancer incidence within a cohort occupationally exposed to asbestos: A study of dose–response relationships. *Occup Environ Med* 2011;68(11):832–6.)

There has been a lot of current interest as to what is a safe level for asbestos. Those that use the linear model feel that the only safe dose is no dose. The scientific evidence overwhelmingly indicates that there is a safe dose for asbestos below which no health hazards will develop. This has been particularly important in regards to the issue of children in schools. There was much concern in the 1980s and 1990s about the risk to school children exposed to small amounts of asbestos from ceiling tiles and other areas of asbestos found in U.S. schools. A large task force to study this question was put together by congress and called the "Health Effects Institute—Asbestos Research," which was an independent, nonprofit organization formed to support research to determine what are the airborne exposure levels prevalent in buildings and what levels are safe. This committee of national figures included Archibald Cox, who was the Professor Emeritus at Harvard Law School; Donald Kennedy, President of Stanford University; and William O Baker, Chairman Emeritus of Bell Laboratories; plus many other well-known scientists. They published the results of their studies in 1991, and concluded that the levels that were commonly found in schools and buildings generally were so low that there was no evidence of any adverse health effects. This work and the *Report of the Royal Commission on Matters of Health and Safety Arising from the Use of Asbestos in Ontario* published in 1984, indicate that there are low levels of exposure at which no adverse health effects can be measured, and that the risk from asbestos exposure is primarily related to the dose of asbestos, as well as the fiber type of asbestos. The dose is measured by the concentration of the asbestos and the duration of exposure.

Rachel Maines has written an excellent book that I recommend to the reader who desires a more thorough review of the historical information about naval and government regulations regarding asbestos safety regulations and usage. (Maines R. *Asbestos and Fire: Technological Tradeoffs and the Body at Risk.* Newark: Rutgers University Press, 2005.)

22

Is there a safe or risk-free level of asbestos exposure?

The question as to whether there is a safe level of asbestos exposure is an oxymoron, or includes contradictory terms and is pointedly foolish, since everyone has had some exposure to environmental asbestos. Everyone has up to 1,000,000 asbestos fibers per gram of dry/wt. of lung tissue in their lungs suggesting therefore that there is a safe level of asbestos exposure. If everyone has asbestos fibers in their lungs, then there must be a safe level of asbestos exposure since the background number of mesothelioma cases is approximately 2–4 per million. The whole issue of what is a safe dose is further complicated by the fact that there is much argument about the methods of measuring dose. The historical measurements that were taken from the mid-1930s through to 1968, were done by measuring the total dose of dust, and then taking a percentage of the total dose of dust, based on the content of the amount of asbestos in the products in the environment, and assuming that the amount of asbestos present in the dust would be represented by a relative percentage of the total dust measured. Actual asbestos fibers in the environment were never measured in these historical studies. Most of the exposure information was obtained by area samples, rather than by personal samplers, which measure the asbestos fiber concentration close to the face or respiratory zone.

The introduction of the membrane filter technique in the mid-1960s, and adopted in 1972 by the National Institute of Occupational Safety and Health (NIOSH) in the United States, was thought to have improved the exposure estimate by actually measuring asbestos fibers in the breathing zone rather than total area dust. However, the criterion for the measurement of fibers was strictly an aspect ratio criterion that the physical dimension of the fiber must be longer than 5 μm with a length-to-diameter ratio of 3:1 or greater. Any fiber seen, using phase-contrast microscopy, was counted as an asbestos fiber, resulting in many cleavage fragments, acicular crystals, and other nonfibrous dusts, being counted as asbestos fibers. Fibers shorter than 5 μm in length have insignificant carcinogenic potential and health risk increases with length. (Case BW, Abraham JL, Meeker G et al. Applying definitions of "asbestos" to environmental and "low-dose" exposure levels and health effects, particularly malignant mesothelioma. *J Toxicol Environ Health* 2011;14:3–39.)

We now recognize that many common non-toxic cleavage fragments of many different types of asbestos-like minerals are counted as pathogenic asbestos fibers using the standard NIOSH-approved light microscopic methodology, although they are not true asbestos fibers and are not hazardous. Furthermore, historical studies looking at hazardous fibers have found that the fibers with diameters of less than 0.25 μm are most likely to cause lung cancer and mesothelioma, but are not visible with the optical microscope. This presents a major problem, in that we are not able to count the fibers that are most hazardous using standard light phase-contrast optical microscopy (PCOM) techniques. Transmission electron microscopy (TEM) is needed to actually count the number of hazardous fibers. Some of these problems were brought up by Ann Wyle in 1984, and later by others. This problem of not actually being able to count the fibers that are really hazardous, produces tremendous bias in interpreting epidemiologic studies, based on using the membrane filter method to estimate the amount of inhaled asbestos.

Risk analysis models need to be made from the number of actual hazardous fibers inhaled, rather than the fiber count made by the membrane filter method. This has been recently supported by the studies of Drs. Dement and Stayner, who have studied the relationship between asbestos fiber diameter and length in the induction of lung cancer in South Carolina asbestos textile factories. Their data, plus other available studies, were summarized in a study commissioned by the Health Council of The Netherlands, which cast doubt on the epidemiological studies that historically have been used to determine relative fiber potency. (Lenters V, Vereulen R, Dogger S et al. A meta-analysis of asbestos and lung cancer: Is better quality exposure assessment associated with steeper slopes of the exposure-response relationships? *Environ Health Perspect* 2011;119(11):1547–55.)

The second problem in fiber counting is that the technique of using light microscopy (PCOM) has changed several times since 1965. Comparison to past measurements is difficult since current techniques for using PCOM result in fiber counts that may be hundreds of times higher than historical measurements. (Rickards AL. Levels of workplace exposure. *Ann Occup Hyg* 1994;38;469–75.)

Bernstein and Hoskins also concluded that

> Across the range of mineral fiber solubilities chrysotile lies towards the soluble end of the scale. Chronic inhalation toxicity studies with chrysotile in animals have unfortunately been performed at very high exposure concentrations resulting in lung overload. Consequently their relevance to human exposures is extremely limited. Chrysotile following subchronic inhalation at a mean exposure of 76 fibers L > 20 micron/cm³ (3413 total fibers/cm³) resulted in no fibrosis (Wagner score 1.8–2.6), at any time point and no difference with controls in BrdU response or biochemical and cellular parameters. (Bernstein DM, Hoskins JA. The health

effects of chrysotile: Current perspective based upon recent data. *Regul Toxicol Pharmacol* 2006;45(3):252–64.)

Bernstein's article resulted in some questioning his credibility and these concerns were answered by Ken Donaldson of the University of Edinburgh, Scotland. (Donaldson K, Oberdorster G. Continued controversy on chrysotile biopersistence. *Int J Occup Environ Health* 2011;17:98–9.)

Short fibers of <5 μm in length do not even reach the pleura. (Schinwald A, Murphy FA, Prina-Mello A et al. The threshold for fiber-induced acute pleural inflammation: Shedding light on the early events in asbestos-induced mesothelioma. *Toxicol Sci* 2012;128(2):461–70.) The long chrysotile fibers were observed to break apart into small particles and smaller fibers. Toxicologically, chrysotile, which rapidly falls apart in the lung, behaves more like non-fibrous mineral dusts, while response to amphibole asbestos reflects its insoluble fibrous structure. Recent quantitative reviews of epidemiological studies of mineral fibers that have determined the potency of chrysotile and amphibole asbestos for causing lung cancer and mesothelioma in relation to fiber type, have also differentiated between these two minerals. The most recent analyses also concluded that it is the longer, thinner fibers that have the greatest potency, as has been reported in animal inhalation toxicology studies. (Bernstein DM, Hoskins JA. The health effects of chrysotile: Current perspective based upon recent data. *Regul Toxicol Pharmacol* 2006;45(3):252–64.)

These findings are nothing new, since they differ little from the findings of Stanton et al. in 1981 that long (>8 μm) and thin (<0.25-μm diameter) fibers are associated with a carcinogenic effect. (Stanton MF, Layard M, Tegeris A et al. Relationship between particle dimension to carcinogenicity in amphibole asbestos and other mineral fibers. *J Natl Cancer Inst* 1981;67:965–75.) Seydou and others have focused on fiber morphology since the long induction time for mesothelioma is more consistent with issues related to fiber morphology than chemical toxicity, and why only long fibers are toxic. (Seydou Y, Chen HH, Harte E, Ventura GD, Petibois C. The role of asbestos morphology on their cellular toxicity: An *in vitro* 3D Raman/Rayleigh imaging study. *Anal Bioanal Chem* 2013;405(27):8701–7.)

Earlier, in 1951, Arthur Vorwald had noted that only long fibers (>20 μm) were fibrogenic and that shorter fibers were not fibrogenic. (Vorwald AJ, Durkan TM, Pratt PC. Experimental studies of asbestosis. *Arch Ind Hyg Occup Med* 1951;3:1–43.) Many authors have concluded that lung cancer incidence with chrysotile exposure is related primarily to those long thin chrysotile fibers seen only with an electron microscope (TEM). The lung cancer-causative fibers were not visible by standard phase-contrast microscopy. (Stayner L, Kuempel E, Gilbert S, Hein M, Dement J. An epidemiological study of the role of chrysotile asbestos fiber dimensions in determining respiratory disease risk in exposed workers. *Occup Environ Med* 2008;65(9):613–9; Berman DW. Comparing milled fiber, Quebec ore, and textile factory dust: Has another piece of the asbestos puzzle fallen into place? *Crit Rev Toxicol* 2010;40(2):151–88.)

More recently, the U.S. Environmental Protection Agency (EPA) has restudied the asbestos-related cancer risk based on mineral size and fiber type. (Berman DW, Crump KS. A meta-analysis of asbestos-related cancer risk that addresses fiber size and mineral type. *Crit Rev Toxicol* 2008;38(Suppl. 1):49–73; Berman DW, Crump KS. Update of potency factors for asbestos-related lung cancer and mesothelioma. *Crit Rev Toxicol* 2008;38(Suppl. 1):1–47.) The authors stated,

> For mesothelioma, the hypothesis that chrysotile and amphibole asbestos are equally potent (relative potency concentration [rpc = 1]) was strongly rejected by every metric and the hypothesis that (pure) chrysotile is nonpotent for mesothelioma was not rejected by any metric. Best estimates for the relative potency of chrysotile ranged from zero to about 1/200th that of amphibole asbestos (depending on metric). For lung cancer, the hypothesis that chrysotile and amphibole asbestos are equally potent (rpc = 1) was rejected (p < or = .05) by the two metrics based on thin fibers (length < 0.4 micron and < 0.2 micron) but not by the metrics based on thicker fibers.

More specifically, Jenifer S Pierce and others evaluated the relative potency of chrysotile asbestos and concluded,

> All of the studies involved cohorts exposed to high levels of chrysotile in mining or manufacturing settings. The preponderance of the cumulative 'no-effects' exposure levels for lung cancer and mesothelioma fall in a range of approximately 25–1,000 fibers per cubic centimeter per year (f/cc-yr) and 15–500 f/cc-yr, respectively, and a majority of the studies did not report an increased risk at the highest estimated exposure. Sources of uncertainty in these values include errors in the cumulative exposure estimates, conversion of dust counts to fiber data, and use of national age-adjusted mortality rates. Numerous potential biases also exist. For example, smoking was rarely controlled for and amphibole exposure did in fact occur in a majority of the studies, which would bias many of the reported 'no-effect' exposure levels towards lower values. However, many of the studies likely lack sufficient power (e.g., due to small cohort size) to assess whether there could have been a significant increase in risk at the reported no-observed-adverse-effects level (NOAEL); additional statistical analyses are required to address this source of bias and the attendant influence on these values. The chrysotile NOAELs appear to be consistent with exposure–response information for certain cohorts with well-established industrial hygiene and epidemiology data. Specifically, the range of chrysotile NOAELs were found to be consistently higher than upper-bound cumulative chrysotile exposure estimates that have been published for pre-1980s automobile mechanics (e.g., 95th percentile of 2.0 f/cc-yr.) an occupation that historically worked with chrysotile-containing

friction products yet has been shown to have no increased risk of asbestos-related diseases. While the debate regarding chrysotile as a risk factor for mesothelioma will likely continue for some time, future research into nonlinear, threshold cancer risk models for chrysotile-related respiratory diseases appears to be warranted.

Pierce and coworkers reviewed the major published epidemiologic studies concerning the dose relationships between asbestos exposure and risk for lung cancer and mesothelioma. They reviewed 350 studies, only 14 of which met their inclusion criteria in which lung cancer risk was stratified by cumulative chrysotile exposure; four such studies were found for mesothelioma. All of the studies involved cohorts exposed to high levels of chrysotile in mining or manufacturing settings. The preponderance of the cumulative "no-effects" exposure levels for lung cancer and mesothelioma fall in a range of approximately 25–1000 fibers per cubic centimeter per year (f/cc-yr) and 15–500 f/cc-yr, respectively, and a majority of the studies did not report an increased risk at the highest estimated exposure. Specifically, the range of chrysotile no-observed-adverse-effects level was found to be consistently higher than upper-bound cumulative chrysotile exposure estimates that have been published for pre-1980s automobile mechanics (e.g., 95th percentile of 2.0 f/cc-yr), an occupation that historically worked with chrysotile-containing friction products, yet has been shown to have no increased risk of asbestos-related diseases. The authors concluded that the debate regarding chrysotile as a risk factor for mesothelioma will likely continue for some time; future research into non-linear threshold cancer risk models for chrysotile-related respiratory diseases appears to be warranted. (Pierce JS, McKinley MA, Paustenbach DJ, Finley BL. An evaluation of reported no-effect chrysotile asbestos exposures for lung cancer and mesothelioma. *Crit Rev Toxicol* 2008;38(3):191–214.)

More recently, Berman compared different protocols for determining risk for cancer. He concluded that the IRIS (Implementing Research Implementation Strategies) risk analysis protocol, used by regulating agencies, seriously underestimates risk from amphibole asbestos exposure when compared to chrysotile asbestos. When fiber size adjustment is made to this protocol, it can be reconciled with the Berman risk protocol. (Berman DW. Apples to apples: The origin and magnitude of differences in asbestos cancer risk estimates derived from using varying protocols. *Risk Anal* 2011;31:1308–26; Berman DW, Crump KS. *Final Draft: Technical Support Document for a Protocol to Assess Asbestos-Related Risk*. EPA# 9345.4-06. Washington, DC: U.S. Environmental Protection Agency, 2003; Berman DW, Crump KS. A meta-analysis of asbestos-related cancer risk that addresses fiber size and mineral type. *Crit Rev Toxicol* 2008;38(Suppl. 1):49–73; Berman DW. Comparing milled fiber, Quebec ore, and textile factory dust: Has another piece of the asbestos puzzle fallen into place? *Crit Rev Toxicol* 2010;40:151–88; Berman DW, Case BW. Quality of evidence must guide risk assessment of asbestos, by Lenters, V; Burdorf, A; Vermeulen, R; Stayner, L; Heederik, D. *Ann Occup Hyg* 2013;57(5):667–9.)

The effect of asbestos exposure due to environmental and low-dose exposures on the risk of mesothelioma remains an important topic of discussion among experts. Experts agree that extrapolation from high to low risk, whether based on inferential statistical (e.g., linear no-threshold models or mode-of-action-based models), is fraught with uncertainty. (Case BW, Abraham JL, Meeker G, Pooley FD, Pinkerton KE. Applying definitions of "asbestos" to environmental and "low-dose" exposure levels and health effects, particularly malignant mesothelioma. *J Toxicol Environ Health B Crit Rev* 2011;14:3–39.)

Some authors have made claims that very low levels of asbestos of <0.5 fibers/mL-years may be associated with an increased risk of mesothelioma. These studies were based on estimates of exposure rather than any measurement of actual exposures, and so are speculative and unreliable. Furthermore, Iwatsubo et al. could not examine mesothelioma risk according to fiber type. It is important to note that historical European data indicate large amounts of amphibole exposure, particularly crocidolite asbestos, as in this French population. (Iwatsubo Y, Pairon JC, Boutin C et al. Pleural mesothelioma: Dose–response relation at low levels of asbestos exposure in a French population-based case–control study. *Am J Epidemiol* 1998;148:133–42.) A German hospital case–control series estimated exposures from work histories. Work histories obtained from hospital records, or from living patients after the diagnosis of a potential asbestos-related disease, are unreliable estimates of actual exposures and greatly overestimate asbestos exposure. (Rodelsperger K, Jöckel KH, Pohlabeln H, Römer W, Woitowitz HJ. Factors for diffuse malignant mesothelioma: Results forma German hospital case–control study. *Am J Ind Med* 2001;39:262–75.) These data were in direct conflict with other epidemiologic studies. Their lung burden studies for chrysotile were not elevated, yet the authors concluded that chrysotile fibers might have caused a mesothelioma, even if not present in lung tissue!

The studies by Iwatsubo and Rodelsperger are limited by small numbers of cases, with unreliable exposure data and a lack of statistical power, and therefore are not useful for generalization to different populations of workers with different exposures, based on intensity and length of exposure to different fiber types with different fiber dimensions. These papers claiming that very low exposures are capable of causing a mesothelioma are contradicted by the animal and epidemiologic studies described earlier and below. The data from a variety of epidemiologic studies have not demonstrated any risk of mesothelioma to amphibole asbestos exposures of less than 5 fiber-years or 0.1 fibers/cc × 50 years.

Hillerdal has claimed that there is no evidence of a threshold dose below which there is no risk of mesothelioma and doubts whether there is a background level of mesothelioma in the absence of some asbestos exposure. The epidemiologic data have overwhelmingly demonstrated a relatively high background to amphibole and chrysotile asbestos contaminated with tremolite exposures without development of mesotheliomas. This study mischaracterizes many exposures and data sets to prove the author's hypothesis. (Hillerdal G. Mesothelioma: Cases associated with non-occupational and low dose exposure. *Occup Environ Med* 1999;56(8):505–13.)

An evidence-based approach to the evaluation of asbestos exposure has been suggested by others. (Marchevsky AM, Harber P, Crawford L, Wick MR.

Mesothelioma in patients with non-occupational asbestos exposure. An evidence-based approach to causation assessment. *Ann Diagn Pathol* 2006;10(4):241–50.)

Figure 22.1 is from an unknown source and distinguishes the actual historical risk data by mixed fiber exposure and demonstrates a threshold for risk as compared to the Occupational Safety and Health Administration (OSHA)/NIOSH risk data, which averages risk from amphibole and chrysotile exposure and assumes no threshold for risk from asbestos exposures to all types, even though there are no data to support adverse effects from low exposures, particularly from chrysotile exposures.

Government agencies extrapolate risk estimates to zero when promulgating the safe exposure dose for workers. While all scientists agree that there are no data on risk from low exposures, government agencies assume a linear model for risk analysis as the most conservative method to protect workers. A linear model assumes that there is no threshold dose for asbestos exposure, in spite of data from all biologic systems that a threshold dose exists. Some nations have threshold limit values for different fiber types. U.S. governmental agencies have chosen to use the risk estimates from data on amphibole exposure, which produce the highest risk, and not chrysotile exposure, to establish risk estimates that provide maximum safety. The estimate of risk when no reliable data for low exposures exist exaggerates the risk from low exposures and that risk is further exaggerated when amphibole data are used to calculate that risk.

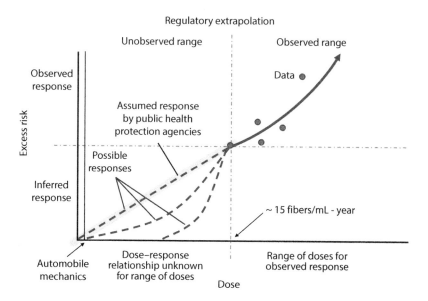

Figure 22.1 Regulators use a linear extrapolation model to calculate risk rather than a logarithmic biological model that assumes a threshold dose and assumes that risk rises as the log of exposure dose, based on actual biological data.

The data from epidemiologic studies that have been used to calculate risk are often flimsy at best, because of the lack of credible exposure assessments where electron microscopy has measured long, thin fibers > 20 μm in length. "In summary, extrapolation from high to low risk, whether based on inferential statistical (e.g., linear no-threshold) models or mode-of-action-based models, is fraught with uncertainty." (Case, BW, Abraham JL, Meeker G, Pooley FD, Pinkerton KE. Applying definitions of "asbestos" to environmental and "low-dose" exposure levels and health effects, particularly malignant mesothelioma. *J Toxicol Environ Health B Crit Rev* 2011;14:3–39.)

No cases of mesothelioma were seen in a group of Australian crocidolite workers with less than 3 months of exposure. (De Klerk NH, Armstrong BK, Musk AW et al. Cancer mortality in relation to measures of occupational exposure to crocidolite at Wittenoom Gorge in Western Australia. *Br J Ind Med* 1989;46:529–36.) No mesotheliomas were seen in North American asbestos workers who were exposed for less than 15 months. (Selikoff IJ, Hammond EC, Seidman H. Mortality experience of insulation workers in the United States and Canada, 1943–1976. *Ann NY Acad Sci* 1979;330:91–116.) Similarly, only one mesothelioma was seen in Rockdale textile workers in whom there was exposure to crocidolite asbestos for less than 10 years and 25 cases were expected. (Peto J, Doll R, Hermon C et al. Relationship of mortality to measures of environmental asbestos pollution in an asbestos textile factory. *Ann Occup Hyg* 1985;29:305–55.) Sluis-Cremer and coworkers studied the mortality and deaths from mesothelioma in South African amphibole miners and noted that mesotheliomas occurred only in men who were exposed for long periods of time, or at least 12 months, but for an average of 15 years. (Sluis-Cremer GK, Liddell FDK, Logan WPD, Bezuidenhout BN. The mortality of amphibole miners in South Africa, 1946–80. *Br J Ind Med* 1992;49:566–75.) Illgren and Browne concluded that a threshold dose of less than 5 fibers/mL-year of amphibole asbestos was unlikely to cause a mesothelioma. (Illgren EB, Browne K. Asbestos-related mesothelioma: Evidence for a threshold in animals and humans. *Regul Toxicol Pharmacol* 1991;18:116–32.)

The incidence of mesothelioma in women (2–4 per million) has remained essentially unchanged over the last several decades as compared to men, with a rate of 10–12 per million. This low incidence suggested that the incidence in women reflects the spontaneous background level of mesothelioma incidence. These data more importantly suggest that there is a threshold dose for mesothelioma. (Price B, Ware A. Mesothelioma trends in the United States: An update based on surveillance, epidemiology, and end results program data for 1973 through 2003. *Am J Epidemiol* 2004;159:107–12.)

The role of amphibole- or tremolite-free asbestos as a cause of mesothelioma continues to be debated, but there is increasing evidence that amphibole-free asbestos does not cause mesotheliomas. To date, there have been no reported cases of mesotheliomas associated with low-tremolite or tremolite-free asbestos exposure in Canadian and South African miners and millers. Amphibole asbestos is the major cause of asbestos-related mesothelioma and lung cancer. However, the debate rages on and others claim that chrysotile asbestos is an important cause of mesothelioma.

The data from wallboard workers exposed to chrysotile asbestos in wallboard mud, as well as brake workers exposed to chrysotile asbestos in brake dust, have failed to reveal mesotheliomas after more than 50 years of follow-up. (Phedka AD, Finley BL. Potential health hazards associated with exposures to asbestos-containing drywall accessory products: A state-of-the-science assessment. *Crit Rev Toxicol* 2012;42:1–27; Finley BL, Pierce JS, Paustenbach DJ et al. Malignant pleural mesothelioma in US automotive mechanics: Reported vs. expected number of cases from 1975–2007. *Regul Toxicol Pharmacol* 2012;64:104–16.) Occasionally, a case report of a few cases of mesothelioma in a wallboard worker or brake mechanic is reported. These types of individual case reports do not prove an association between the work exposure and these asbestos products without lung fiber analysis. Many workers are incidentally exposed unknowingly to amphibole asbestos and isolated cases reports have no probative value. (Dahlgren J, Peckham T. Mesothelioma associated with use of drywall joint compound: A case series and review of literature. *Int J Occup Environ Health* 2012;18(4):337–43.)

Quantification of asbestos fiber translocation from the lung reveals that amosite amphibole asbestos fibers translocate quickly (within 7 days) into the pleura and produce an inflammatory response. In contrast, chrysotile asbestos fibers are quickly cleared from the lung and do not produce a significant inflammatory response, nor enter the pleural space. (Bernstein DM, Rogers RA, Sepulveda R et al. Quantification of the pathological response and fate in lung and pleura of chrysotile in combination with fine particles compared to amosite asbestos following short-term inhalation exposure. *Inhal Toxicol* 2011;23:372–91.)

The argument among experts often centers on whether a chrysotile asbestos worker was also exposed to amphibole asbestos, invalidating the claim that there are many examples of mesotheliomas caused by amphibole-free asbestos. (Kanarek MS. Mesothelioma from chrysotile asbestos: Update. *Ann Epidemiol* 2011;21:688–97; Lin S, Wang X, Yu I et al. Cause-specific mortality in relation to chrysotile-asbestos exposure in a Chinese cohort. *J Thorac Oncol* 2012;7:1109–14.) Yano published a report of mesotheliomas found in what was thought to be amphibole-free chrysotile asbestos exposure in China. (*Am J Epidemiol* 2001;54:538–43.) Subsequent studies have identified tremolite amphibole asbestos as a contaminant of Chinese chrysotile asbestos in varying amounts in a range of 0.02%–0.310% in six Chinese chrysotile mines. Lin et al. stated that Russian and Canadian chrysotile asbestos was imported into China as well as local chrysotile. The authors found two mesotheliomas out of 259 deaths. (Lin SL, Wong X, Yu I et al. Cause-specific mortality in relation to chrysotile-asbestos exposure in a Chinese Cohort. *J Thorac Oncol* 2012;7:1109–14.) Asbestos exposures have historically been very high in China, at 415 mg/m^3 in the 1960s and a range of 0.1–12.6 fibers/mL in 2001. The prevalence of asbestosis in various Chinese epidemiologic studies has ranged from 10% to 30%, indicating high exposures in the past. (Courtice MN, Lin S, Xiaorong W. An updated review on asbestos and related disease in China. *Int J Occup Environ Health* 2012;18:247–53.) The claims that Chinese chrysotile is amphibole free have not been proven. Table 22.1 gives

Table 22.1 Summary statements of quantitative mesothelioma risks from asbestos exposure at different levels of cumulative exposure

Risk of mesothelioma data

Risk summary for cumulative exposures between 10 and 100 fibers/mL/year

Crocidolite: best estimate about 400 deaths per 100,000 exposed for each fiber/mL-year of cumulative exposure. Up to twofold uncertainty

Amosite: best estimate about 65 deaths per 100,000 exposed for each fiber/mL-year of exposure. Two to fourfold uncertainty

Chrysotile: best estimate about two deaths per 100,000 exposed for each fiber/mL-year of exposure. Up to threefold uncertainty

Risk summaries for cumulative exposures of 1 fiber/mL-year

Crocidolite: best estimate about 650 deaths per 100,000 exposed. Highest arguable estimate: 1500; lowest: 250

Amosite: best estimate about 90 deaths per 100,000 exposed. Highest arguable estimate: 300; lowest: 15

Chrysotile: best estimate about 5 deaths per 100,000. Highest arguable estimate: 20; lowest: 1

Risk summaries for cumulative exposures of 0.1 fibers/mL-year

Crocidolite: best estimate about 100 deaths per 100,000 exposed. Highest arguable estimate: 350; lowest: 25

Amosite: best estimate about 15 deaths per 100,000 exposed. Highest arguable estimate: 80; lowest: 2

Chrysotile: risk probably insignificant. Highest arguable estimate: 4 deaths per 100,000 exposed

Risk summaries for cumulative exposures of 0.01 fibers/mL-year

Crocidolite: best estimate about 20 deaths per 100,000 exposed. Highest arguable estimate: 100; lowest: 2

Amosite: best estimate about three deaths per 100,000 exposed. Highest arguable estimate: 20; lowest: insignificant

Chrysotile: risk probably insignificant. Highest arguable estimate: 1 death per 100,000 exposed

Source: Hodgson and Darnton.

an estimate of risk of mesothelioma based on fiber types. (Hodgson JT, Darnton A. The quantitative risks of mesothelioma and lung cancer in relation to asbestos exposure. *Ann Occup Hyg* 2000;44(8):565–601.)

HOW DO WE DEFINE RISK?

The word risk implies the possibility of something unpleasant occurring. The greater the possibility of some adverse event, the greater the risk. The only way to understand risk is by comparison with risks most people take every day, such

Table 22.2 Estimated lifetime risk of mesothelioma per 100,000 in relation to chrysotile asbestos by Hodgson and Darnton (HD) or Berman and Crump (BC) models and cumulative exposure

Cumulative exposure (fibers/mL-year)	HD	BC	HD?BC
10.0	25 (5–70)	10	2.7
1.0	5 (1–20)	1	4.8
0.01	1 (1–5)	<1	8.4
0.010	<1 (<1–1)	<1	15
0.001	<1 (<1–1)	<1	18

Source: Modified from Darnton A. WATCH paper (Table 1). Chrysotile Asbestos Expert Panel, 2007, p. 24.

as driving a car, playing sports, or something more remote, such as being struck by lightning. Life is full of risks and individual and government agencies have to determine what constitutes an "acceptable risk." The term "acceptable" is a term that changes with the norms of different societies, largely due to socio-economic considerations. India and China still manufacture asbestos products, which have been banned in most Western nations. When Dreesen did his textile plant study, it was understood that the proposed standard did not protect all workers. The Fleischer–Drinker study found three cases of asbestosis among 1074 workers, or 0.28% of workers. That low incidence was thought to be acceptable at the time and deemed "safe"! Today, three cases of asbestosis out of 1074 pipe fitters or one out of every 358 workers would be considered hazardous and unsafe. As society evolves, consideration of what is safe or relatively risk free also changes. What was thought to be safe in the 1960s is not thought to be safe today. The term safe can only be understood in the context of contemporary societal standards at the time the term was used (see Table 22.2; Figures 22.2 and 22.3).

From 1940 to 1975, asbestos exposure, particularly in shipyards and asbestos manufacturing, would be more likely to be the cause of a mesothelioma, and later exposures would be unlikely as a cause. The relative contribution of any

---

Everything is a poison

- The basic principle of toxicology elucidated in the 1547 manuscript by Paracelsus is: "What is that is not a poison? All things are poison and nothing is without poison. It is the dose only that makes a thing not a poison."

Figure 22.2 Risk is related to dose and every American has been exposed to asbestos, but only those few Americans with heavy exposure will develop disease. (From Ottoboni MA. *The Dose Makes the Poison a Plain Language Guide to Toxicology*, 2nd Ed, New York: Van Nostrand Reinhold, 1991.)

Examples of safe but potentially deadly common substances	
Water	Water intoxication
Oxygen	Oxgen toxicity
Alcohol	Alcohol poisoning
Arsenic	Arsenic poisoning
Silica	Silicosis
Tobacco	Chronic obstructive pulmonary disease (COPD), oral and lung cancer
Asbestos	Cancer, mesothelioma

Figure 22.3 We are all exposed to a variety of potentially toxic substances.

year of exposure gradually falls with time since it is always the early exposures that are more likely to be the cause of irreparable changes in cell biology that lead to tumorigenesis. Today, it is most common to find mesothelioma latency times of 50 or more years. This is thought to be due to the effect of lower exposures resulting in longer latency. Very few individuals have had high exposures to amphibole asbestos since most manufacturers removed asbestos from their products by 1975.

In summary, risk for asbestos-related mesothelioma is related not only to fiber type, fiber size, and fiber length, but also iron content, fiber durability, latency, intensity, and duration of the initial exposure. Early exposures have the major impact on causation.

Today, we know that everyone has some significant background environmental exposure to asbestos, based on the measurement of the background level of asbestos in never-exposed human lungs. (Churg and Wiggs 1986; Churg 1993.) Individuals who live near the asbestos mines of Quebec, with background levels at 100 times the normal urban level, have no elevated risk of mesothelioma. Only those individuals with much higher exposures are at risk of mesothelioma. (Camus et al. *Ann Occup Hyg* 2002;46:95–8; Case et al. *Ann Occup Hyg* 2002;46:128–31.)

The basic principle of toxicology, elucidated in the 1547 manuscript by Paracelsus, is "What is that is not a poison? All things are poison and nothing is without poison. It is the dose only that makes a thing not a poison." (Ottoboni, MA. *The Dose Makes the Poison—A Plain Language Guide to Toxicology*, 2nd Edition. New York: Van Nostrand Reinhold, 1991.) Toxicology focuses on the adverse effects of potential toxic substances, with the focus being determining *adverse effects*. Everything is potentially toxic, including the air we breathe and the water we drink. Excessive inhalation of oxygen will cause oxygen toxicity, and excessive ingestion of water causes water intoxication, which can be lethal. Excessive exposure to various asbestos fibers may be injurious and cause asbestos-related disease. The basic question is how much asbestos exposure is dangerous, or what level of exposure, based on fiber size and fiber type, is necessary to cause an adverse effect? The answer to that question has been referred to governmental agencies such as the ACGIH, NIOSH, and EPA to answer. Over time, new information has been

> **Threshold dose**
>
> • All biological processes and information on toxic effects of chemicals, drugs, poisons, dusts, fumes, smoke, etc., reveal that small doses of toxic products are harmless.
>
> • Government agencies calculate risk by a process of back extrapolation to zero in an effort to overestimate risk and to protect the public.

Figure 22.4 Asbestos burden in the general population. (From Churg A. Chrysotile, tremolite, and malignant mesothelioma in man. *Chest* 1993;3:621–8.)

published in the scientific literature concerning the safe dose of asbestos exposure, beginning in 1971, when the federal government assumed the rule-making from the states. Over 23 years, the OSHA has gradually lowered the permissible exposure limit from 12 fibers/cc in 1971 to 0.1 fibers/cc in 1994, where it remains today (see Figure 22.4). (Martonik JF, Nash E, Grossman E. The history of OSHA's asbestos rulemakings and some distinctive approaches that they introduced for regulating occupational exposure to toxic substances. *AIHAJ* 2001;62:208–17.)

There is no such thing as zero risk, so government agencies must decide what risk is acceptable. The current standard on asbestos exposure of 0.1 fibers/cc accepts that this exposure limit reduces the risk of mesothelioma to an "acceptable level" of one death in 10,000 people. (Hughes JM, Weill H. Asbestos exposure—Quantitative assessment of risk. *Am Rev Respir Dis* 1986;133(1):5–13; Weill H, Hughes JM. Asbestos as a public health risk: Disease and policy. *Annu Rev Public Health* 1986;7:171–92; Weill H, Hughes JM, Jones RN. Asbestos: A risk too far? *Lancet* 1995;346(8970):304; Morawetz JS. Tales of acute risk assessment: Health effects made out of whole cloth. *Am J Ind Med* 2005;47:370–5; Slovic P. Perception of risk. *Science* 1987;236:280–5; The methodology of worker (risk) notification, special issue. *Am J Ind Med* 1993; 23:1–229; Ames BN. What are the major carcinogens in the etiology of human cancer? Environmental pollution, natural carcinogens, and the causes of human cancer: Six errors. *Important Adv Oncol* 1989:237–47.)

To gain perspective on relative risks, please evaluate the following table. A lifetime risk of 1 in 100,000 is equivalent to an annual risk of 1 in 1,000,000.

SOME COMMONPLACE RISKS FOR DEATH

All cancers	1 in 4
Cigarette smoking	1 in 3
Air pollution, Eastern United States	1 in 50
Automobile accident, motorist or passenger	1 in 80
Home accidents	1 in 120

Motor vehicle accident (pedestrian)	1 in 400
Electrocution	1 in 3000
Acceptable risk (NIOSH) from asbestos exposure	1 in 10,000
Death in automobile accident	1 in 10,000
Being hit by meteorite	1 in 25,000
Death by murder in the United States	1 in 25,000
Drinking water with EPA (limit of chloroform)	1 in 50,000
Rate of mesothelioma, U.S. population 2003–2008	1 in 100,000
Playing high school football, annually	1 in 100,000
EPA definition of no risk is less than	1 in 100,000
Being hit by falling aircraft	1 in 200,000
Spontaneous mesothelioma in women	2–3 in 1,000,000

There is no such thing as "no risk." Risk relative, and therefore the definition of "what is safe," must use everyday life experiences, as shown above, to make comparisons for determining what is safe. According to Nicholson, the EPA, Food and Drug Administration, and Consumer Product Safety Commission made the decision not to regulate products unless the risk of death is >1 in 100,000. The lifetime risk from continuous exposure to asbestos at a level of 0.1 fibers/cc for both lung cancer and mesothelioma has been estimated to vary between 0.6 and 4.2–11.2 deaths/100,000, which is roughly one death in 10,000 if the highest estimated value is used to calculate risk. Government agencies commonly use the highest risk estimation to set the maximal tolerable, or safe dose, of a toxic substance, in order to adequately protect the general public. (Nicholson WJ. Airborne mineral fiber levels in the non-occupational environment. Non-occupational exposure to mineral fibers. *IRAC Pub* 1989;90:239–61.)

I have been asked many times to opine on whether a given exposure was excessive. This line of questioning is problematic, since it is the role of government agencies, and not scientists, to determine what constitutes a safe dose of any toxin.

A good example of the difficulty in establishing a safe standard is the government response to arsenic. Arsenic at levels of >100 μg/L is known to produce cancers of the lung, bladder, and skin. Arsenic at levels pf >50 μg/L probably also causes cardiovascular disease, respiratory disease, and diabetes.

High environmental arsenic levels have long been recognized as correlating with higher risk of cardiovascular disease, but a secondary analysis of data from a recent study, now shows that even at the low levels commonly found in rural communities across the United States, arsenic exposure is strongly related to cardiovascular risk and mortality in a dose-dependent fashion, using data from the Strong Heart Study, a population-based cohort study of cardiovascular disease in three Native American communities in rural Arizona, Oklahoma, and the Dakotas. For their analysis, Ms. Moon and her colleagues measured arsenic species concentrations in stored urine samples from 3575 men and women with no cardiovascular disease at enrollment during 1989–1991. These study subjects, aged 45–75 years at baseline, were followed for cardiovascular outcomes for 17–19 years.

A total of 1184 subjects developed cardiovascular disease during follow-up, with 846 incident coronary heart disease events and 264 incident strokes. A total of 439 subjects died from cardiovascular disease, including 341 who died from coronary heart disease and 54 who died from stroke. Urinary arsenic concentrations at baseline correlated with the development of cardiovascular disease. Compared with men and women who had the lowest arsenic levels, those in the highest quartile were more likely to develop cardiovascular disease (hazard ratio [HR]: 1.32), coronary heart disease (HR: 1.30), and stroke (HR: 1.47). The association between arsenic levels and cardiovascular risk was strongest among men and women who had diabetes, a subgroup of the population that has not been evaluated in previous studies of arsenic exposure. This finding "needs to be interpreted cautiously and requires replication in other populations," the researchers said. The EPA has estimated that 13 million Americans are chronically exposed to arsenic in drinking water, and many millions more are exposed to arsenic in food. It is possible that mitigating these exposures could reduce the burden of cardiovascular disease in the United States and across the globe, the authors added.

Urinary arsenic levels at baseline also correlated with cardiovascular mortality. Compared with men and women who had the lowest levels, those in the highest quartile were more likely to die from cardiovascular disease (HR: 1.65), coronary heart disease (HR: 1.71), or stroke (HR: 3.03). (Moon MA, Guallar E, Umans JG et al. Association between exposure to low to moderate arsenic levels and incident cardiovascular disease: A prospective cohort study. *Ann Intern Med* 2013;159(10):649–59.)

Millions of people worldwide are exposed to arsenic in drinking water, and many are likely co-exposed to other agents that could substantially increase their risks of arsenic-related cancer. Very high lung and bladder cancer odds ratios (ORs), and evidence of greater-than-additive effects, were seen in people exposed to arsenic concentrations >335 µg/L, and who were tobacco smokers (OR: 16, 95% CI: 6.5–40 for lung cancer; OR: 23, 95% CI: 8.2–66 for bladder cancer; Rothman Synergy Indices: 4.0, 95% CI: 1.7–9.4; and 2.0; 95% CI: 0.92–4.5, respectively). Evidence of greater-than-additive effects were also seen in people co-exposed to arsenic and second-hand tobacco smoke and several other known or suspected carcinogens, including asbestos, silica, and wood dust. (Ferreccio C, Yuan Y, Calle J et al. Arsenic, tobacco smoke, and occupation: Associations of multiple agents with lung and bladder cancer. *Epidemiology* 2013;24(6):898–905.) These findings suggest that people co-exposed to arsenic and other known or suspected carcinogens have very high risks of lung or bladder cancer. There have been no epidemiological studies of cohorts with asbestos exposure, smoking, and arsenic exposure.

The current government standard is 10 µg/L of arsenic. This level may be exceeded by certain foods such as apple, grape, and pear juice, rice, and chicken meat. Arsenic may contaminate drinking water. It is difficult to promote public safety, and at the same time, not establish onerous standards that could destroy parts of the food industry, without offering significant reductions in risk from adverse health effects to the general population. If the arsenic level was reduced to 1 µg/L, it would shut down the rice, poultry, and orchard industry, as well as close most community and local water systems that rely on well water. Thousands of people would become unemployed and many lives would likely be lost from depression, alcohol, drugs, suicide, and other causes related to poverty and unemployment. Food costs would soar for everyone. The determination of what is a safe standard is very complex, requiring a delicate balance between allowing acceptable levels of adverse health effects and other social, environmental, and governmental considerations. Government must determine what constitutes an acceptable risk for exposure to all potentially toxic substances. The scientific/medical/government community attempts to reduce risk of negative health effects from all toxins to a relatively safe standard, but there is always a possibility of some very remote risk that a toxin such as asbestos or arsenic remains. Scientists do not use the term *never*, since science does not speak in absolute terms. Public agencies and attorneys want risk definitions in absolute terms which science cannot deliver. (Navas-Acien A, Nachman KE. Public health responses to arsenic in rice and other foods. *JAMA Int Med* 2013;173:1395–96.)

Most toxins, such as asbestos and arsenic, can never be entirely eliminated, since they are naturally present in the earth, the air we breathe, the food we eat, and the water we drink. Modern industrial hygienists recognize the concept of hormesis or a biphasic, U-shaped, or J-shaped analysis of risk assessment. Many minerals that cause adverse health effects in high doses cause salutary effects in low doses. For instance, copper in low doses is needed for certain vital human enzymatic processes. Excessive copper causes liver disease. Iron is needed to make functioning hemoglobin in red blood cells, but excessive iron causes cancer and liver disease. (Calabrese EJ, Baldwin LA. Hormesis: The dose response revolution. *Annu Rev Pharmacol Toxicol* 2003;43:175–97.)

Misconceptions about the health risks of asbestos abound. There is anxiety about any exposure to asbestos, such as working in an area where asbestos products were used in the past or encapsulated. Hopefully, this book has reduced the general concern about casual exposure to asbestos such as from building dust during the New York 9/11 World Trade Center, building implosions. Low-level exposures are common in the environment and only substantial time-weighted amphibole asbestos exposures above 0.1 fibers/cc are associated with health risk.

In summary, everyone is exposed to environmental asbestos, so what counts?

1. Some say any asbestos exposure is significant. This is wrong! Everyone has some asbestos exposure due to environmental exposure. Individuals in Quebec with background levels that are 100 times the ambient level in urban America have no risk of asbestos-related mesothelioma or lung cancer. (Camus M, Siemiatycki J, Meek B. Nonoccupational exposure to chrysotile asbestos and the risk of lung cancer. *N Engl J Med* 1998;338:1565–71.)

2. One fiber can kill you. This is wrong! Adults normally have up to 1 million asbestos fibers per gram of dry lung.

3. There is no safe dose of asbestos exposure. This is wrong! Only heavy exposures to long, thin fibers in the breathing zone based on fiber type and size are hazardous.

4. Any mesothelioma in a worker with any asbestos exposure is causally related to that exposure. This is wrong! There are many causes of mesothelioma, and *only* amphibole asbestos fibers of appropriate size, in high doses, and for prolonged periods cause mesothelioma. Some 20%–40% of mesotheliomas are idiopathic in males and the majority of mesotheliomas in women have no known cause.

5. What is an acceptable risk? Risk is always present from a variety of causes. There is no such thing as "zero risk." The societal question as to what an acceptable risk is from asbestos exposure can only be determined when available data are based on fiber type, fiber length, and fiber diameter, using improved analytical methods such as TEM. Many of the historical epidemiologic studies have lacked critical information on respirable dose, including duration of exposure, peak exposures, fiber type, asbestos product type, accurate job exposure description, and description of place of employment and job safety requirements. Information simply based on job title is inadequate to accurately describe risk.

There are competing interests in the academic community about the health effects of asbestos. Fear-mongering and exaggerated claims about the risks of asbestos exposure create a demand for more research and funding. This book provides the reader with a balanced view of the literature and the risks from asbestos exposure. It covers the important issues and has provided sufficient bibliographic references for the reader who wants to develop a deeper understanding of asbestos health effects.

Glossary

Acicular: The very long and very thin, often needle-like shape that characterizes some prismatic crystals. (Prismatic crystals have one elongated dimension and two other dimensions that are approximately equal.) Acicular crystals or fragments do not have the strength, flexibility, or other properties often associated with asbestiform fibers.

ACGIH: American Conference of Governmental Industrial Hygienists.

Actinolite: An amphibole mineral in the tremolite–ferroactinolite series. Actinolite can occur in both asbestiform and nonasbestiform mineral habits. The asbestiform variety is often referred to as actinolite asbestos.

Amphibole: A group of minerals composed of double-chain SiO_4 tetrahedra linked at the vertices and generally containing ions of iron and/or magnesium in their structures. Amphibole minerals are of either igneous or metamorphic origin. Amphiboles can occur in a variety of mineral habits including asbestiform and nonasbestiform.

Amosite: An amphibole mineral in the cummingtonite–grunerite series that occurs in the asbestiform habit. The name amosite is a commercial term derived from the acronym for Asbestos Mines of South Africa. Amosite is sometimes referred to as brown asbestos.

Anthophyllite: An amphibole mineral that can occur in both the asbestiform and non-asbestiform mineral habits. The asbestiform variety is referred to as anthophyllite asbestos.

Asbestiform: A specific type of mineral fibrosity in which crystal growth is primarily in one dimension and the crystals form as long, flexible fibers. In minerals occurring in asbestiform habit, fibers form in bundles that can be separated into smaller bundles and ultimately into fibrils.

Asbestos: A generic term for silicate minerals occurring in the asbestiform habit, usually used to refer to those minerals that have been commercially exploited as asbestos, including chrysotile in the serpentine mineral group and tremolite asbestos, actinolite asbestos, anthophyllite asbestos, cummingtonite–grunerite asbestos (amosite), and riebeckite asbestos (crocidolite) in the amphibole mineral group. *See also* Covered mineral.

Asbestos body: A thin individual asbestos fiber with beaded appearance covered with an iron coating found predominantly in lung tissue.

Aspect ratio: The ratio of the length of a particle to its diameter.

BAL: Bronchoalveolar lavage; used in bronchoscopy to sample for asbestos bodies.

Bio-persistence: The ability to remain in the lung or other tissue. Bio-persistence of mineral fibers is a function of their fragility, solubility, and clearance.

B-Reader: A certified physician who has passed an examination based on the proper interpretation of chest x-rays according to the ILO standard.

CAP-NIOSH: College of American Pathologists–NIOSH diagnostic criteria for the pathological diagnosis of asbestosis, updated 2010.

Chrysotile: A mineral in the serpentine mineral group that occurs in the asbestiform habit. Chrysotile generally occurs segregated as parallel fibers in veins or veinlets and can be easily separated into individual fibers or bundles. Often referred to as "white asbestos," chrysotile is used commercially in cement or friction products and for its good spinnability in the making of textile products.

Cleavage fragment: A particle formed by comminution (i.e., crushing, grinding, or breaking) of minerals, often characterized by parallel sides. In contrast to a fiber from an asbestos mineral, EMPs in a population of cleavage fragments are generally wider and shorter, have generally lower aspect ratios, and do not exhibit fibrillar bundling at any level of examination.

Countable particle: A particle that meets specified dimensional criteria and is (to be) counted according to an established protocol. A countable particle under the NIOSH asbestos fiber definition is any acicular crystal, asbestiform fiber, prismatic crystal, or cleavage fragment of a covered mineral that is longer than 5 μm and has a minimum aspect ratio of 3:1 based on a microscopic analysis of an airborne sample using NIOSH Method 7400 or an equivalent method.

Covered mineral: Minerals encompassed under the existing NIOSH REL (recommended exposure limit) for Airborne Asbestos Fibers and Related Elongated Mineral Particles, which includes minerals having the crystal structure and elemental composition of the asbestos varieties (chrysotile, riebeckite asbestos [crocidolite], cummingtonite–grunerite asbestos [amosite], anthophyllite asbestos, tremolite asbestos, and actinolite asbestos) or their nonasbestiform analogs (the serpentine minerals antigorite and lizardite, and the amphibole minerals contained in the cummingtonite–grunerite mineral series, the tremolite–ferroactinolite mineral series, and the glaucophane–riebeckite mineral series).

Crocidolite: An asbestiform amphibole mineral in the glaucophane–riebeckite series. Crocidolite, commonly referred to as "blue asbestos," is a varietal name for the asbestiform habit of the mineral riebeckite.

Durability: The tendency of particles to resist degradation in lung fluids.

Elongated mineral particle (EMP): Any particle or fragment of a mineral (e.g., fibril or bundle of fibrils, or acicular, prismatic, or cleavage fragments) with a minimum aspect ratio of 3:1, based on a microscopic analysis of an airborne sample using NIOSH Method 7400 or an equivalent method.

Elongated particle (EP): A particle with a minimum aspect ratio of 3:1, based on a microscopic analysis of an airborne sample using NIOSH Method 7400.

EPA: U.S. Environmental Protection Agency.

Erionite: A noncommercial asbestiform zeolite mineral fiber that is the most mesotheliogenic fiber known and originally discovered in Turkey, but is also found widely in the Western United States.

FEV1: Forced expiratory volume in the first second after a maximal exhalation preceded by a maximal inhalation.

Fiber: "Fiber" can be used in a regulatory context or in a mineralogical context. In the regulatory context, a fiber is an elongated particle equal to or longer than 5 μm with a minimum aspect ratio of 3:1. The dimensional determination is made based on a microscopic analysis of an air sample using NIOSH Method 7400 or an equivalent method. In the mineralogical context, a fiber is an elongated crystalline unit that resembles an organic fiber and that can be separated from a bundle or appears to have grown individually in that shape. This regulatory definition includes cleavage fragments and nonpathologic dust. It does not count small pathologic fibers.

f/cc: Fibers per cubic centimeter of air deposited on a membrane filter averaged over 8 hours.

f/cc/years (f/cc-yr): Cumulative exposure calculated by multiplying the average exposure in f/cc over a 40-hour week and averaged over 50 weeks × years of exposure to calculate total lifetime exposure.

Fibril: A single fiber of asbestos that cannot be further separated longitudinally into thinner components without losing its fibrous properties or appearances.

Fibrous: A descriptive characteristic of a mineral composed of parallel, radiating, or interlaced aggregates of fibers, from which the fibers are sometimes separable.

Fragility: The tendency of particles to break into smaller particles.

FVC: The total volume of expired air after a maximal inhalation.

HPV: Human papilloma virus.

HRCT: High-resolution computerized tomography.

IARC: International Agency for Cancer Research.

ICOERD: International Classification of Occupational and Environmental Respiratory Diseases. An international instrument for classification of HRCT films from occupational exposures such as asbestos.

ILO: International Labor Office classification of interpreting chest x-rays.

IPF: Idiopathic pulmonary fibrosis.

LA: Libby, Montana, amphibole fiber; a combination of amphiboles including actinolite, winchite, richterite, and tremolite-contaminating vermiculite.

LDCT: Low-dose computerized tomography.

mppcf: Million particles of dust per cubic foot. mppcf is roughly equivalent to 6 f/cc using PCOM and membrane filters or roughly 185 particles of dust per cc.

NIOSH: National Institute for Occupational Safety and Health; regulatory arm of OSHA.

NOAEL: No-observed-adverse-effects level.

Nonasbestiform: Not having an asbestiform habit. Nonfibrous forms of the asbestos minerals have the same chemical formula and internal crystal structure as the asbestiform variety, but have crystal habits in which growth is more equivalent in two or three dimensions instead of primarily one dimension. When milled or crushed, nonasbestiform minerals generally do not break into fibers/fibrils, but rather into fragments resulting from cleavage along the two or three growth planes. Often cleavage fragments can appear fibrous.

OSHA: Occupational Safety and Health Administration; enforcement arm of the U.S. Department of Labor.

PCOM: Phase-contrast optical method of counting fibers according to NIOSH Method 7400.

PEL: Permissible exposure limit.

Refractory ceramic fiber (RCF): An amorphous, synthetic fiber produced by melting and blowing or spinning calcined kaolin clay or a combination of alumina (Al_2O_3) and silicon dioxide (SiO_2). Oxides (such as zirconia, ferric oxide, titanium oxide, magnesium oxide, and calcium oxide) and alkalies may be added.

SEM: Scanning electron microscopy.

SIR: Standard incidence ratio.

SMR: Standard mortality ratio.

Solid solution series: A grouping of minerals that includes two or more minerals in which the cations in secondary structural position are similar in chemical properties and size and can be present in variable but frequently limited ratios.

Synthetic vitreous fiber (SVF): Any of a number of manufactured fibers produced by the melting and subsequent fiberization of kaolin clay, sand, rock, slag, etc. Fibrous glass, mineral wool, ceramic fibers, and alkaline earth silicate wools are the major types of SVFs, also called man-made mineral fibers or man-made vitreous fibers.

TEM: Transmission electron microscopy.

Thoracic-sized particle: A particle with an aerodynamic equivalent diameter that enables it to be deposited in the airways of the lung or the gas exchange region of the lung when inhaled.

TLV: Threshold limit value.

Tremolite: An amphibole mineral in the series tremolite–ferroactinolite. Tremolite can occur in both fibrous and nonfibrous mineral habits. The asbestiform variety is often referred to as tremolite asbestos. Due only to changes in the International Mineralogical Association's amphibole nomenclature, subsets of what was formerly referred to as tremolite asbestos are now mineralogically specified as asbestiform winchite and asbestiform richterite.

Zeolites: Aluminosilicate solids bearing a negatively charged honeycomb framework of micropores, which can have fibrous forms such as erionite.

Index

Printed and bound by CPI Group (UK) Ltd, Croydon, CR0 4YY

24/10/2024

01778301-0012